Each Little Bird That Sings

Jayantika Davé has been a passionate birder for over fifty years, having been introduced to this fascinating hobby at a very young age by her learned ornithologist grandfather K.N. Davé. She is the author of *100 Indian Garden Flowers*, and lives in Gurugram and Shyamkhet, Uttarakhand. In her professional life, Jayantika is an advisor on human resource strategy and has led the human resources function in global organizations.

Each Little Bird That Sings

Discover India's Birds and Their Myths and Legends

Jayantika Davé

Published by
Rupa Publications India Pvt. Ltd 2025
7/16, Ansari Road, Daryaganj
New Delhi 110002

Sales centres:
Bengaluru Chennai
Hyderabad Jaipur Kathmandu
Kolkata Mumbai Prayagraj

Copyright © Jayantika Davé 2025

The views and opinions expressed in this book are the author's own and the facts are as reported by him which have been verified to the extent possible, and the publishers are not in any way liable for the same.

All rights reserved.

No part of this publication may be reproduced, transmitted, or stored in a retrieval system, in any form or by any means, electronic, mechanical, photocopying, recording or otherwise, without the prior permission of the publisher.

P-ISBN: 978-93-6156-618-9
E-ISBN: 978-93-6156-374-4

First impression 2025

10 9 8 7 6 5 4 3 2 1

The moral right of the author has been asserted.

Printed in India

This book is sold subject to the condition that it shall not, by way of trade or otherwise, be lent, resold, hired out, or otherwise circulated, without the publisher's prior consent, in any form of binding or cover other than that in which it is published.

Contents

- Birds have been grouped by a predominant colour.
- Within each colour they have been grouped by size, from the smallest to the largest.
- The index at the back of the book lists all the birds covered, and the page number on which they occur.

Foreword 7
Note from the Author 8–9
How to Use This Book 10–11
About Birds and Starting Your Birding Journey 12–13

Black 14–49

Grey 178–205

Black and White ... 50–79

Multi-coloured ... 206–217

Blue 80–89

Red 218–231

Brown 90–153

White 232–243

Duck & Geese ... 154–163

Yellow 244–253

Green 164–177

Bibliography 254
Acknowledgements 255
Index 256–258

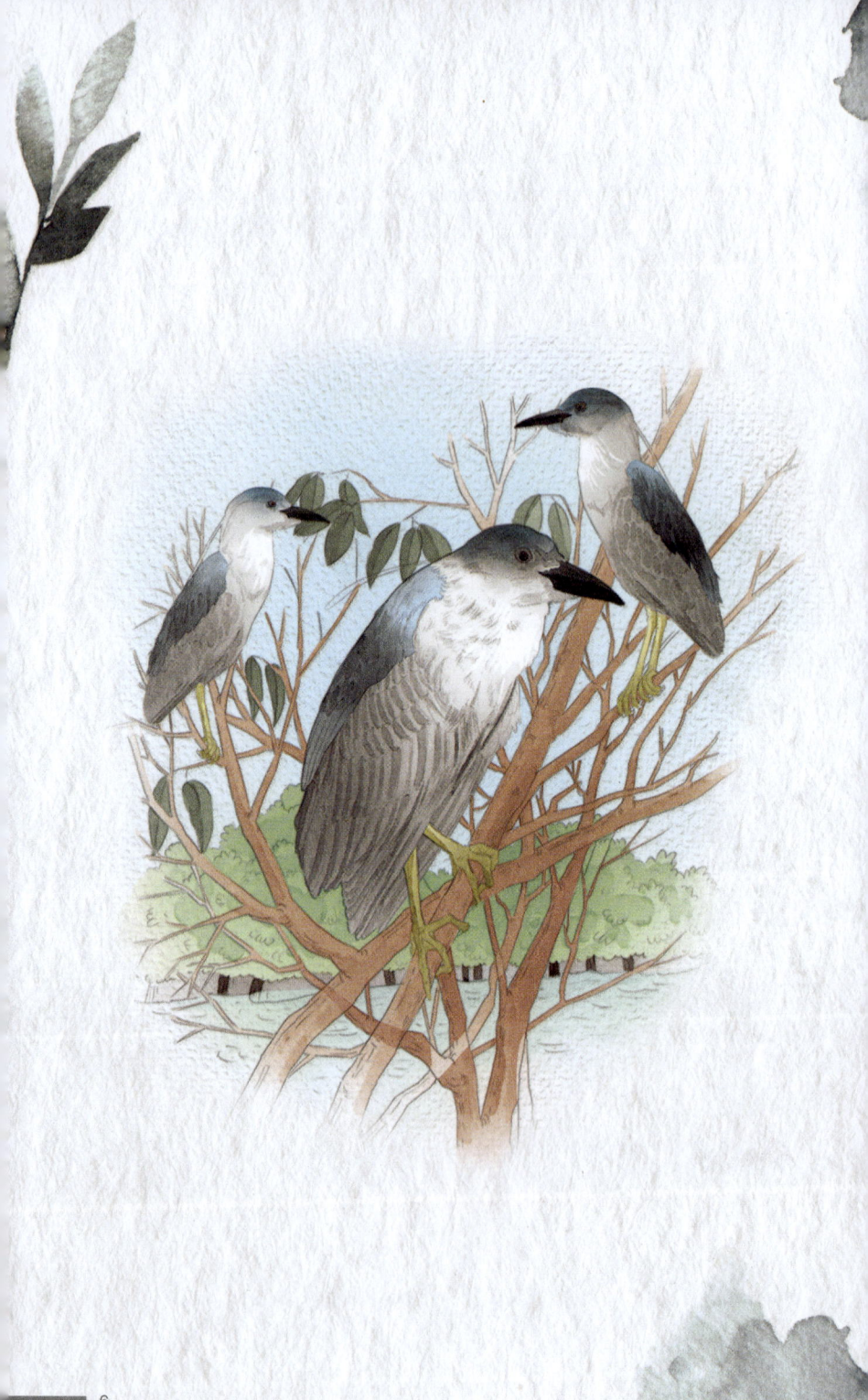

Foreword

In a democracy such as ours, nature conservation can only succeed if the upper echelons in power desire it and, more importantly, if the people themselves demand it. Currently, we remain mega-mammal-centric and go to national parks mainly to see lions, tigers, elephants and rhino, missing out on the colourful chirping birds, the scents and sounds of the wilderness itself, and on communion with nature.

The true purpose of wildlife literature is twofold: to enhance knowledge and to advance an empathy for nature. Scientists from Stuart Baker to Salim Ali have written comprehensive technical treatises on the birds of India. But we need to popularize birds with the common man to win converts to the cause of nature conservation. We need layman 'wildlifers' to identify birds by their song, size and colour, to understand, appreciate and admire them.

Jayantika Davé has done nature conservation a favour by writing this volume. She has covered 250 of our most common and captivating birds, enriched with personal observations of their habits and behaviour. For ease of identification, she has grouped birds by their predominant colour and by size, reducing the struggle that beginners have with scientific names and classifications.

She has covered a very diverse cross-section of both resident and migratory birds, from the Paradise Flycatcher to Pelicans, from Cranes to the Cormorants, and covered birds that require special attention to save them from extinction – the Great Indian Bustard, the lesser florican, and others.

I hope you enjoy reading this book as much as I did.

— M.K. Ranjitsinh

Note from the Author

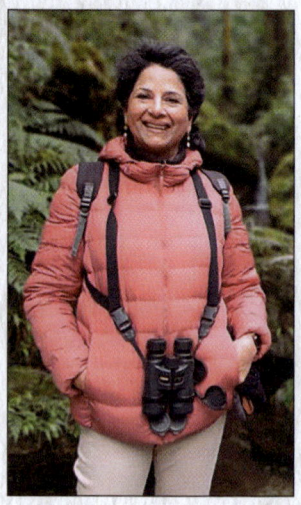

I grew up in a bungalow in Lodhi Estate, with a large garden, surrounded by old trees – ideal bird habitat! My grandparents would periodically visit us from Jabalpur, and my grandfather would walk the garden with me – pointing out shrikes creating insect larders in the shrubbery, placing a sheet of cardboard on a defunct light and attracting doves to nest on it, and sharing spell-binding tales of keeping a Sarus as a pet, and a Racquet-tailed Drongo that could whistle the whole reveille! So, my journey as a birder started young, with my paternal grandfather, K.N. Davé, being this magical personality who knew so much about birds and flowers! He went on to write his acclaimed study, *Birds in Sanskrit Literature*, which, till today, is deemed to be the definitive work in this field. I also inherited his fascinating library of bird books, written by erudite ornithologists who had roamed our forests since the 1800s.

My father, A.K. Davé, furthered this interest by taking us out every Sunday, with a packed picnic lunch, to areas surrounding Delhi, where the highlights were the birds that he would point out to us – our own private birding family gang of my mother Smita Davé, my sister Amrita, my brother Uttam, and me!

My journey continues, with my husband, Himanshu Jani, who has been my keystone – always up for a birding trip no matter how tough, and who has been my sounding board through the writing of this book; my children, Vedika and Rushali – companions in all my adventures; my sons-in-law Aditya and Gaurang, always interested in our tales; my brother Uttam – the eager explorer; and the Mehta and Davé families who have been my backbone and cheered for me every step of the way!

Another key figure for me while I was still very young was Dr Salim Ali, whose book on Indian birds had an index by predominant feature or colour, which was a thought that stayed with me, and that I have now used, in an even simpler way, for this book. I wrote to him twice, at the tender age of 12, with some bird enquires, and he was kind enough to reply, which fuelled my passion further!

Birding trips expanded when Nikhil Devasar re-energized the Delhi Bird group, which Bikram Garewal had initially started, and soon my dear friend Jasjit Mansingh and I were regulars again. Nikhil has stayed a dear friend, mentor and guide, and my birding journey has been enriched by wonderful friends who have made each birding trip so special – Ankit Vohra, Anita Mani, Drs Rajiv and Mona Khanna, Kavi Nanda, Neelam & Satish Khosla, Pia Sethi, Pragya Taneja, Rajat and Jyotsna Sethi, Sheila Chhabra, Sanjay Tiwari, Suneeta Sharma, Satie Sharma;

knowledgeable and caring bird guides Arka Sarkar, Chandramouli Ganguly, Rakesh Ahlawat and Rattan Singh; Ruvina and Ramindar Singh who encouraged me when I struggled; and the warm, wonderful and encyclopaedic Lavkumar Khachar.

This book came about after some non-birder friends wanted to get initiated into birding, and were looking for a way to do that more easily. At the same time, I was reading my grandfather's book about birds in our scriptures, as well as tales of yore told by the knowledgeable birders of the 1800s, and wishing that some of those stories could be read more widely. The lockdown created the mind-flash about writing this book, with birds grouped by colour and size, and enriched with tales and mythology!

The mythology has been drawn from my grandfather's knowledge and writings from our scriptures. He identified birds in our scriptures, with tales starting from the Rigveda, which mainly concerned itself with the mystic Soma cult; to the Atharvaveda and its mentions of birds of prey; the Samhitas of the Yajurveda (1000 BCE), when the Indo-Aryans had become familiar with a lot more birds and were beginning to teach them to repeat human words; the Yajus Samhita and its mention of about 60 birds while reciting the verses about horse sacrifice; and the Puranas and other books describing the practice of divination from the ways and movements of birds and animals. I have tried to bring these tales to life.

I hope this book ignites the passion for birding in new birders, and provides enriched reading for experienced birders too!

I close with a hymn to the wonder of nature, written by Mrs Cecil Frances in 1848, which led to this title for my book...
Each Little Bird That Sings.

> *Each little flower that opens,*
> ***Each Little Bird That Sings,***
> *God made their glowing colours,*
> *He made their tiny wings.*
>
> > *Yes, all things bright and beautiful,*
> > *All creatures great and small,*
> > *All things wise and wonderful,*
> > *The Lord God made them all.*

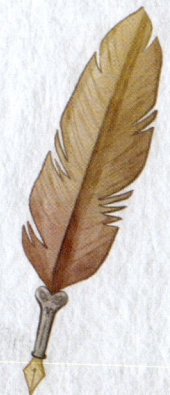

May you always live in wonder!
—Jayantika Davé

How to Use This Book

This book has been written to facilitate ease of identification of birds in the field, while enriching identifications with mythology, tales and trivia that help the bird come alive in the eyes of the viewer. The English name and species are listed, together with the Hindi or the most common colloquial name, as well as the Sanskrit name where available.

To facilitate ease of identification, particularly for a new birder, the birds have been grouped first by the most predominant colour of that bird, and within each colour group, by size, from the smallest to the largest. So, for example, if you see a black bird that is not too large, turn to the 'black tab' section of the book, look towards the middle, and you should find your bird!

The bird is accurately represented by a photograph, and the mythology, tales and trivia are richly illustrated by hand.

Within each colour, we have the birds organized from the smallest to the largest, each having the following sub-heads: **Description; Habits; Call; Mythology, Tales & Trivia.**

The colour classifications by predominant colour are:

- Birds whose predominant colour is **Black**
- Birds whose predominant colour is **Black and White**
- Birds whose predominant colour is **Blue**
- Birds whose predominant colour is **Brown**
- **Duck & Geese** have been grouped together here, as they will often be seen together
- Birds whose predominant colour is **Green**
- Birds whose predominant colour is **Grey**
- **Multi-coloured** birds have been grouped here
- Birds whose predominant colour is **Red/Orange**
- Birds whose predominant colour is **White**
- Birds whose predominant colour is **Yellow**

India is home to more than 1,200 species of birds, and this book covers approximately 250 of the more common or the more spectacular ones. The female in the bird family is often dull, and so the classification is based on the more definitive colouring of the male bird.

Species name

English name

Colour tab

Great Barbet

Scientific name: *Psilopogon virens* Size: 33 cm
Hindi name: *Traiho*
Sanskrit name: *Pippal*

Sanskrit name

Hindi name

Bird photograph

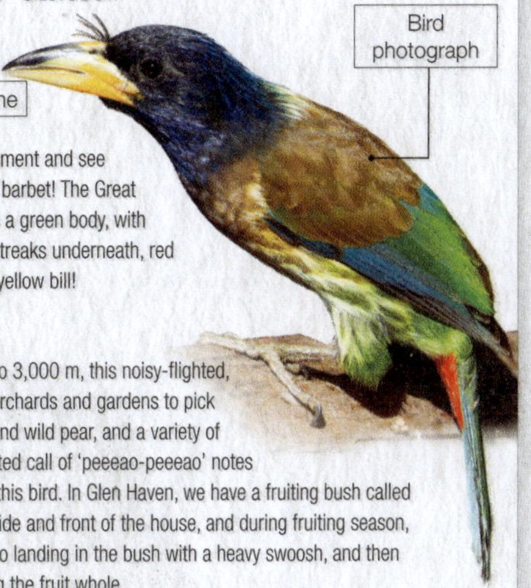

Description

So, it seems that God decided to experiment and see how many colours he could put on one barbet! The Great Barbet, which is our largest barbet, has a green body, with a dark-blue head, brown back, yellow streaks underneath, red under the tail, and a really large heavy yellow bill!

Habits

A resident of our Himalayas, found up to 3,000 m, this noisy-flighted, purely arboreal bird comes to forests, orchards and gardens to pick figs, berries, flowers of rhododendron and wild pear, and a variety of insects. The incessant, endlessly repeated call of 'peeeao-peeeao' notes are what will draw your eye to look for this bird. In Glen Haven, we have a fruiting bush called Tushar growing in the gaderas on the side and front of the house, and during fruiting season, there will be large numbers of the Traiho landing in the bush with a heavy swoosh, and then disappearing into it, plucking and eating the fruit whole.

The courtship is quite lovely, with tail-spreading and wagging, low head-bowing, and vociferous singing often together in chorus!

Call

One bird will start with the resounding, melancholy 'peeeao-peeeao' notes, and soon every other Great Barbet in the vicinity will join to form an endless chorus!

Hand illustrations for mythology

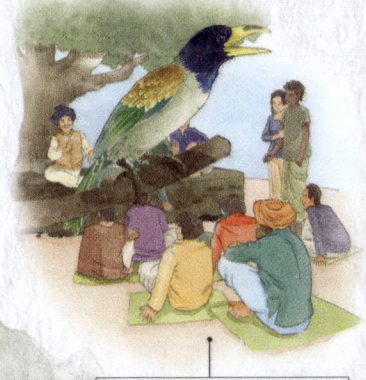

Mythology, Tales & Trivia

There is a hill-people story that the Great Barbet is the incarnation of the soul of a suitor who died of grief, since he could not be with the love of his life, as his request was turned down by the Panchayat. His soul now resides in the Great Barbet, and unceasingly cries out 'Anyaaya, Anyaaya' meaning 'injustice'!

About Birds and Starting Your Birding Journey

As you start on your birding journey, it is important to understand the basic anatomy of a bird, so that you can describe it accurately, or look up and understand the description better from whichever bird book you are using. Here is a simplified version of the anatomy of a bird.

The Parts of a Bird

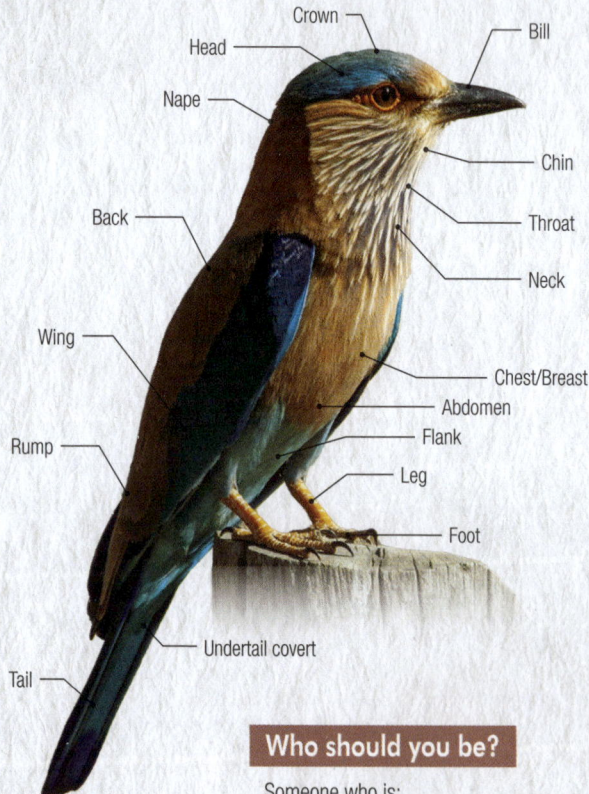

Who should you be?

Someone who is:

Patient – a good sighting takes time
Quiet – don't frighten away the birds
Observant – watch for bird movements
A Good Listener – notice and differentiate between bird calls

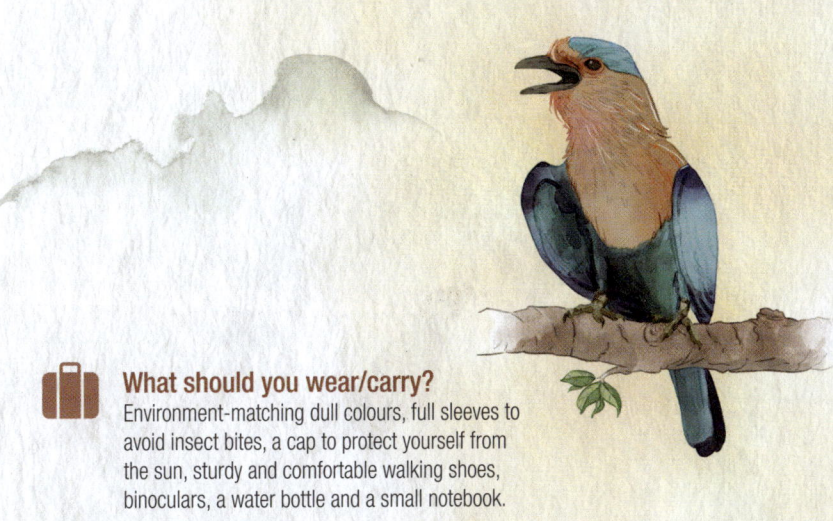

What should you wear/carry?
Environment-matching dull colours, full sleeves to avoid insect bites, a cap to protect yourself from the sun, sturdy and comfortable walking shoes, binoculars, a water bottle and a small notebook.

When should you bird?
Early mornings are the best – ideally just after first light. If you are not an early bird, then early evening is another time to catch bird activity.

Where should you bird?
To keep up the interest, find out about spots where you can see a variety of birds, and where the birds could be easier to see – for example, a water body. Your garden, or apartment complex, or a nearby park are great places to start.

With whom should you bird?
It is sometimes easier to join a local bird club or group. A quick search on the internet will definitely throw up a local group. Often, it is very rewarding to just start on your own.

Equipment
A **good pair of binoculars** is a great investment to increase the pleasure of birding. Anything from a **8 (magnification) × 40 (field)** to a 10 × 50 is good. A higher magnification makes it difficult to keep the binoculars steady. You can start with a lower-end Olympus or Nikon, move on to a mid-cost Zeiss or Nikon Monarch, and invest in the higher-end, more expensive ones once you have found your feet.

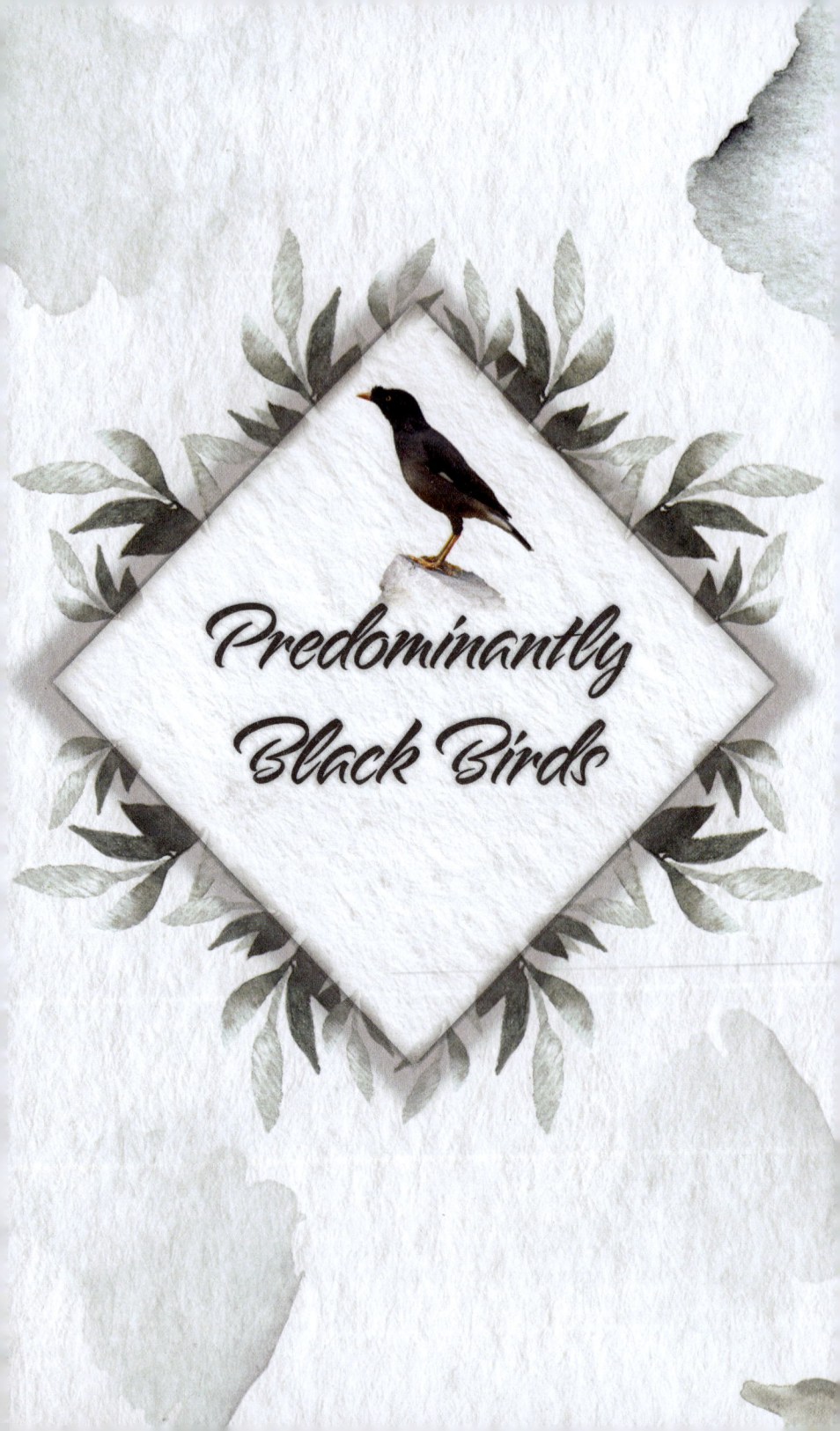

Dusky Crag Martin

Scientific name: *Ptyonoprogne concolor*   Size: 13 cm
Hindi name: *Chatan Ababil*
Sanskrit name: *Kutidooshak, Nakuti, Nahikuti*

Description

Many of us live in tall apartments in our cities, and you may have been curious about this tiny, very dark bird, with a short square tail, that can be seen flying in a slow and deliberate way around the buildings. This is the Dusky Crag Martin, which often flies in the company of swallows, but is distinguished from them by being smaller, uniformly dark, and much more leisurely in its movement.

A very similar-looking bird, but with a white throat and rump, is the **Little Swift**. In the *Som Vartika*, the continuous flight of the Little Swift is depicted as the nature of the *aatmaan*, which is in a state of ecstatic happiness, stays only in a high spiritual plane, and rarely descends to the ground…a lovely analogy!

Habits

The Dusky Crag Martin gets its name from the fact that in its natural surroundings, it is a lover of tall wild crags and caves – the famous Ajanta and Ellora caves are alive with them! They feed on insects in flight, and due to their quick turns, they are very successful feeders close to crag faces.

The Dusky Crag Martin belongs to the mud nest-builder group and builds a neat half-cup of mud, with a soft lining, placing it under a ledge, on a cliff face or old fort, or the urban equivalent of cliffs – our tall apartment buildings!

Call

A cheerful soft chi-chi or a soft twittering!

Mythology, Tales & Trivia

The scientific name is derived from a combination of two words – the Greek *ptuon*, which means fan and refers to the fan-shaped tail, and *procne*, which comes from the legend of a mythological girl who was turned into a swallow-like bird to escape the anger of her husband.

Jayantika Davé

Purple Sunbird

Scientific name: *Cinnyris asiaticus*   Size: *10 cm*
Hindi name: *Shakar Khora, Phool Soongni*
Sanskrit name: *Bhringrol, Madhukar*

Description

A tiny, glossy, purple-black bird with a long curved beak, restlessly flitting around your purple kachnar, or other nectar-filled flowers, singing its cheery refrain of 'ching-ching, chikee, chikee, chikee', as if it could not contain its happiness in its tiny frame – the Purple Sunbird! The males look almost black, but when the sunlight hits them, you will see a beautiful purple-greenish sheen.

A very similar bird is **Loten's Sunbird**, which is seen only in the southern part of India. The main differentiator is a bill that is longer and more deeply arched, and a maroon band across the breast.

Habits

They are seen in pairs or very small groups, and are very restless, flicking their wings constantly, moving from one flower to another, sometimes perching, sometimes hanging upside down, but always sticking their long beaks and tubular tongues into the depths of a flower to drink its nectar. As the name Shakar khora denotes, they mainly live on nectar, though sometimes they catch insects too.

The nest is an untidy elongated structure of small strips of leaves, grass or bark, all bound together by cobwebs, and built by the female and male together. It is often built very close to our homes, as the birds sense safety in human presence. Once built, the hen bird settles down to her maternal duties, with her chin resting on the windowsill, watching the world go by!

Call
Chwit, wich.

Mythology, Tales & Trivia
In the *Vayu Purana* 36.5, interesting descriptive words like Shinjijarika (to describe their tinkling call), or Madhukar, based on their habit of collecting nectar, have been used.

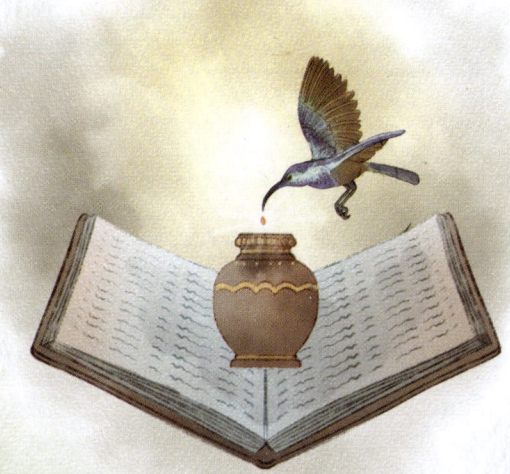

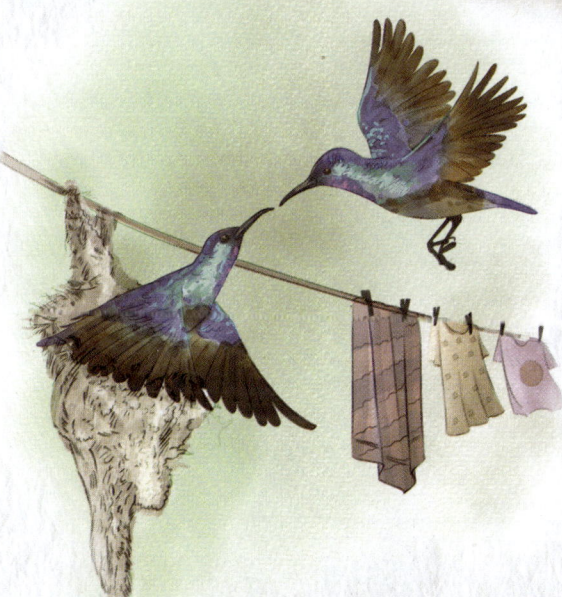

In our home in Delhi, we had two nesting pairs, which came back every year to the same place. One would build their nest anchored to a thin wire hanging right outside my bedroom window. The second pair was even more fearless and loved to nest at one end of a clothesline that was used daily!

Jayantika Davé

Black Redstart

Scientific name: *Phoenicurus ochruros*   Size: *15 cm*
Hindi name: *Thirthira, Thar-thar Kampa*
Sanskrit name: *Kapekshuk = kap (tremble) + ikshu (blade of grass)*

Description

It's winter, and you see a sparrow-sized black and bright rufous-red bird, constantly flicking its tail, and dipping and bowing…you can almost imagine that it has arrived at the theatre in its black-and-red tuxedo and is bowing low and greeting all new arrivals!

The Black Redstart has made its dramatic entrance!

The **White-capped Redstart** is very similar to the Black Redstart, with a few key differences – the white priest's cap, the shocking rufous-red tail, and its presence in or alongside a mountain stream in the Himalayas. Often called the Dhobin or washerwoman due to its habit of being near the edge of a stream, and also because the bright white head can be likened to a bundle of washed white clothes!

Habits

The Thirthira is a busy, industrious bird, and forages for grubs, worms and fruit on the ground, occasionally jumping up into a short flight to catch insects. Perching on a low bare rock or stone, the constant flirting of the tail and the body-shiver are a dead giveaway! When it descends to the plains in winter, it is a delightfully friendly, confiding bird, and can often be seen in the shady parts of our gardens.

It nests in the high mountains of Kashmir, Nepal and Tibet, building a small cup-shaped nest of grass and hair, and placing it in old stone walls or in Tibetan chortens.

Call

A squeaky tsip…tsip…delightfully described by Salim Ali as 'the squeaking of an unoiled bicycle wheel, revolving at a moderate speed'!

Mythology, Tales & Trivia

The genus name is self-descriptive, and means red-tailed (phoenix = red, ouros = tailed). The Hindi and Sanskrit names are of course beautifully descriptive of the habits of this bird.

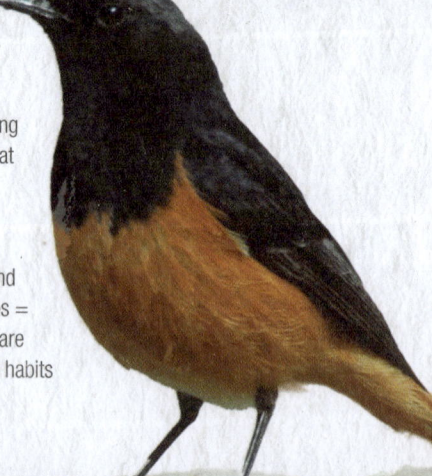

Indian Robin

Scientific name: *Saxicoloides fulicatus*   Size: *19 cm*
Hindi name: *Kalchuri*
Sanskrit name: *Krishnashakuni, Krishnapakshi*

Description

A smart, perky, glossy black-and-brown bird, with a cheekily cocked tail displaying a bright chestnut-rufous patch, and a white badge of honour on its wings…our very own resident robin! Hugh Whistler quotes these as an example of how the East and West are diametrically different – the Indian Robin wears its red under the tail rather than on its breast!

Habits

Resident, and non-migratory, the Kalchuri is very comfortable amongst human habitation, and is seen around our homes and gardens, often perched on rooftops. Robins like open dry scrubland, and will not be found in thick forest or high rainfall areas. They are industrious feeders, rising early with a cheery song to take insects, and, unlike other birds, they also work late into the evening to catch insects clustering around lights, while continuing to sing cheerfully. The males are very noticeable and aggressive during the breeding season, with their incessant singing, and display of lowering and spreading their tail feathers, and then raising them and fluffing up their undertail rufous patch, defending their territory strongly.

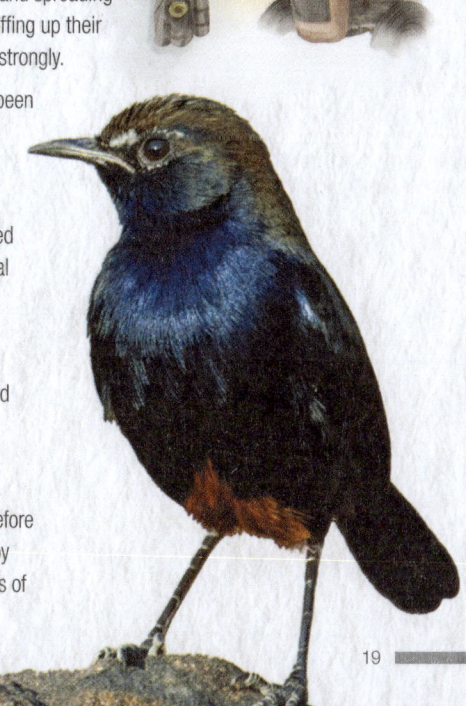

Robins nest in unusual places, and nests have been found in shoes, coal pockets, tractors and even under car bonnets and the baskets of scooters!

Douglas Dewar describes how the nests are sometimes decorated with buntings and coloured foil if the nesting season coincides with a festival and these scraps are easily available!

Call

A high-pitched warbling song, which is short and repeated often!

Mythology, Tales & Trivia

The robin was treated as a bird of augury, and before asking it any questions, it had to be addressed 'by several flattering epithets consisting of the names of the goddess Parvati', according to K.N. Davé.

Jayantika Davé

Barn Swallow

Scientific name: *Hirundo rustica*   Size: 18 cm
Hindi name: *Ababil*
Sanskrit name: *Chatak, Poojni, Bhaandeek*

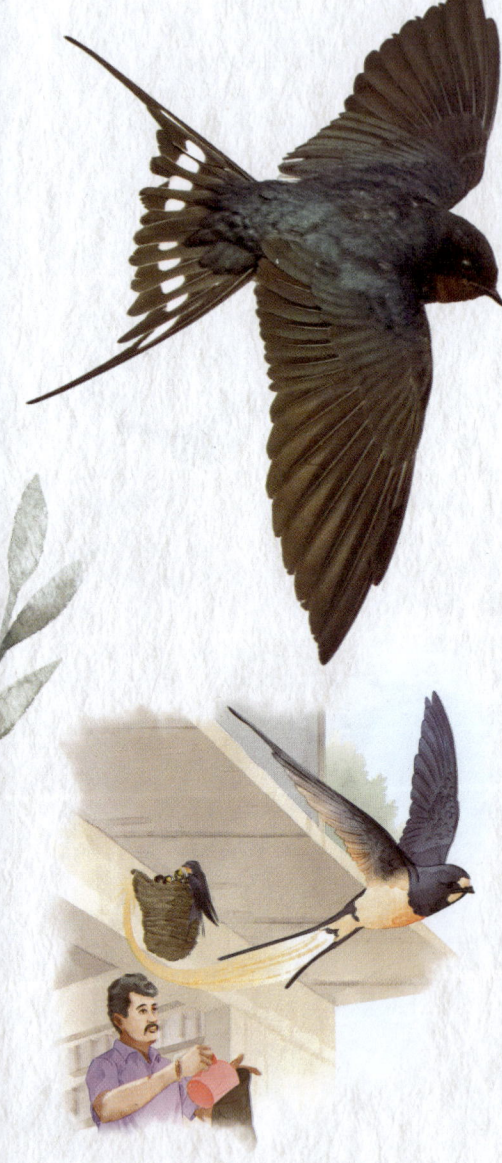

Description

As the saying goes – 'One swallow doth not a summer make'…but the appearance of swallows definitely heralds the approach of summer! As the weather warms, this distinctive swallow, with a steel-blue back, a lovely rich rufous forehead, chin and throat, and a deeply forked tail, appears.

Two other lovely residents are the **Wire-tailed Swallow,** with a chestnut cap and two long, thin wire-like feathers extending from its tail, and the **Red-rumped Swallow,** which has a clear chestnut rump and hind collar.

Habits

In winter, the Barn Swallow is seen across India, on electric wires, roof edges and bare branches, usually in close proximity to habitation.

The nest is a neat cup of mud and grass, stuck to the underside of buildings and rafters, with it being re-used often for 10–15 years, and once for a record 48 years! In our local market in the hills, there is a provision shop where the same pair has been nesting for years, placing their nest in the rafters just above the shopkeeper's head, and fearlessly flying in and out, building their nest and feeding their young!

Call

A variety of twitters and a clear vit-vit are most common!

Mythology, Tales & Trivia

There is a belief that if a swallow's nest is damaged, the home where this happened would cease to prosper!

The Barn Swallow's annual migration journey is around 11,000 km or more. So, interestingly, sea mariners used swallow tattoos to ensure their safe return from sea, and to indicate how far they have travelled. Nine thousand kilometres at sea meant a single swallow tattoo, and a second tattoo could only be added after completing 18,000 km!

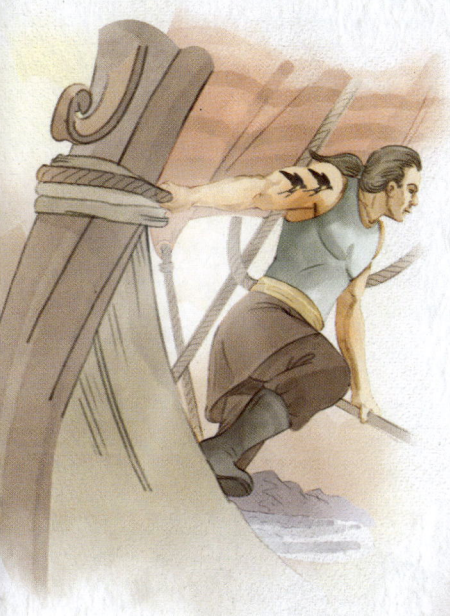

Barn Swallows are also the most picturized birds on postage stamps all over the world!

The longer the tail streamers of the male swallow, the more attractive is the suitor to the female!

A number of famous poets and playwrights have written about swallows – John Keats in 'To Autumn', Oscar Wilde in 'The Happy Prince', and William Shakespeare in *Richard III*.

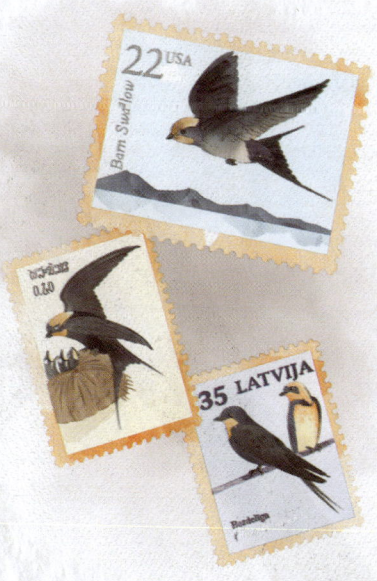

Jayantika Davé

Red-vented Bulbul

Scientific name: *Pycononotus cafer*   Size: 20 cm
Hindi name: *Kala Bulbul, Bulbuli*
Sanskrit name: *Pench*

Description

A jaunty, dark-brown-black bird, with an upright stance, a partially crested black head, an elegant waistcoat with scales of brown, and red on the seat of its trousers! Please meet the lovely Red-vented Bulbul!

Habits

Its cheerful call and bright, energetic habits make it a spirit-lifting visitor to all gardens. Its name originates from the Persian word *bolbol* meaning 'nightingale', because of its cheery sweet voice. The Red-vented Bulbul loves its feast of fruit, insects, flower petals and nectar. A fruiting Banyan is a particular favourite, termite swarms after a rain shower provide a special treat, and freshly growing peas absolutely have to be eaten! Its beautifully woven, cup-shaped nest is often placed trustingly close to human habitation.

Call

A lovely 'ginger beer' call, interspersed with 'pick', draws attention to this bird; its constant vigilant eye and harsh alarm screeches are immediately respected by all birds in the vicinity!

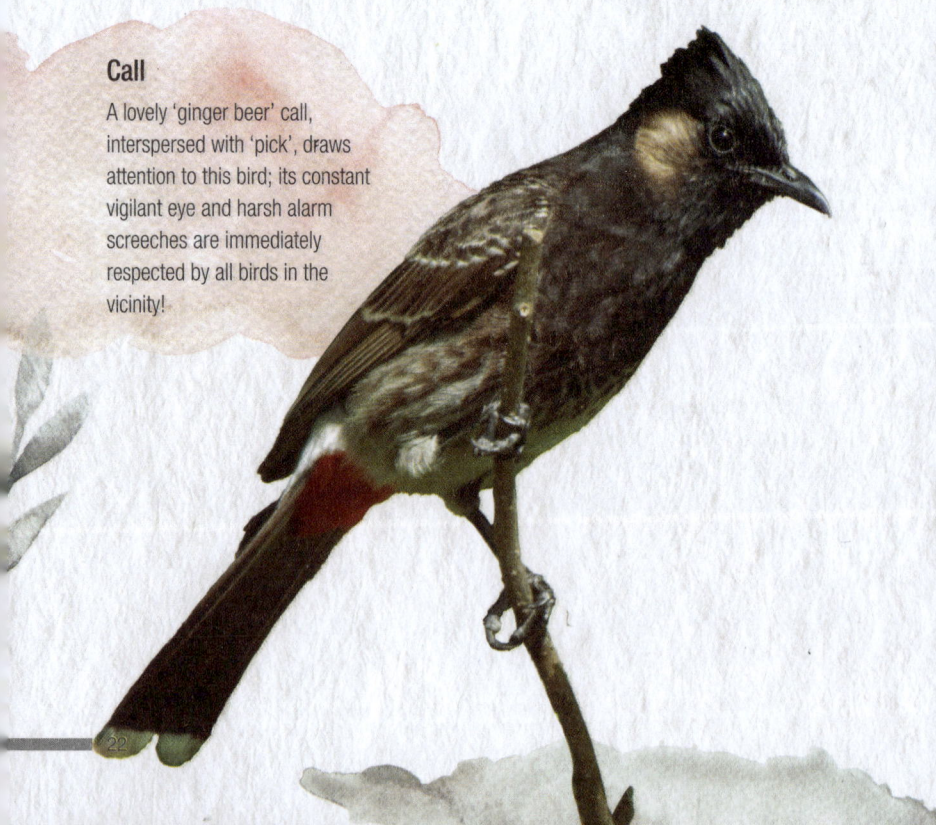

Mythology, Tales & Trivia

Manusmriti 8.166 tells the story of the Vedic singer Vats who went through the fire ordeal to prove his Brahmanic parentage, and later the sage ascended to heaven, but he left the Red-vented Bulbul as his mark on earth – a bright, cheerful singer with the mark of the fire as a red patch under the tail.

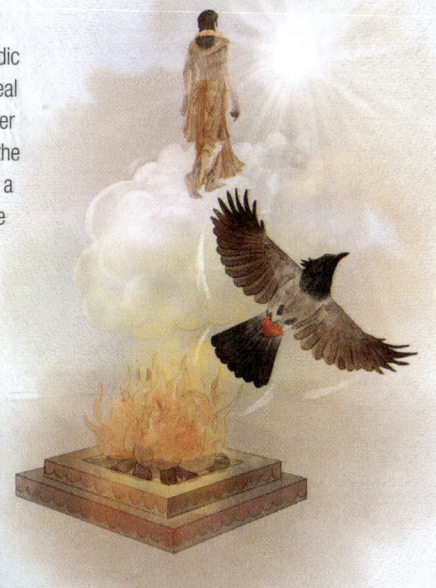

Whistler describes that in the old days people were so fond of the Bulbuli that they would carry it around, tied to their finger with a little string or tied to a jewel-encrusted little perch.

They are pugnacious by nature, and Bulbul fights were organized where the aim was to pluck out as many of the 'red seat' feathers of their opponent as possible, with Dewar quoting Rs 500 as the cost of a good fighter, which was a lot of money in those days!

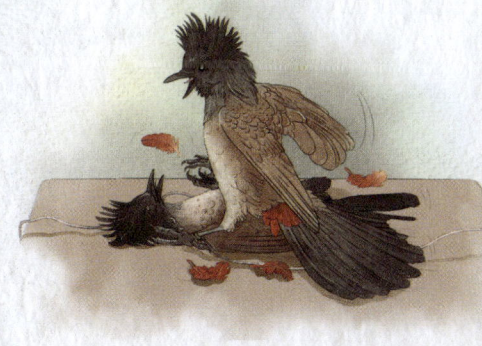

The bright-red feathers were also used by the rajahs to embellish the white-beaded neck-bands of their polo ponies.

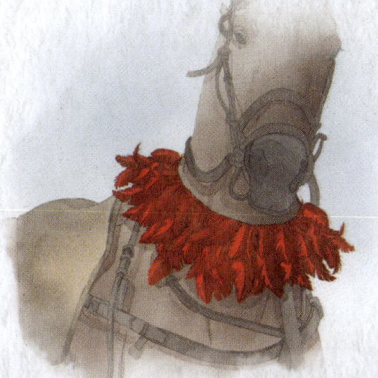

Jayantika Davé

Common Starling

Scientific name: *Sturnus vulgaris*   Size: 21 cm
Hindi name: Tilyer Myna, Kusnai, Tilora, Nakshi Tilyer
Sanskrit name: *Parushan* = spotted, *Tailpak* = covered in oil

Description

In winter, the Common Starling makes its appearance in our parks and gardens. You will notice them as flocks of myna-sized birds, with oily-looking iridescent feathers glossed with purple or green, and spangled with white. The flocks are large, noisy, squabbly ground feeders. The new black feathers have white tips, which give rise to the visual appearance of spots!

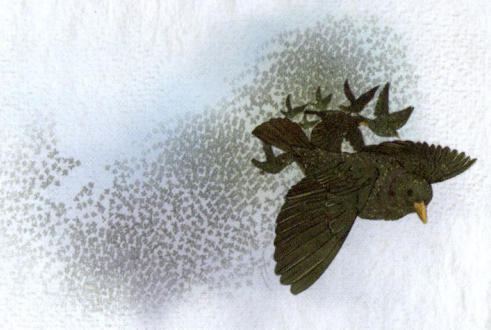

Habits

The Tilyer Myna is a busy feeder, stabbing into the ground repeatedly with its beak at every step, and walking in a very hurried and strangely zig-zag fashion! These birds practise 'roller feeding', where the birds at the back continuously rise in a wave to the front to try to get at the best food, and remain at the front, till the next 'roller wave' arrives. They eat insects, grains, fruits and seeds.

Another very recognizable habit is 'murmuration', where the flock suddenly takes to the air, flying in dense tight flocks, in very complex formulations that constantly expand and contract, and wheel and change direction. A mesmerizing sight, since each bird keeps its distance from only its 'neighbour' birds, and therefore, despite the sharp and quick twists and turns, no bird collides with another!

In the evenings, they crowd into trees to roost, arguing, pushing, chattering and squabbling, and covering anything below the tree in lots of birdshit!

Call

A starling is a great mimic, and can include the calls of up to 20 birds in its repertoire! The older it gets, the more it learns, and the more complex its call becomes!

Mythology, Tales & Trivia

In the *Manusmriti*, an oil thief is said to be reborn as a starling in his next life!

Starlings have very refined taste buds! In experiments, it was found that they can differentiate between salt, sugar, and citric and bitter tastes!

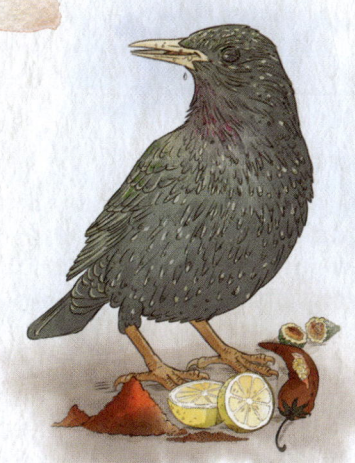

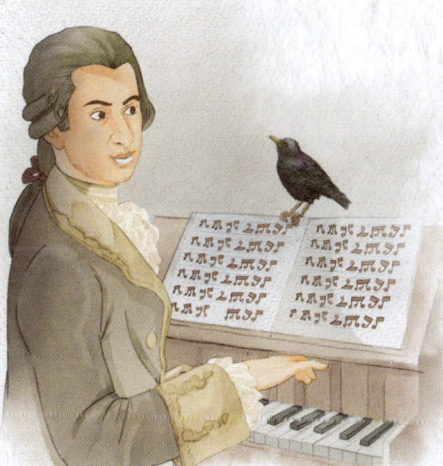

Mozart had a pet starling, which could sing his piano concerto in G major!

To attract a female, the male adorns the nest with a few bright green leaves, sometimes a flower, and most importantly, sweet-smelling herbs!

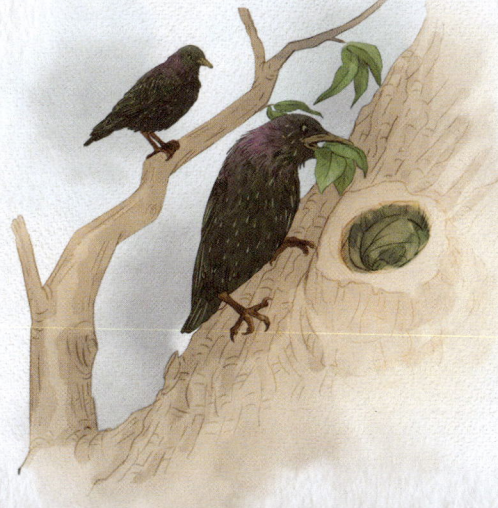

Jayantika Davé

Rosy Starling

Scientific name: *Pastor roseus*   Size: *21 cm*
Hindi name: *Gulabi Myna*
Sanskrit name: *Madhusarika, Suvarnasarika*

Description

The lovely black, white and pink combination of the Rosy Starling always make me think of a smart priest, with a black head of somewhat untidy hair, a black cassock and a lovely pink waistcoat! The glossy head, pale orange legs, and a constant chattering complete the picture of this winter visitor to India.

Habits

These highly gregarious birds form large noisy chattering flocks, devouring grasshoppers, insects, fruits and grains, though their absolute favourite is the nectar they can get from flowers. During a Goa holiday, it was a treat to see a tall semul tree resplendent with large fleshy red flowers, and the site of much squabbling and aggression between the Rosy Pastors and other Mynas who also wanted a feed! Evenings are the time to swarm, congregate and roost, with showy flypasts, and twists and swirls in a cloud of pink, white and black, all the while keeping up a constant chattering.

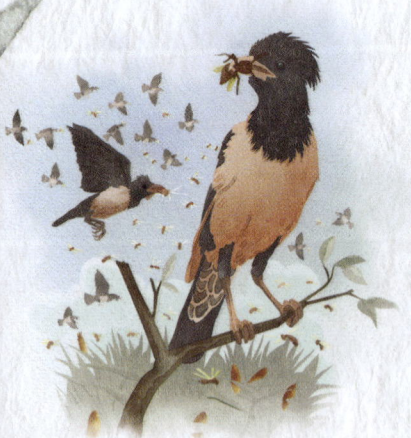

Call

A very typical starling call…a mixture of rough rattles, squeaks, chirps, with a lot of wing trembling, almost like a young one!

Mythology, Tales & Trivia

In China, in 1980, an expert thought of introducing and attracting the Rosy Starlings to a locust-infested farming area. Since then, the locusts are completely under control, and the use of pesticide has dramatically dropped!

The stark black-and-white combination of the bird gave rise to the name Pastor for its priestly appearance, with the addition of Rosy, for its lovely rosy-pink waistcoat.

Jungle Myna

Scientific name: *Acridotheres fuscus*   Size: *23 cm*
Hindi name: *Jungli Myna*
Sanskrit name: *Jaantsaarik, Haholika*

Description
This slightly demented-looking grey-black myna is easily recognized by its aggressively forward-slanting bristled forehead feathers, giving it a strangely annoyed look, as if someone woke it up too early, and it has just tumbled out of bed! Its angry dishevelled appearance always make me chuckle! Yellow or blue eyes, and a bright-yellow bill and legs complete the distinctive look. In flight, the large white wing patches show up clearly.

Habits
Typically found in the more forested areas of the Himalayas, the Northeast and the Western Ghats, they are omnivorous feeders, eating insects, fruits and seeds. They love the berries from trees and bushes, the nectar from flowering trees, and often descend to the ground to eat seeds. In cultivated areas, they follow farmers ploughing the fields to pick off insects, and also perch on grazing mammals to eat their parasites. Like other mynas, they roost communally.

Call
A noisy collection of whistles, and a harsh 'chak chak'!

Mythology, Tales & Trivia
While taking nectar from large flowers such as the Erythrina, they inadvertently pollinate the flowers too, with their head-tuft feathers acting as brushes.

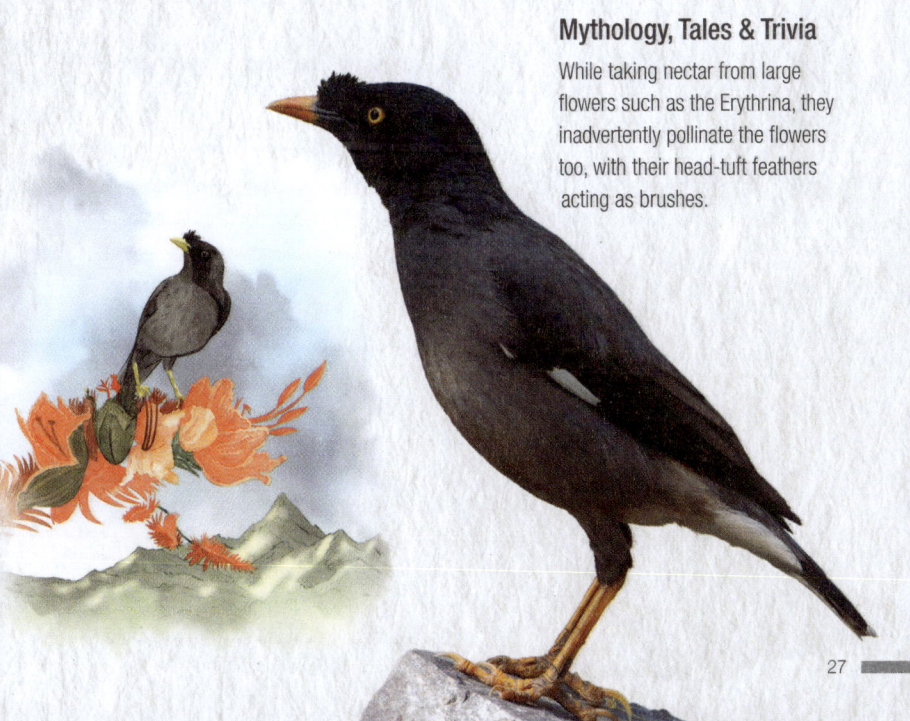

Jayantika Davé

Black Bulbul

Scientific name: *Hypsipetes leucocephalus*   Size: 25 cm
Hindi name: *Kala Bulbul*
Sanskrit name: *Vanbakra, Karniyak, Govatsak*

Description

When you are in the Himalayas, and the fruit is ripe on the tushar or pangar trees, and a noisy brood of black, untidy and crested, medium-sized birds arrives, they are most likely to be the Black Bulbuls! This noisy, conspicuous, slate-grey and black bulbul with a ragged crest, a deeply forked tail, and bright orange-red beak and legs is quite a lovely sight!

Habits

The Kala Bulbuls arrive in small groups onto a fruiting tree, announcing their arrival with loud, grating mewing calls. They are very fond of berries, and the local chestnut or pangar is an absolute favourite in the fruiting season. They also make aerial sallies to catch insects. Very gregarious, the Kala Bulbul moves in groups of at least 15–20 birds. The noisy mewing, calling and feeding continues for a while, and then the group moves on to another tree to continue the same racket.

In the Western Ghats, you will see a very similar bulbul, the **Square-tailed Bulbul**. It is much darker though, almost uniformly black, without any of the grey that highlights the northern Black Bulbul. But the striking red beak and legs, and untidy messy crest remain the same!

Call

A strangely cat-like mewing, though very grating, call!

Mythology, Tales & Trivia

Tribal folklore has a quaint story about how the Black Bulbul gets its colouring! As the tale goes, once there was a big flood, and the tribe had to quickly move to higher grounds. In the hurry, their fire got left behind! All paths were blocked, and no one from the tribe could return to quickly salvage their fire. But the Black Bulbul volunteered to fly there and get them a burning piece of wood. So off it went, and returned, as promised, with a glowing ember. But the fire had burnt all its feathers black, and its beak and feet were burnt red!

Grey-winged Blackbird

Scientific name: *Turdus boulboul*   Size: 28 cm
Hindi name: *Kala Kastura*
Sanskrit name: *Kalvink, Kasturi, Kaalchatak*

Description

The resident Grey-winged Blackbird is elegant in black, with distinct silvery, shining, light-grey wings. Its bright orange bill and eye rings stand out in the dark foliage in which this bird normally sits.

Its counterpart in the peninsular hills of India is the **Indian Blackbird** – a very similar-looking dark stocky bird, with a bright orange lipstick bill, a matching eye-ring and a small, teardrop-shaped patch of bare orange skin around the eye.

Habits

This is a quiet, shy bird, moving around mainly in the trees, but it also forages in the forest understorey, with rapid hops and stops, turning over leaves and eating insects, grubs, earthworms and caterpillars. When it is bringing up its young, this shy bird becomes really bold, and follows me fearlessly around the garden as I am overseeing the tilling of the soil, filling up its beak with lines of earthworms, reminiscent of the way fish line up in a puffin's beak! In our hill home, they have also learnt that easy food is to be had when I am putting out food for our dogs Buddy and Shogun. So, as soon as I emerge with their bowls, the Grey-winged Blackbirds will arrive on the neighbouring trees, waiting for the dogs to abandon some food, which they quickly finish off!

Call

A lovely and loud melodious song, with each phrase ending in a little twitter; though, as Whistler puts it, 'individuals vary a good deal in the merits of their performance'! In the old days, this beautiful song resulted in a number of birds being caught and sold as cage birds!

Jayantika Davé

Black Drongo

Scientific name: *Dicrurus macrocercus*   Size: 28 cm
Hindi name: *Kotwal*
Sanskrit name: *Goprerak (rider on cow's back), Dhoomyat (unafraid of smoke — since it flies in and out of smoke to pick off insects disturbed by forest fires!)*

Description

The glossy black silhouette, shot with blue and green highlights, of a long, slender, upright bird; with a distinctive, deeply forked tail, is a familiar sight on wires and fences all over India. A noisy, chattering, pugnacious species, it is resident across all of India, and is seen in open areas, forest edges, wetlands and fields.

Habits

It is an early riser, starting to call well before dawn, and forages well into twilight. It perches on high vantage points, sallying forth to catch insects on the wing.

The Kotwal ('guard'), as this bird is appropriately named in Hindi, is very aggressive near its nest, around which it establishes a 'sphere of influence', as described by Edward Hamilton Aitkin (E.H.A.); and the crow, being a notorious poacher of questionable character, is forbidden to enter that, at the peril of a 'bolt from the blue' attack by the drongo!

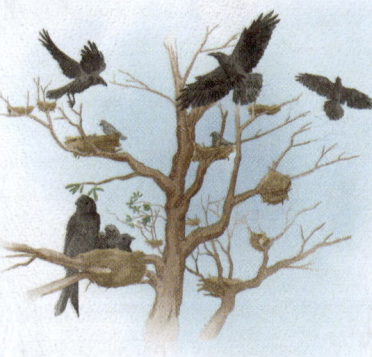

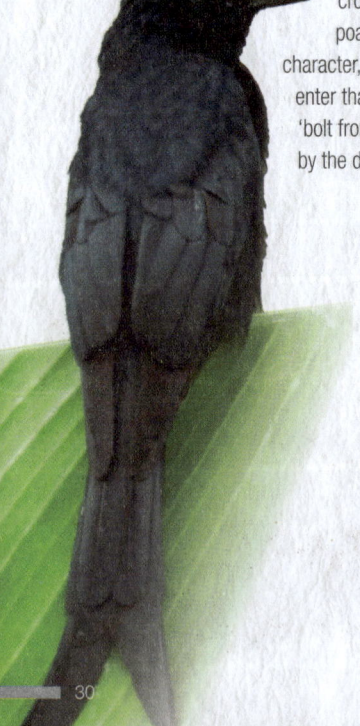

Smaller birds often nest in the same tree as the drongo, as they know their nests will be protected too!

Dewar describes the making of the nest thus — once the basic shape is made, each parent takes turns to sit in it, and turn round and round, shaping it into a beautiful cup, in much the same way as a potter handles clay!

Call

The most common is a 'tee-hee' very similar to the **Shikra**, interspersed with harsh cackles and a great deal of mimicry of other birds too!

Each Little Bird That Sings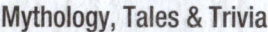

Mythology, Tales & Trivia

According to K.N. Davé, in the Mahabharata, Duryodhana is said to have adopted the brave aggressive ways of the Kulinga (Black Drongo), to worry the Pandavas and drive them away from their kingdom.

In parts of Punjab, it is revered because of the belief that it brought water to Husayn Ibn Ali, who is revered by Shi'a Muslims.

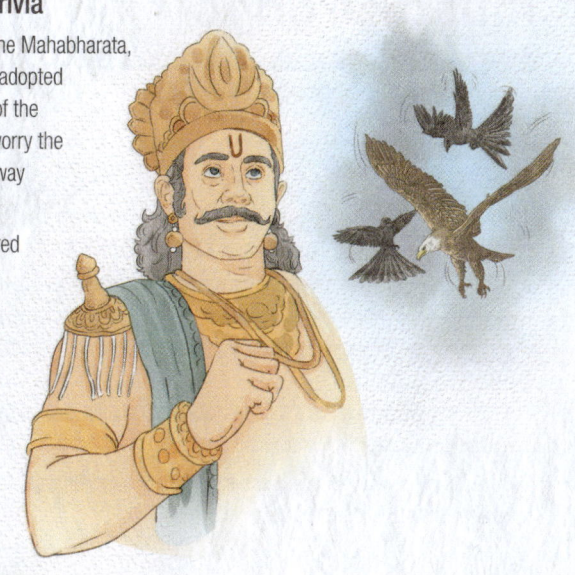

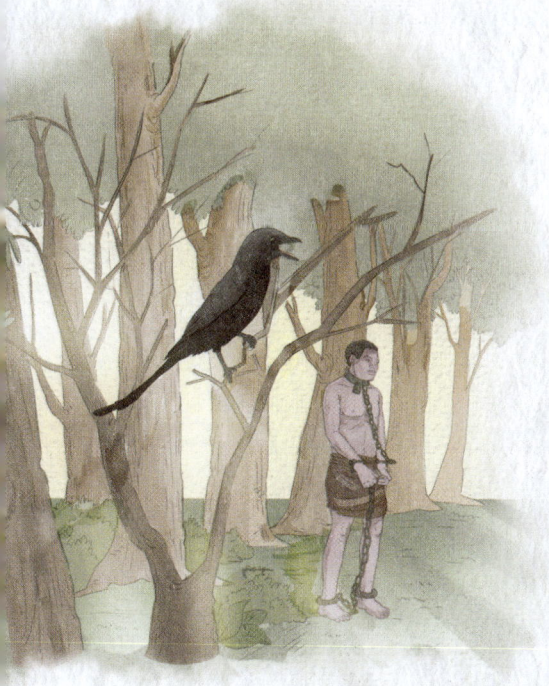

There is a lovely little story called 'The Drongo Bird' by Adella Gautier, in which a drongo started mimicking the sounds of chains and copying a strange language, which alerted the local people of Madagascar to the arrival of slave traders. The people quickly melted into the forests and avoided being captured!

Jayantika Davé

Greater Racquet-tailed Drongo

Scientific name: *Dicrurus paradiseus*   Size: *32 cm*
Hindi name: *Bhimraj, Bhringaraj*
Sanskrit name: *Bhringaraj*

Description

This large, distinctive black drongo with a blue-green gloss, and a distinctive crest of curled feathers, is seen in forested areas in the Himalayan foothills and across India. It is characterized by two long wire-like streamers attached to its tail, ending in broad spatulas.

As Salim Ali says, it looks as if a large black bird is being chased by two large black bees!

A smaller, similar version is the **Lesser Racquet-tailed Drongo**, which however is seen only in the Himalayan foothills.

Habits

There is nothing shy about these drongos. They draw attention to themselves by perching in the open in forests, and with their variety of calls and mimicry. They feed almost entirely on the wing, swooping from their high perches, doing an adept catch and returning to the perch.

The Bhimraj indulges in an elaborate courtship display consisting of hops and turns and dropping leaves to be picked up in mid-air. These birds are said to mate for life.

Call

Very varied calls with whistles, metallic sounds, sequence of notes and complex imitations of other birds. They are clever enough to mimic raptor calls to panic other birds into abandoning their prey!

Mythology, Tales & Trivia

The *Bhagavata Purana* has a pretty verse that says that when a devotional song is sung, a noisy congregation immediately quiets. Similarly, the whole forest goes silent in admiration when the Bhimraj starts singing! The Ramayana and the Mahabharata also have mentions of the Bhimraj as a superb mimic and a beautiful songbird.

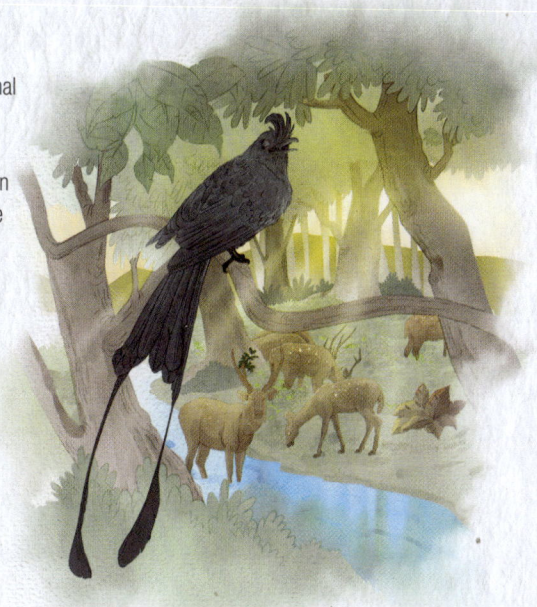

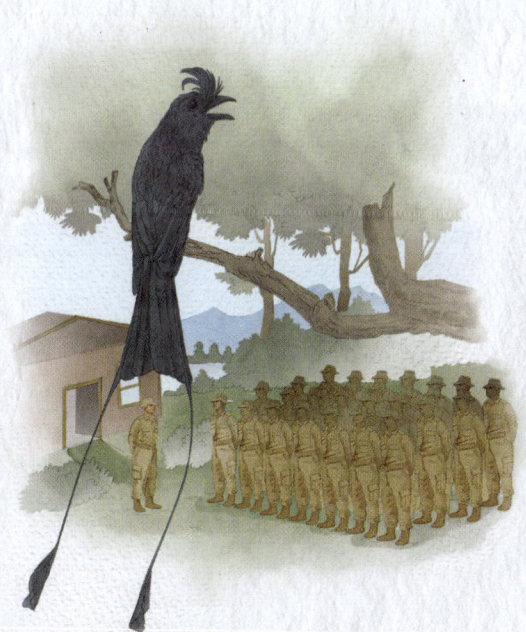

According to K.N. Davé, in the *Vaijayanti Kosa* it has been described as *budhimaan* (intelligent), and in the *Kalpadru Kosa* as *satyavaak* (perfect mimic).

Stuart Baker related how in one army battalion, there was a lovely Greater Racquet-tailed Drongo that sounded the reveille, every morning, 'with absolute correctness and punctuality'! The reveille consists of 3 parts of 20 notes each, with 2 parts being identical, but the third part being different… so a truly complicated composition to copy exactly!

Jayantika Davé

Bronze-winged Jacana

Scientific name: *Metopidius indicus*   Size: 30 cm
Hindi name: *Jal Pipi*
Sanskrit name: *Jal Kapot (water dove/pigeon)*

Description

So, 'walking on water' is the phrase for doing the impossible…which the Jacana does with great ease, giving it the name Lily Trotter or Lotus Bird! So, when you see a tall leggy bird walking on leaves across water, it is highly probable that you are seeing a Jacana. The Bronze-winged Jacana has an overall dark-black appearance, with a long, striking white stripe extending over the eye, a russet patch under its flicked tail, and lovely green-bronze highlights on its wings when the sun hits them.

Habits

They are most often seen singly or in pairs, walking on aquatic vegetation and feeding off insects and other invertebrates found on the leaf surfaces. If you come too close and the Jacana is unable to run away, it lies down with its neck stretched out and half-submerges itself, so that it is almost invisible!

In this species, what is very interesting is that the female is truly the queen! She is larger, maintains a harem of males to incubate the various clutches of her eggs, feed and raise them, and designates the 'best' male amongst them to be the defender of her territory.

Call

Grunts and a seek-seek.

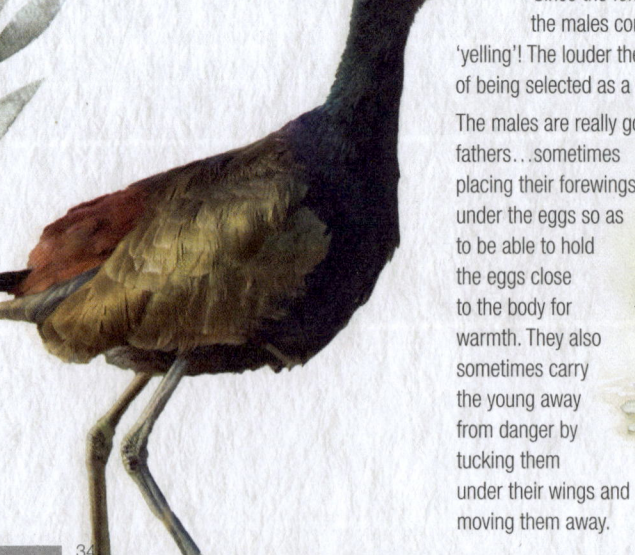

Mythology, Tales & Trivia

Since the female is truly the queen, the males compete for attention by 'yelling'! The louder the yell, the more chances of being selected as a mate!

The males are really good fathers…sometimes placing their forewings under the eggs so as to be able to hold the eggs close to the body for warmth. They also sometimes carry the young away from danger by tucking them under their wings and moving them away.

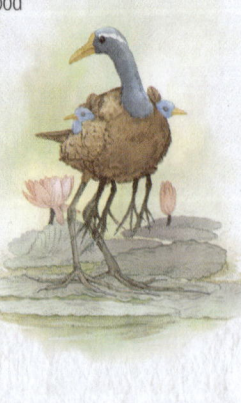

Blue Whistling Thrush

Scientific name: *Myophonus caeruleus*   Size: 33 cm
Hindi name: *Hazaar Dastaan (in Kashmiri)*
Sanskrit name: *Shreevad*

Description

This dark thrush is seen across the Himalayas, and as it appears, you wonder…is it black?…no, it is purple!…looked like it had spots, but can't see them now?! All a trick of the light! Its true appearance of deep purple-blue, with metallic violet-blue spots, can be seen only in bright light. In all other light it looks a glossy black. The bright yellow bill, however, is unmistakable. A friend of ours, Atul Bakshi, practises Agnihotra (worship of the rising and setting sun), and during the Brahma Muhurat, which is the first light of the sun, it is always the Blue Whistling Thrush that is singing – so he has named it the 'Brahma Muhurat class monitor'!

Habits

4.45 a.m. in the morning, and the first song I hear is the prolonged melodious whistling of the Blue Whistling Thrush. It is dark all around, and the Blue Whistling Thrush pours out its heart in this beautiful series of tumbling notes! No wonder the Kashmiri name for it is Hazaar Dastaan…a thousand stories to tell!

They are seen singly or in pairs in the temperate and moist forests of the Himalayas, appearing with a quick hop onto a rock, a quick spurt of a run and a noisy strong flight. Constantly turning over leaves and rocks as they look for insects, grubs and snails, they are somewhat shy, and move quickly into deeper cover in the trees, where they spread and droop their tails if they are alarmed.

In our hill home, they ousted a pair of pigeons from the bird house and built their nest there – an interesting volcano-shaped edifice, made of moss, roots and mud!

Call

A host of beautifully melodious phrases, interspersed with clear resounding whistles, and with mimicry woven in too! Often, the first song you hear before dawn, and the last one at the onset of night!

Mythology, Tales & Trivia

It is also called the Brahma Muhurat bird, as it is the first bird that is singing at that time of the morning.

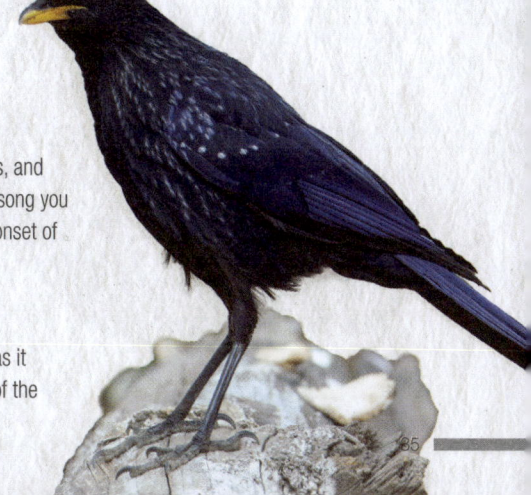

Jayantika Davé

Black Francolin

Scientific name: *Francolinus francolinus*   Size: *34 cm*
Hindi name: *Kala Teetar*
Sanskrit name: *Krishna Teetar*

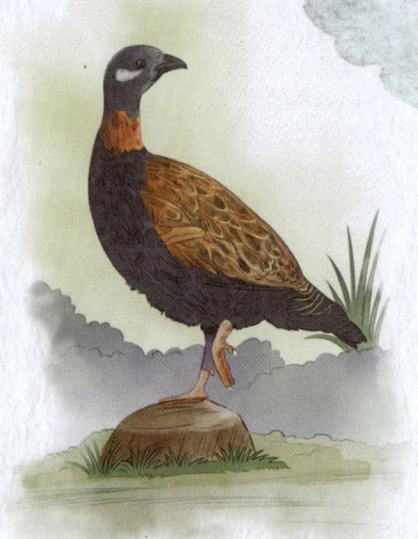

Description

This is a bird you will hear before you see it! A strident 'kik-kik-keekarik' or *Subhan teri qudrat*, as it is prettily annotated, is repeatedly uttered in an open field or hillside. The bird itself will, at that time, be typically perched on top of a small stone, tossing its head back so that its call can be heard for miles! The Black Francolin is a strikingly smart bird with a predominantly black appearance, but once it is in binocular range, the gorgeous combinations of black, rich brown, rich russet and white, punctuated with bars and spots, show up!

Habits

A lover of scrubby habitat, forest edges and cultivated crops, the Black Francolin prefers thick vegetation, often near water. While it has a strong direct flight punctuated by glides, it prefers to quickly skulk away through undergrowth, and the habitat it chooses facilitates this. It eats grass seed, grain, berries, insects and some plants and leaves. It looks like a typical partridge, and hence its local Hindi name of Kala Teetar. Black Francolins mate for life.

Call

Its strident kik-kik…keekarik call can be heard early mornings and evenings, and often echoes with birds calling back from all directions. Prettily described as '*Subhan teri qudrat*' or '*lehsun pyaz adrak*' or 'Paan bidi cigarette'! As Whistler says, it has a cheery 'ring of pride and well-being'!

Common Moorhen

Scientific name: *Gallinula chloropus*
(gallinula = chicken + chloro = green + pus = feet)   Size: 34 cm
Hindi name: *Jal Murghi, Murghaabi*
Sanskrit name: *Krishna Jal Kubchut*

Description

In water bodies across India, you can see this resident large and dumpy, charcoal, grey-black bird, with white slashes all along its side, flashing white undertail, yellow legs and a distinctively bright-red frontal shield.

Habits

It swims like a duck, pushing its head forward, and yet is able to walk on top of vegetation due to its large spread-out feet that balance its weight on lily pads. These birds tend to swim near and amongst vegetation, only very occasionally venturing out into open water.

On land, they walk in a somewhat crouched, careful fashion, watching where they gently place their feet, and constantly flicking their tail up, showing off the white beacon-light tail feathers. When startled into flight, they fly awkwardly with their long legs hanging, and quickly find cover and land. They forage on vegetable material, and on small aquatic creatures, which they find by flipping floating leaves.

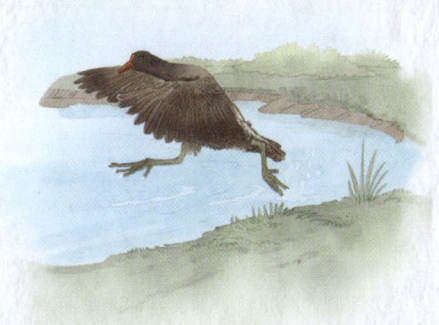

Call

The Common Moorhen is often heard before it is seen! A noisy bird, with a loud kirrik-crek-rek-rek, and a variety of loud, harsh and gurgling calls, often as a chorus. The call is so loud that an unfamiliar observer might think that there is a large, dangerous, somewhat crazy animal lurking in the vegetation!

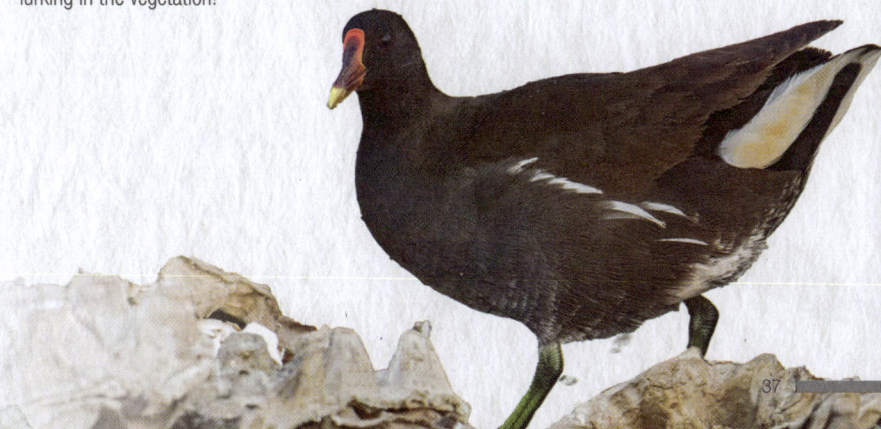

Jayantika Davé

House Crow

Scientific name: *Corvus splendens* Size: 40 cm
Hindi name: *Kowwa*
Sanskrit name: *Balipushtkaak, Bhasmachavikaak*

Description

One of our commonest and most noisy of birds, this tramp in black and grey is a consummate thief, equipped with great intelligence, daring and an insatiable curiosity. It is an easy bird to spot, with its bright beady eye, and its complete comfort around human habitation. With its loud raucous caw-cawww…who can miss the Kowwa!

Habits

The House Crow is an omnivorous scavenger and hangs around homes, garbage dumps, and anywhere where food has been left unattended!

It is a highly intelligent, multi-skilled bird, which has been known to use tools and sequential intelligence to complete a series of tasks to gain that prized bit of food. The Koel regularly tricks it into bringing up her young! The nest itself is a tinker's delight – with one of the most creative ones made from spectacle frames discreetly stolen from an optician in Fort, Mumbai.

They mob, they bully, they sidle, they steal, and yet…there is much that is attractive about this bright, intelligent bird with its beady eye!

Call

A harsh kaaaw-kaaaw, with the throat feathers puffed up with the effort, and the tail depressed with each call!

Mythology, Tales & Trivia

Lord Shanidev, who is the protector of property and who controls thievery, has the crow as his *vahan*.

In the *Padma Purana*, Jayanta, the son of Indra, assuming the form of a crow, insulted Sita, and Rama punished him by depriving him of one of his eyes. Since then the crow is supposed to have only one eye, which is why the crow continually turns his head from one side to the other.

During *shradha*, crows are fed as it is believed that they carry food to the departed souls of one's ancestors.

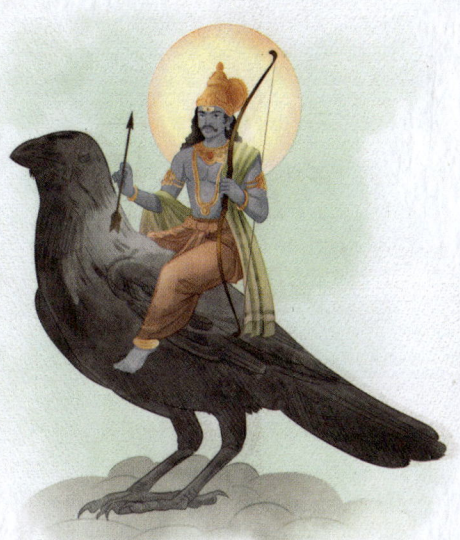

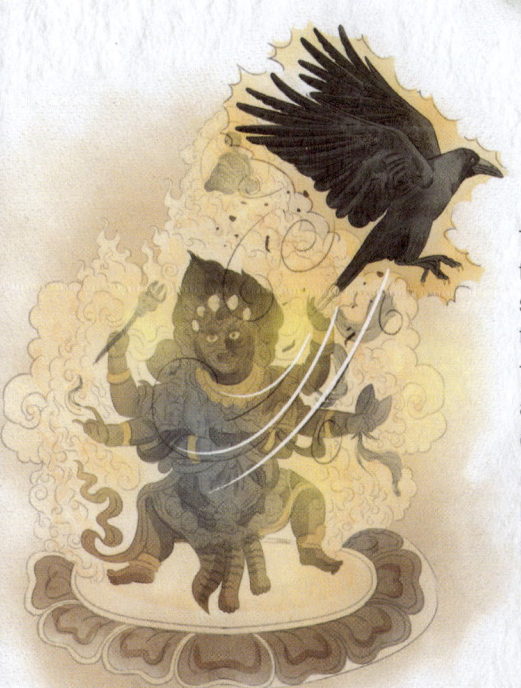

They throw hard nuts into traffic, wait for them to be crushed, and then synchronize their retrieval with the traffic lights!

There are many stories in the Ramayana and other legends about the crows' devotion to Lord Rama.

In Buddhism, the crow is believed to be the incarnation of the Mahakala, the protector of the monasteries in Tibet.

Jayantika Davé

Eurasian Coot

Scientific name: *Fulica atra*   Size: 37 cm
Hindi name: *Dasari, Dasarni*
Sanskrit name: *Sumukh (contrasting white beak and shield with black face)*

Description

On lakes and water bodies across India, this plump slaty-black bird, with a gleaming white bill and white forehead shield, is easy to spot. The proverb 'bald as a coot' arose from this hairless white forehead! It is most often seen running across the water, or swimming in large flocks. Out of water, its disproportionately large feet are distinctive.

Habits

The Eurasian Coot's favourite habitat is water bodies with submerged aquatic vegetation or mats of floating weed or hyacinth or lily leaves, amongst which it forages for algae, leaves, seeds and small live prey. It bobs its head as it swims, and periodically dives under water, with a little jump up before plunging in. Preferring not to fly, it runs across the water with much splashing, and needs a long run-up to even take off on a relatively weak flight. While mainly diurnal, on moonlit nights it continues to forage well into the night.

Call

A noisy bird with its most typical call being a throaty short 'kow' or 'kowk', sometimes combined together into a 'kow-kowk'.

Mythology, Tales & Trivia

Emperor Jehangir, in his memoirs, refers to the coot by the Persian name of Qashq-ul-dagh, with Qashq meaning the white sandalwood mark that the Brahmins wore on their foreheads.

The Dasari used to be so numerous in the early 1900s that Whistler describes their presence as a 'herd', and says that their numbers used to be estimated by the square mile! And when the whole 'herd' would take off, the sound was like 'the noise of great waves breaking on a shingle beach'!

Native hunters used to catch them by submerging into water up to their necks, placing a duck-like object on their heads, and thereby approaching close enough to grab them.

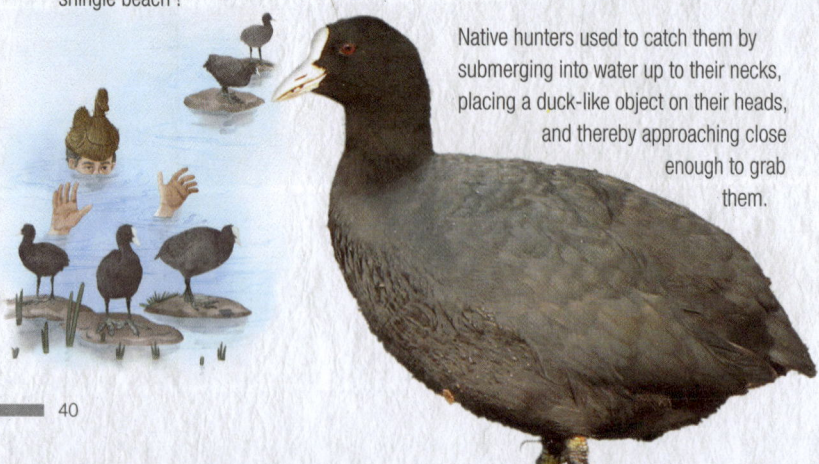

Jungle Crow

Scientific name: *Corvus (macrorhynchos) culminatus*   **Size:** 41 cm
Hindi name: *Kala Kowwa, Jungli Kowwa*
Sanskrit name: *Krishnakaak*

Description
This all-black crow, with uniformly purple-glossed plumage, is easy to distinguish from the House Crow because of its all-black appearance, its not so intrusive nature, and the hoarse caww-caww call – like a House Crow with a bad cold! It is very similar in appearance to the **Large-billed Crow** found higher up in the Himalayas.

Habits
A widespread resident across India, it is a versatile feeder. It feeds from the ground and from the trees, and will eat anything, whether alive or dead, and whether it is a plant or an animal. It has a heavy-winged flight, and is quite bold in urban areas, though less frequently seen as compared to the House Crow.

During the nesting season, the Asian Koel does its parasite trick here too, but less frequently than it does with the House Crow.

Call
The call is a very harsh kaaw-kaaw, interspersed with chuckles, gurgles and croaks! The throat is puffed up and the tail dips with each call!

Mythology, Tales & Trivia
According to the Mahabharata and our Puranas, the punishment for stealing fish or flesh is rebirth as a Jungle Crow.

Whistler writes that in the early 1900s, he saw the Jungle Crow audaciously settling on the packs of mule trains crossing the high Himalayan passes and tearing holes in the packs, to get the grains within!

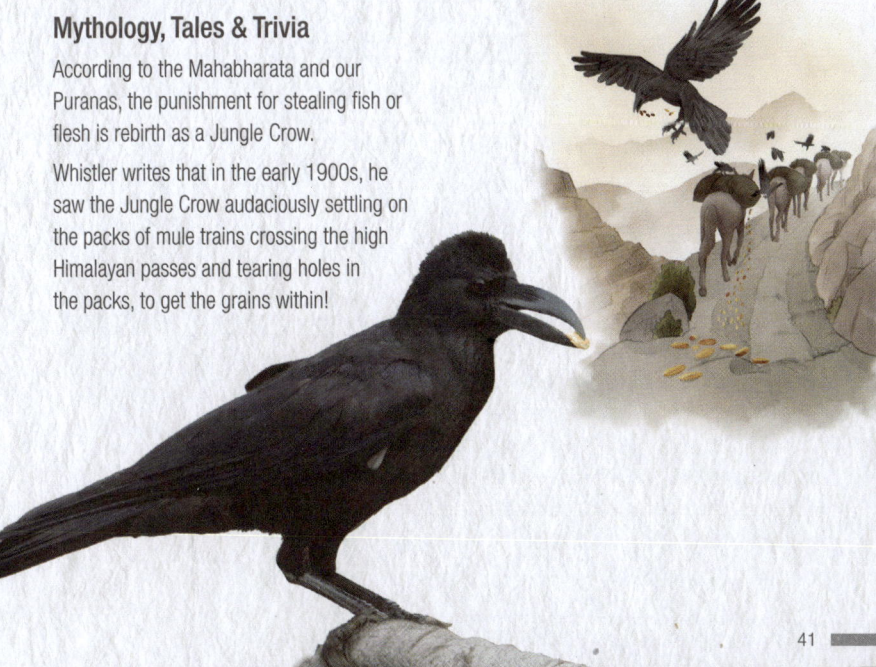

Jayantika Davé

Asian Koel

Scientific name: *Eudynamys scolopaceus*   Size: 43 cm
Hindi name: *Koel*
Sanskrit name: *Krishna Kokil*

Description

This large and glossy bluish-black cuckoo, with a pale grey bill and a bright red eye, is present in open woodlands all across India, and draws attention to itself with its loud, liquid, melodious 'ko-el ko-el', ku-ooo ku-ooo' call, rising in cadence with each call.

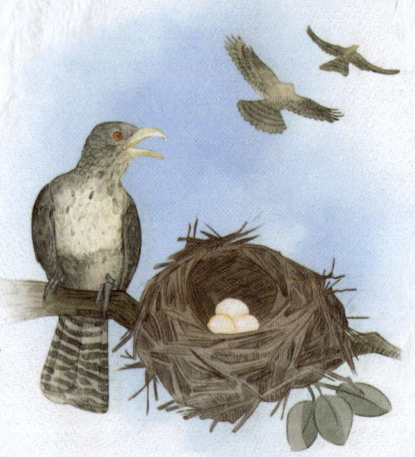

Habits

Koels are primarily fruit lovers, and while they also eat insects, caterpillars, eggs and small animals, they are primarily seen around fruit trees. They skulk in dense foliage, and often swallow fruit whole, and then regurgitate the seeds at different places.

It is a parasitic cuckoo, and lays its eggs in the nests of medium-to-large birds, though its favourites are the Jungle and the House Crow. So the way it works is this…the male koel approaches a nest where a female crow is sitting and harasses it and chases it away. As soon as this happens, the female koel sneaks in, and quickly lays its egg in the now vacant nest. Sometimes the cuckoo nestling will tip out the crow babies to ensure they get all the food…not a nice tenant to have!

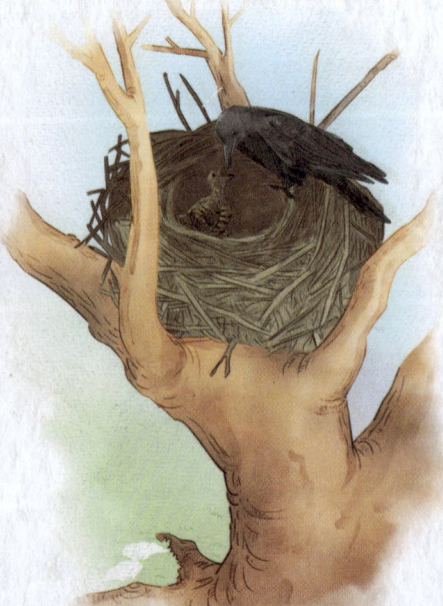

Call

Ku-ooo, ku-ooo or ko-el ko-el, with a great sense of excitement to the call, rising to a fever pitch by the seventh or eighth call…and breaking off, to start all over again, periodically interspersed with kik-kik-kik.

Mythology, Tales & Trivia

The Sanskrit name of Kokila is often used for someone who sings or writes sweet verse, calling to mind the melodious call of the koel. In the *Manusmriti*, it was decreed that the Kokila should be protected from all harm.

K.N. Davé talks about how in one of our scriptures, the koel is referred to as the crow's aunt – Kaakpitrasvsa – because in India, a sister who comes across hard times often leaves her children to be brought up in her brother's house.

As many as 11 koel eggs have been found in one House Crow nest!

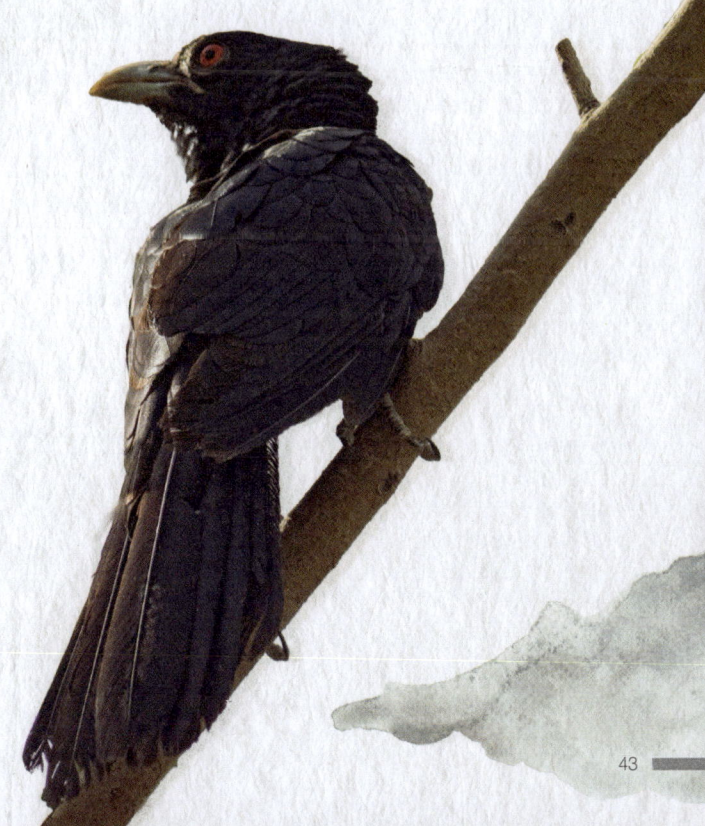

Jayantika Davé

Little Cormorant

Scientific name: *Microcarbo niger* Size: *51 cm*
Hindi name: *Paan Kowwa, Jograbi*
Sanskrit name: *Paaniyakaakika*

Description

This relatively small all-black duck-like bird is seen on water bodies throughout India, with the very apt Hindi name of Paan Kowwa or water crow! With a strangely flat head, and a very sharply hooked bill, it swims with most of its body below the waterline. A quick flick, and it disappears below the water for some time, reappearing some distance away.

The very similar **Indian Cormorant** is larger, has a more rounded head, a blue iris, and a whiter throat with a yellow throat pouch.

Habits

Inhabitants of both inland and coastal water bodies, these active birds are found singly, in pairs or in small groups. They are expert underwater divers and swimmers, and feed on fish, frogs and crustaceans, diving quickly underwater, catching their prey and then surfacing to swallow it. Opportunistic grabbers like other cormorants, gulls, egrets or storks try to do a quick steal at that time! A rest break consists of perching on a rock next to the water, and spreading out its wings for a complete dry-out.

They are gregarious breeders, making their nests on small trees in or near the water, together with herons or egrets.

Call

Very vocal around their nests and while roosting, they make continuous low-pitched ah-ah-ah and kok-kok-kok calls!

Mythology, Tales & Trivia

Young cormorants are fed heartily by their very hardworking parents, and so their bellies are always full of small fish. If these young cormorants are startled or suspicious, their first response is to regurgitate up their food, resulting in a stream of newly caught fish descending on the unsuspecting observer!

The Paan Kowwa is a bird with submarine-like habits, and when alarmed, it is able to submerge its body completely, only leaving its head out like a periscope!

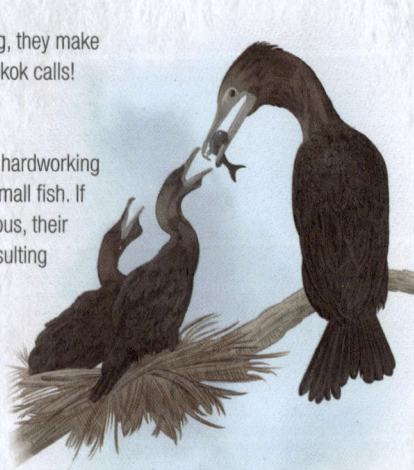

Each Little Bird That Sings

Red-naped Ibis

Scientific name: *Pseudibis papillosa*   Size: 68 cm
Hindi name: *Kala Baza*
Sanskrit name: *Raktasheersh Aati, Bhu-kaak*

Description
A tall black bird, with a downcurved bill, a bright red, warty, featherless head and a white wing patch…the Red-naped Ibis! The wing and tail feathers have a lovely blue-green gloss, and it is typically seen in open dry fields, in small groups of not more than 10 birds.

Habits
Widely distributed across India, it is found on irrigated farmlands, other open and dry lands, and also near marshes. An omnivorous feeder, it takes insects, frogs, small animals as well as grain, often following tillers to feed on disturbed insects and grubs. The action is one of walking and continually probing into the soft ground. These birds are increasingly being seen in large parks and gardens, near water bodies. They roost communally on trees and on islands, and fly into and from them, in a V formation.

Call
They are typically fairly silent, but have a descending loud braying, grating call during breeding or on the wing!

Mythology, Tales & Trivia
During British times, the Red-naped Ibis was hunted for good eating as well as for sport, using the Shaheen falcon.

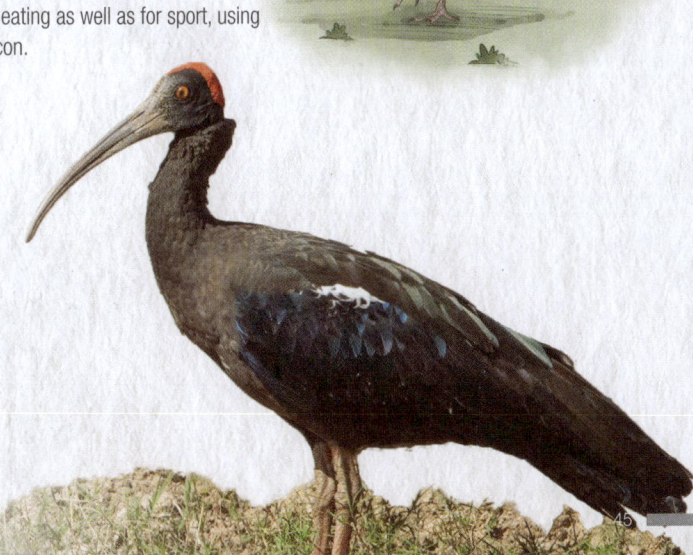

Jayantika Davé

Great Cormorant

Scientific name: *Phalacrocorax carbo*   Size: 90 cm
Hindi name: *Ghoghur, Maha Jal Kaak (Sanskrit)*
Sanskrit name: *Abhiplav*

Description

This is the largest cormorant we see in India and is a winter visitor across most of the country. Its black plumage has a blue gloss, with very characteristic bare-yellow skin on the face and throat region. It is often seen perched on rocks or tall bare trees with its wings outspread.

Habits

They are seen in both inland and coastal water. Fish is their main food, and they dive effortlessly, catching and eating smaller fish even underwater, whereas the larger ones are brought up and swallowed whole. They are clumsy fliers, preferring to take off only when very threatened, and even then, they push off with both feet together, barely skimming the surface of the water, looking for the closest place to settle back again. After each long fishing bout, they like to emerge from the water, perching on an exposed elevated position, and following a whole process of shaking off water – undulating the wings, shaking the body, shaking the head and wagging the tail, in that order!

They are gregarious while roosting or breeding, often with heron and ibis. In Jamnagar, Gujarat, they decided that the scaffolding to restore an old Jamnagar palace had been erected only for them to nest!

Call

While normally silent, it produces a variety of deep, guttural calls at nesting sites, and at roosts!

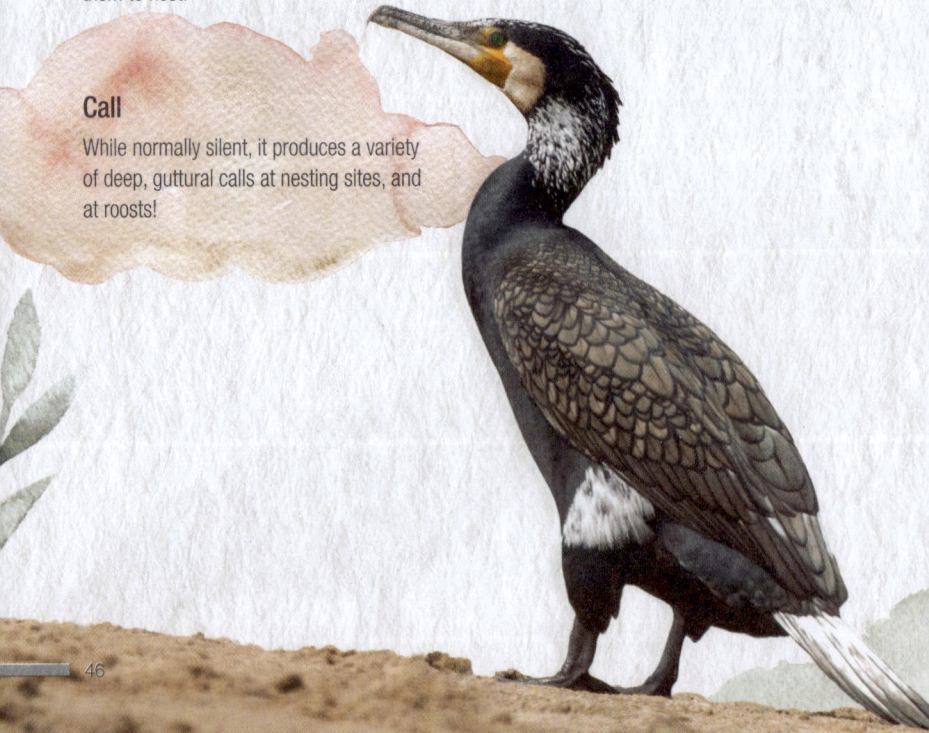

Mythology, Tales & Trivia

In China and Japan, fishermen use cormorants to fish for them, and place a neck ring or tight line around their necks, so that they cannot swallow the fish they have caught, and which the fisherman then take from them.

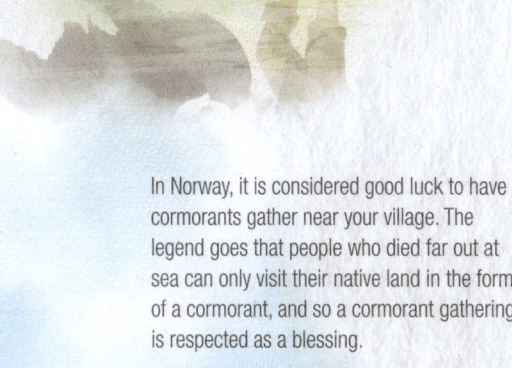

In Norway, it is considered good luck to have cormorants gather near your village. The legend goes that people who died far out at sea can only visit their native land in the form of a cormorant, and so a cormorant gathering is respected as a blessing.

Jayantika Davé

Darter

Scientific name: *Anhinga melanogaster* Size: 92 cm
Hindi name: *Panwa, Sanpoli Pandubbi*
Sanskrit name: *Madgu (water snake)*

Description

'Is that a snake you say?!… Or is it a bird?!… But I can't see the body!' So, when that's your confusion, what you are seeing is the Darter! The Darter is seen primarily on water, and has a very thin, long, snake-like neck and a long pointed bill. When it swims, its body stays completely submerged, and the curved neck sways this way and that, giving it the colloquial name of Snakebird!

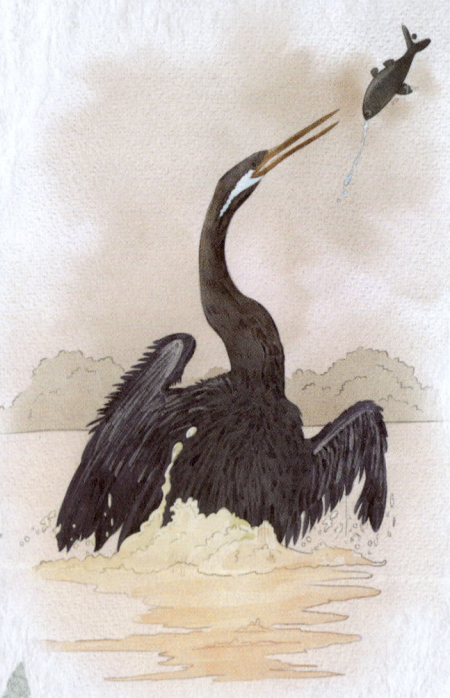

Habits

The Panwa lives mainly on freshwater lakes and streams, swimming with its body submerged, and its webbed feet moving the body forward. The neck moves jerkily, and is used to dart forward and into the water, to impale a fish. Fish are chased and speared, often underwater, then tossed into the air, landing head first into its open bill! Often seen together with cormorants, they also share the habit of spreading out their wings to dry when perched on rocks or small scrubby trees next to the water.

Call

Normally silent!

Mythology, Tales & Trivia

The Sanskrit name for the Darter is Madgu, which is also the name for the water snake – this is so apt, as the Darter has a very snake-like neck!

K.N. Davé mentions how in the Ramayana 3.47.47, when Ravana offers Sita his love, she insults him by comparing him to a mean-looking Darter, whereas the one she admires is like the princely peacock and the graceful goose.

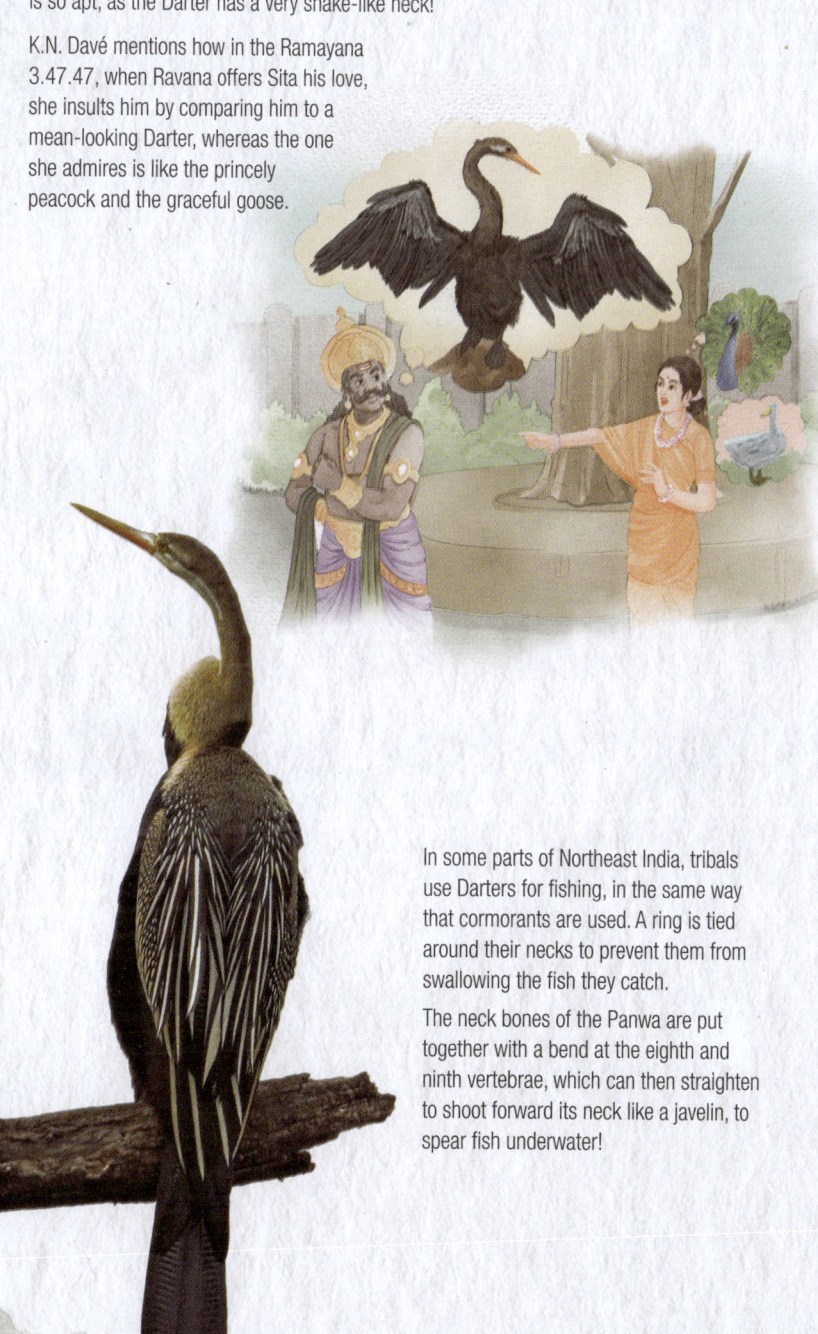

In some parts of Northeast India, tribals use Darters for fishing, in the same way that cormorants are used. A ring is tied around their necks to prevent them from swallowing the fish they catch.

The neck bones of the Panwa are put together with a bend at the eighth and ninth vertebrae, which can then straighten to shoot forward its neck like a javelin, to spear fish underwater!

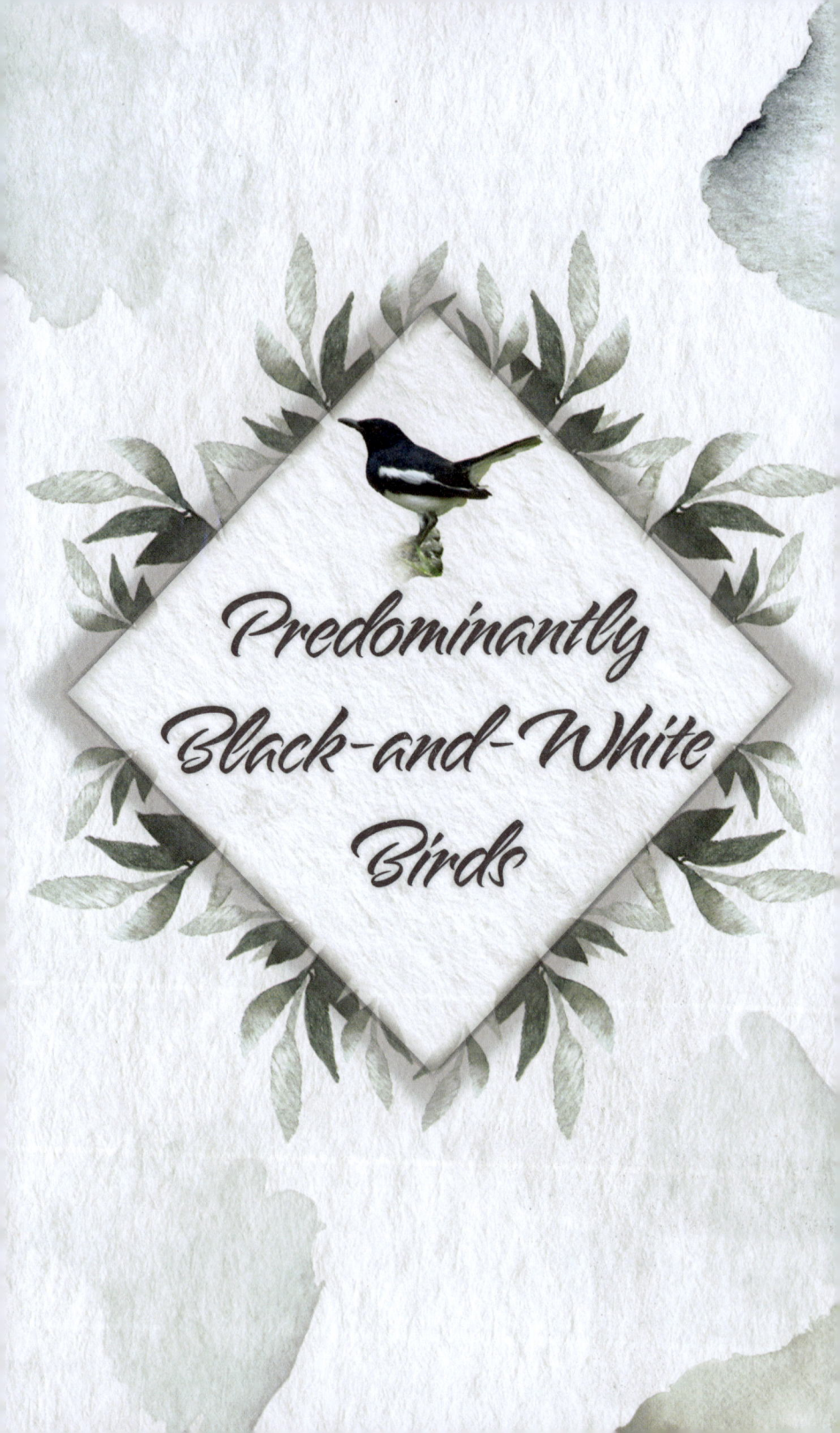

Pied Bushchat

Scientific name: *Saxicola caprata* Size: *13 cm*
Hindi name: *Kala Pidda*
Sanskrit name: *Pidu, Paidu*

Description
The resident plump Pied Bushchat, with an alert, upright look to it, is very visible on exposed perches in open habitats. The male is a glossy black, with a white slash on the wings, and that, together with its white lower stomach, makes it quite distinctive.

Habits
The Kala Pidda is a familiar bird of open grasslands, and likes being near villages and cultivation. It is found perched on top of a scrubby tree, from where it makes a quick dart to the ground to pick up an insect, and then quickly back onto its lookout point.

It has a lovely courting display, with the male whistling a pretty song, holding its wings high, flying slow and puffing up the undertail white feathers. At the sight of a rival, the display turns menacing, with the wings dropped to show the white slashes more clearly, and the neck stuck out threateningly. Quite amusing to see this small bird trying to look dangerous!

Call
A whee and a chruk normally, accompanied by a full song during breeding!

Mythology, Tales & Trivia
Among one of the indigenous tribes in the Nilgiris, there is a story about how the Pied Bushchat got its white wing slash. Once, there was a priest who was churning buttermilk to extract butter. He stopped for a rest, and a watching Bushchat scolded him. The priest got annoyed, and flicked the butter from his hands, and it white-streaked the Bushchat's black wing!

It is often careless about where it builds its nest, with even the footprint of a bullock serving the purpose of a depression, and a tuft of grass providing a little shelter!

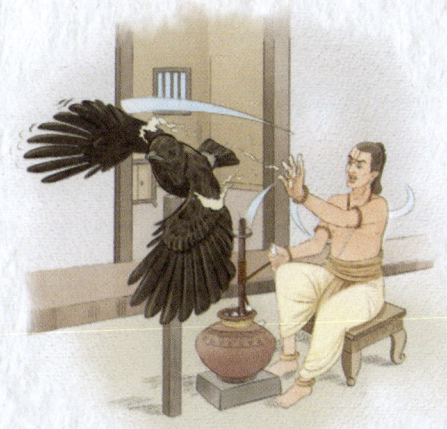

Jayantika Davé

White-browed Fantail Flycatcher

Scientific name: *Rhipidura aureola*   Size: 18 cm
Hindi name: *Machharya, Nachan, Chakdil*
Sanskrit name: *Latva, Bindurekhak*

Description

This resident, cheerful, restless dark flycatcher can be seen all over India. Its most striking feature is its dark, white-tipped tail, which it constantly cocks and spreads out like a fan, with its wings drooping to the side. The Hindi name of Nachan talks to the 'never sit still' dancing movements of this lively little bird, bobbing, pirouetting, graceful!

The similar **White-throated Fantail Flycatcher** is visible mainly in the Northeast and the Himalayas, and has a white throat and dark belly, while the pretty **White Spotted Fantail Flycatcher** has a spotted necklaced throat and a white belly, and is seen primarily in Peninsular and South India.

Habits

Usually seen in ones or twos, these birds flit about tirelessly in the low and mid-levels of trees and shrubs, endlessly flicking and spreading their tail, constantly bowing to the observer! Whistler beautifully describes the Fantail Flycatcher as having an 'inimitable joi-de-vivre'! They are very comfortable around human habitation, gardens and secondary forests, and are not shy of humans. They are very adept at catching insects in the air.

Call

A short, harsh chuck-chuck, or a lovely clear whistling song!

Mythology, Tales & Trivia

Whistler wrote beautifully about this bird: 'It turns from side to side with restive, jerky movements; like a ballet dancer trying out new steps in front of a mirror.' Also, 'The dainty round fan of the tail is opened and closed and flirted with all the coquetry and grace of a beauty of Andalusia'!

EHA's description is equally pretty: 'So buxom, blithe and debonair; I am tempted to ask – Prithee, why so gay?'

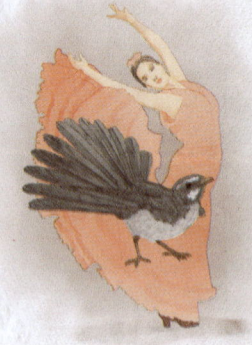

Each Little Bird That Sings

Yellow-crowned Woodpecker

Scientific name: *Dendrocopos mahrattensis*   Size: 18 cm
Hindi name: *Katphora*
Sanskrit name: *Darvaghaat, Kaashtthkukut*

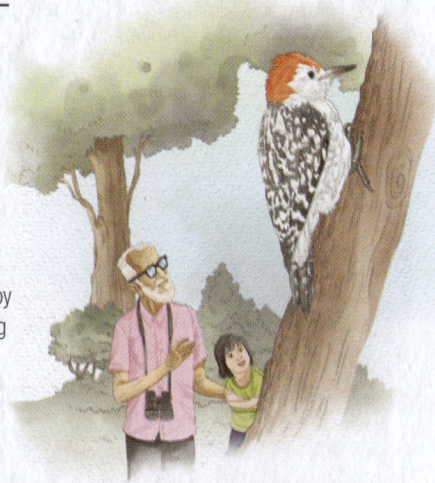

Description

This pretty and small black-and-white woodpecker has a special memory for me! When I was only 13, I saw this woodpecker (which at that time used to be called the Mahratta Woodpecker) but I was confused about its identity. So I wrote to Dr Salim Ali, asking him what I was seeing! And imagine my joy when he took the trouble to write back, explaining that what I was seeing was a female Yellow-crowned Woodpecker!

Resident across India, this is a busy little bird, constantly moving up and down tree trunks.

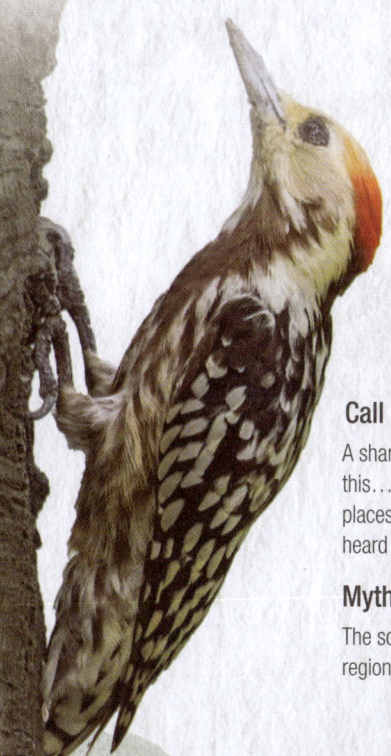

The very similar **Brown-fronted Woodpecker** is seen mainly in the Himalayas, and is distinguished from the Yellow-crowned Woodpecker by a brown, instead of yellow, forehead.

Habits

The Yellow-crowned Woodpecker avoids dense evergreen forest, preferring more open woodland. It is seen singly or in pairs, busily flying from trunk to trunk, landing low and scuttling up in jerks, directly or in spirals, halting to tap on the bark or putting its head on one side to peer into crevices for lurking insects. It rarely descends to the ground and is often seen clinging upside down to investigate a particularly grub heavy piece of bark.

Call

A sharp chik chik and a chickk–r–r–r…sounding like 'This… this…and thitherrrr', as if it is pointing out good grub-hiding places to its mate! Its drumming on hollow trunks can be heard far away!

Mythology, Tales & Trivia

The scientific name *mahrattensis* came from the Mahratta region of Maharashtra, where it was most commonly seen.

Jayantika Davé

White-browed Wagtail
(Large Pied Wagtail)

Scientific name: *Motacilla maderaspatensis*   Size: 21 cm
Hindi name: *Khanjan, Dhobin, Mamula*
Sanskrit name: *Ashvakhya*

Description
Built like a typical wagtail…very horizontal to the ground, with a tail that never stops wagging, this is the largest of the wagtails we see in India, and is easily identifiable!

Habits
The Khanjan, or eye-shaped bird, is most often found near water bodies, and around urban environments where water is easily available. Seen in pairs or very small groups, these birds are quite comfortable around humans and are not shy. They perch and walk extensively on the ground and are also strong fliers, with the flight a beautifully drawn pattern of undulating dips and rises. Mainly insectivorous, they have a varied diet of caterpillars, spiders, and a variety of other bugs and beetles.

S.C. Law also describes the mighty singing contests that occur during the breeding season, when many males vie for the hand of one uninterested female, by singing a vigorous and many-noted song, till she is captivated by one individual's prowess. He likened it to a *swayamvara*!

Call
The usual call is a soft 'wheech', while the song itself can be long and loud with a number of different variations!

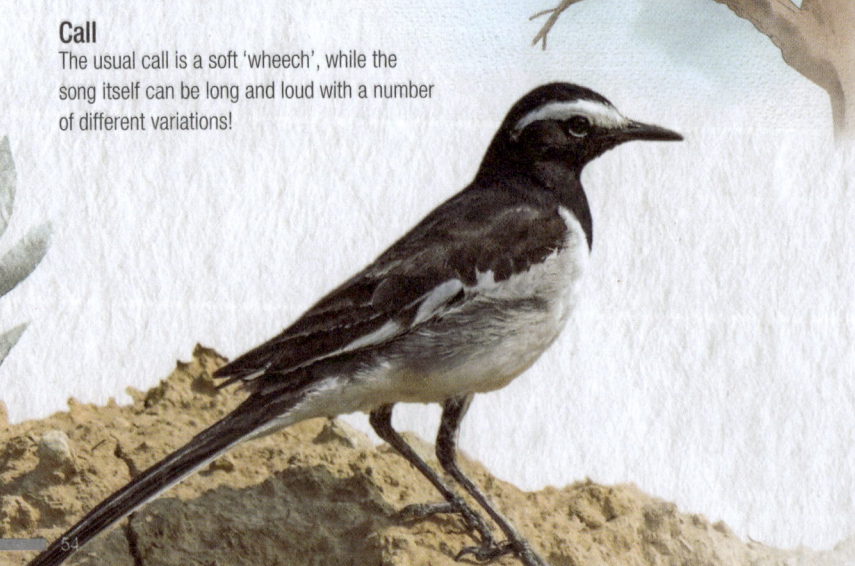

Mythology, Tales & Trivia

Dewar tells of a pair of these birds which built their nest on a ferry boat that went across the Jamuna. This boat was not often used, but when it was, the female wagtail would continue to sit on its nest, and the male would sit on the edge of the boat and continue to sing!

Another interesting nest site was in an iron ring, attached to a buoy in the middle of the Jamuna at Agra!

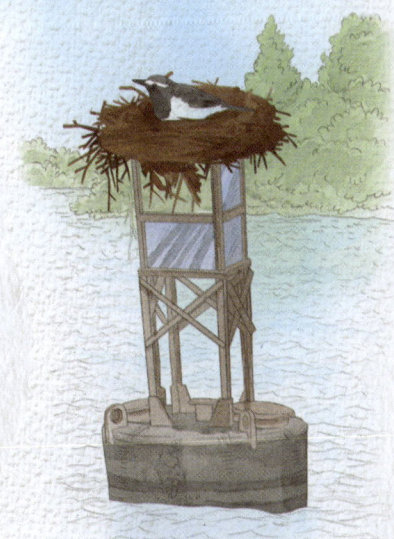

Jayantika Davé

Oriental Magpie-robin

Scientific name: *Copyschus saularis*   Size: 20 cm
Hindi name: *Dahiyar, Dhaiyal, Sau Lari*
Sanskrit name: *Kalvidak*

Description

One of my father's favourite birds! The Oriental Magpie-robin is a dapper, glossy blue-black and white bird, with a smartly cocked tail. It is a quiet, unobtrusive bird, happy to be near people, sitting on a wall, and interestedly watching what its humans are doing! An early riser, and a cheerful hard worker, the Dahiyar forages and sings from dawn to dusk.

Habits

With a clear preference for open woodlands, gardens or cultivated areas near human habitation, the Magpie-robin cheerfully forages amongst leaf litter, all the time holding its cocked tail aloft and uttering a soft 'swee'. Mainly insectivorous, these birds also drink the nectar from large-flowered trees like the seemul and the Erythrina.

During the breeding season, it completely lives up to its colloquial name of Sau Laria – meaning 'the 100-note song'! Its long, continuous, sweet and very varied song pours forth from its uplifted beak, accompanied by a lot of flicking and opening of its tail, puffing of its chest, and strutting about!

Call

A soft swee-swee normally, with a long and very varied song during the breeding season!

Mythology, Tales & Trivia

It used to be kept in captivity for the sweetness of its song, and its ability to learn a few short phrases. L.J. Mackintosh has heard one bird singing *Nabizee rozi da do* – 'give us this day our daily bread!'

The Indian name of Dhayal and Sau Lari has led to some funny confusions! Eleazar Albin in 1737 used the Indian name Dhayal, and others thought he was saying 'sun dial'. Meanwhile, Linnaeus interpreted Sau Lari and sundial as something to do with the sun, and therefore added solaris to the name! It was only much later that people realized that Sau Lari referred to the 100-notes song! So, finally the scientific name was corrected to saularis.

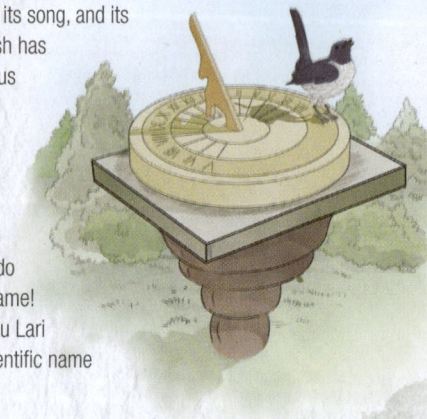

Asian Pied Starling

Scientific name: *Gracupica contra*   Size: 23 cm
Hindi name: *Ablaki Myna*
Sanskrit name: *Chitrangi, Kunpi*

Description

The Asian Pied Starling is a strikingly marked black-and-white myna, with a yellow bill and bare red skin around the eye. It used to be known as the Pied Myna in my youth! It is a relatively shy myna, with a sweet call, and is seen around cities and villages, though its numbers are fewer as compared to its vigorous Common Myna cousins.

Habits

The Ablaki Myna likes areas with scattered trees and access to open water, and is widespread across the north and middle of India. They are very comfortable around human habitation, though they don't enter into our verandahs or perch on our terraces. They feed in small groups on lawns, on open ground and on trees, mainly on fruits like figs and lantana, grains, insects and worms. They feed like other starlings, pushing their beak into the ground, and then strongly forcing it open to unearth worms. Roosting time is a noisy communal affair, with many birds clamouring together on one tree.

The nest is a big, untidy, loose mass of grass, paper, string and cloth, with many messy paper and grass bits trailing off it, placed high in a tree.

Call

A liquid warbling call, also with sharp warning calls, and mimicking of other birds!

Mythology, Tales & Trivia

The Asian Pied Starling is a good mimic and can mimic humans as well as other birds. The Sema Nagas will not eat this bird because they believe that it is a human reincarnated as a bird.

The eyes are so placed that they almost act as binoculars, looking down the bill and being able to see clearly what is being unearthed as it is plunged into the ground.

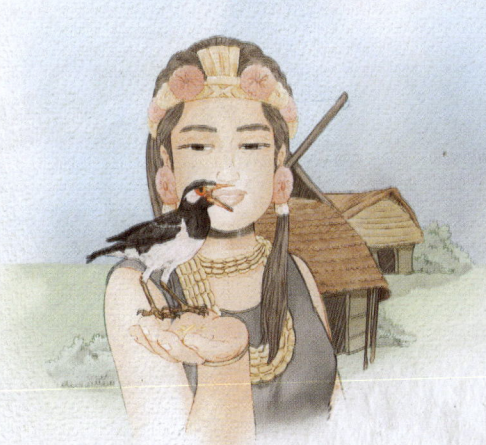

Jayantika Davé

Pied Kingfisher

Scientific name: *Ceryle rudis*   Size: *25 cm*
Hindi name: *Kaudiala Kilkila*
Sanskrit name: *Kshatrak = open umbrella*

Description

The Hindi name is the perfect descriptor for the distinctive Pied Kingfisher. *Kaudiala* = coins; *kilkila* = referring to its laugh-like call – so the bird with coin-like spots and a laughing call! Look out for this medium-sized black-and-white kingfisher near streams and ponds, with its lovely swept-back crest and black necklace! This is a kingfisher of the plains, and is replaced by the very similar-looking, though larger and bigger crested, **Crested Kingfisher** in the Himalayas.

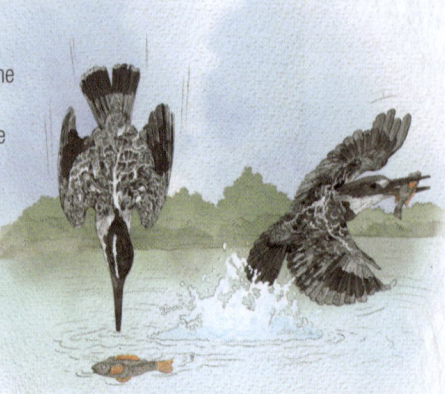

Habits

The Pied Kingfisher is resident across India, up to heights of 1,800 m. Lakes, rivers, ponds and coastal lagoons are all good haunts, so long as the area around is open and not dense forest. It can be seen perched on trees alongside the water, with a typical bobbing motion of its head and a flicking of its tail, as it surveys the water for its favourite prey – fish, aquatic insects, crabs, frogs and molluscs. Once prey is spied, it launches itself, hovering above the spot, pointing its beak downwards as if it is taking aim, folds its wings and plunges in fearlessly! If it has been successful, it emerges with the fish in its beak, cackling with triumphant joy, and flies straight back to the same perch it left from.

These birds dig out and nest in long tunnels near water, which end in a broader egg chamber.

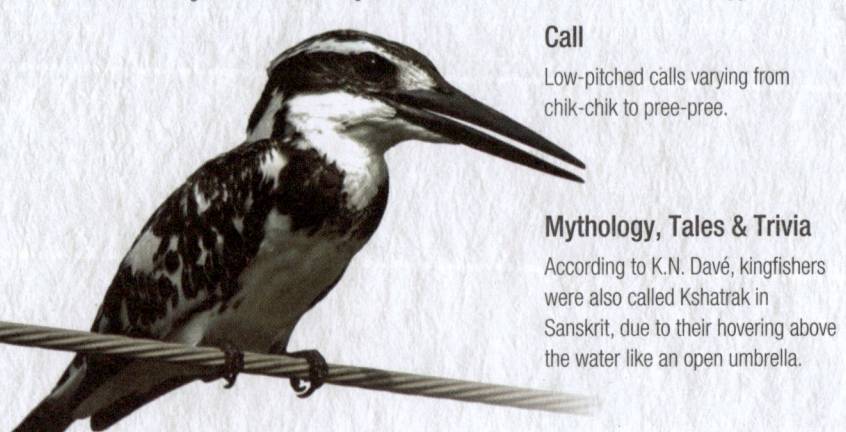

Call

Low-pitched calls varying from chik-chik to pree-pree.

Mythology, Tales & Trivia

According to K.N. Davé, kingfishers were also called Kshatrak in Sanskrit, due to their hovering above the water like an open umbrella.

Spotted Forktail

Scientific name: *Enicurus maculatus*   Size: 28 cm
Hindi name: *Khanjan Pidda*
Kashmiri name: *Shakhel Lot*

Description
Daintily picking its way through well-shaded forest streams in the Himalayas, you see the shy Spotted Forktail – a vision in black and white, with a long, deeply forked tail. A shining white head and dense star-like white spotting on its black upper back complete the fairytale!

Habits

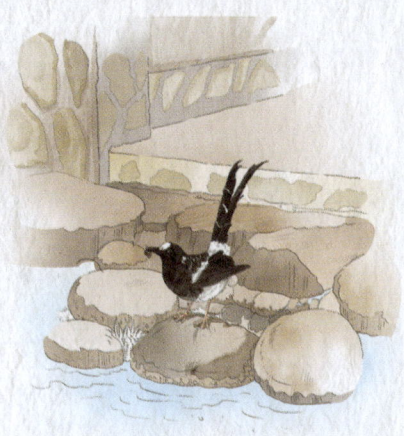

A picture-book habitat of sheltered streams, small rivulets, dotted rocks to perch on, waterfalls and shadowed banks thick with fern in the Himalayan foothills and higher, is where you will most often see the Khanjan Pidda, looking for aquatic insects, molluscs, larvae and caterpillars. Despite having such a striking colouration, the fact that it stays in shadowy spaces, with tumbling water, often makes it difficult to see. A dainty traveller, it does little runs up a stream, often pirouetting and turning sideways with its lovely, forked tail constantly swaying up and down – almost as if it were the show-stopper in a fashion show!

While it is shy and reclusive, in our mountain home, one year, a pair picked a set of moist moss-covered steps as their happy hunting ground, and to our utter delight, arrived every day for a couple of weeks!

Call
A soft, sweet whistling swhee call!

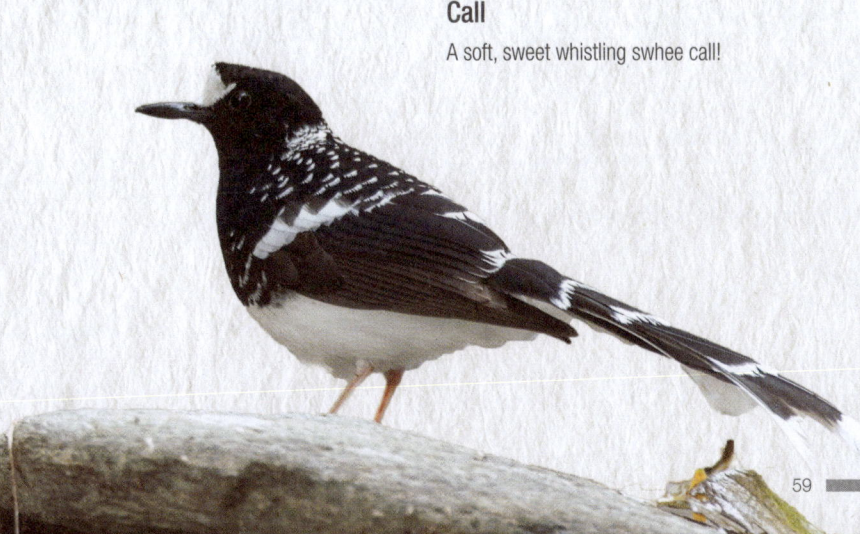

Jayantika Davé

Pheasant-tailed Jacana

Scientific name: *Hydrophasianus chirurgus*   Size: *31 cm*
Hindi name: *Piho, Pihuya*
Sanskrit name: *Jalmanjaur, Jalshikhandin*

Description

In the rainy season, look around for the Pheasant-tailed Jacana on water bodies with a lot of lily or lotus pads, on which it walks with ease. At this time it comes into its breeding plumage, with long tail streamers, held high in a lovely arch. A chocolate-brown body, a white face and a beautiful golden nape are the identifiers, even during non-breeding time. No wonder then that in Assam, it is known as the Rani Didao Gophita, or 'little white water princess'!

Habits

While their preference is for walking on top of water, they often swim or wade into the water while foraging for their prey. They forage for insects, invertebrates and some seeds and plant material, sometimes separately or in groups, and are not shy of humans.

The female literally rules the roost! She is larger, selects different males by doing a courtship display herself, and can mate with up to 10 males, moving to the next mate after laying eggs, and leaving the male in charge of the eggs!

Call
A mewing mee-awnp 'angry cat' call!

Mythology, Tales & Trivia

The males are very good fathers, and can push the nest to safety, or move the eggs themselves by holding them between their bill and their breast, or between the wings and their body.

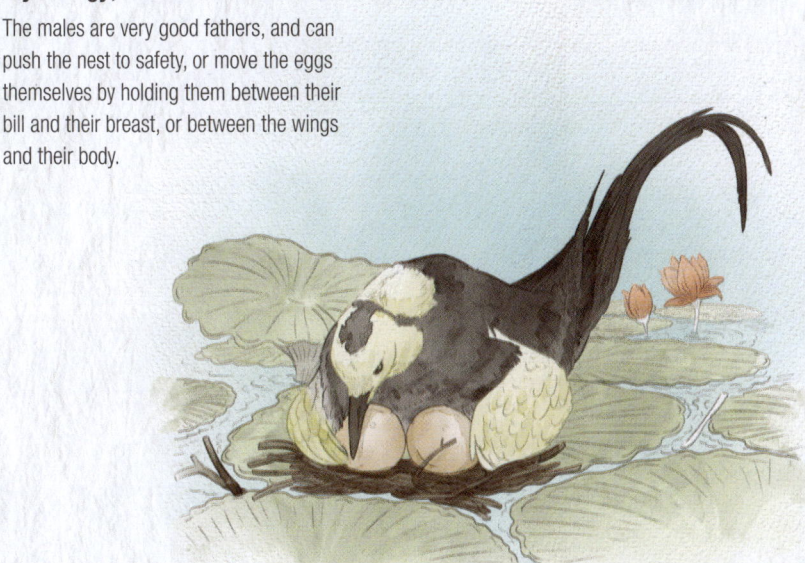

This bird was first described by French explorer Pierre Sonnerat in 1776 as the Surgeon of Luzon, since he felt its breeding tail feathers looked like the lancets used by surgeons of that time for blood-letting!

The scientific name *Hydrophasianus* means water pheasant, as the bird in breeding looks like a miniature pheasant!

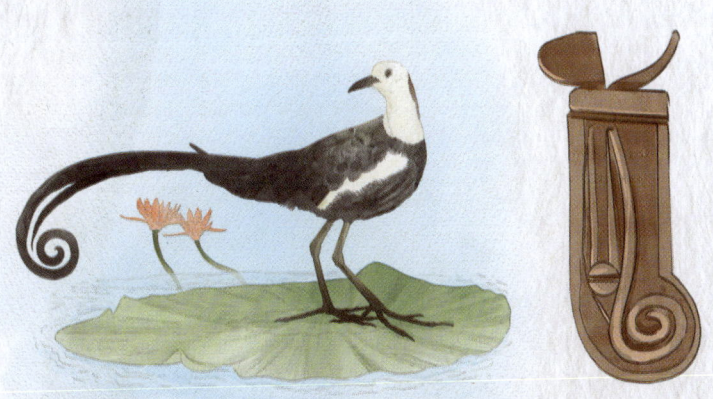

Jayantika Davé

Jacobin Cuckoo

Scientific name: *Clamator jacobinus*   Size: 32 cm
Hindi name: *Papiya, Kala Papiya, Chatak*
Sanskrit name: *Sarang Chatak, Divaukas*

Description

The slim and elegant Jacobin Cuckoo, dressed in glossy black-and-white priestly Jacobin robes, with a black, somewhat flattened, though very noticeable, crest, makes its appearance in India with the onset of the monsoon season. Its beautiful, liquid, ringing call of 'piu-piu pee pee piu' always makes my heart lift at the thought that the monsoons are near!

Habits

It frequents open woodlands and scrub and also plains and gardens in the cities, and avoids thick forest or very dry areas. Primarily insectivorous, it enjoys grasshoppers, termites, caterpillars, snails and also the eggs of the host birds who it parasitizes to lay its own eggs. It stays true to its scientific name *Clamator*, and is clamorous in its calls, often calling late into the night.

A parasitic cuckoo, it chooses babblers and bulbuls to be foster parents for its young.

Call

The lovely 'see you-see you-see you' notes descend in scale, followed by a faster series of rising 'quick-quick-quick' notes!

Mythology, Tales & Trivia

In Indian mythology and poetry, it has been referred to as the Chatak, which is represented as a bird with a deep longing for rain to quench its thirst. K.N. Davé talks about how Kalidasa, in his beautiful *Meghadoota*, uses the Chatak as a metaphor for yearning for love.

Interestingly, the eggs laid match the colour of the host bird. So they are blue when laid in a babbler's nest, but whiter if laid in the nest of a Red-vented Bulbul!

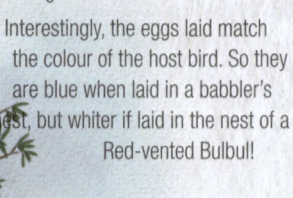
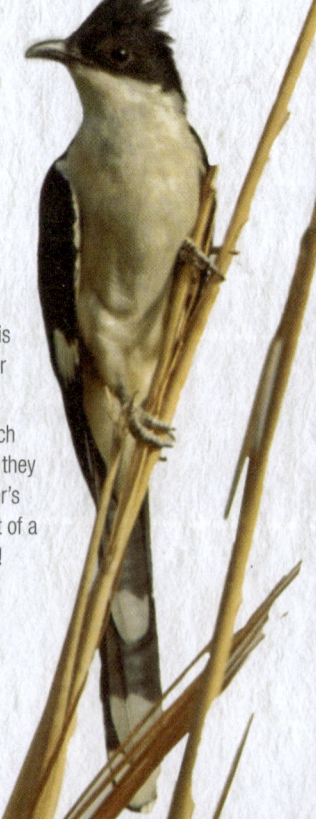

White-breasted Waterhen

Scientific name: *Amaurornis phoenicurus*   Size: 32 cm
Hindi name: *Jalmurghi, Dawak, Dahak, Dauk*
Sanskrit name: *Daatyauh*

Description

Looking as if they have just received their sparkling white shirt back from the dhobi, the White-breasted Waterhen is often seen around water bodies or marshes in villages or large residences. This smart, upright, jaunty bird is a leggy combination of dark grey-black, with a white face and stomach, and a tail that is continually flicked up and down, doing a traffic-light rufous flash!

Habits

The Jalmurghi is fairly bold around human habitation, doing a quick run when it feels threatened, but rarely taking to flight. These birds are resident across India, and are most often seen in the plains, singly or in pairs, feeding along the edges of a water body, looking for insects, crustaceans, worms, seeds, and even little fish.
According to Hugh Whistler, from June to October courtship starts with bowing and rubbing of bills, and 'loud harsh roars which might have been elicited from a bear by roasting it slowly over a slow fire.'

Call

A loud call comprised of a variety of croaks, grunts and harsh rolls, followed by a kru-ak, kru-ak, kru-ak-a-wak-wak.

Mythology, Tales & Trivia

When I was around 12 years old, we lived in a government house with a large garden, at the foot of which would be a thick hose pipe, which brought in water from the Jamuna, resplendent with silt. In the evenings, I would hear this call, like the rattling of the wooden spool of a 'chik' (a bamboo screen) being rolled down. I could never see what made it, so I wrote to Salim Ali asking him what that sound could be. Pat came his letter – go to the water point in your garden in the evening…you should see a White-breasted Waterhen! And how right he was!

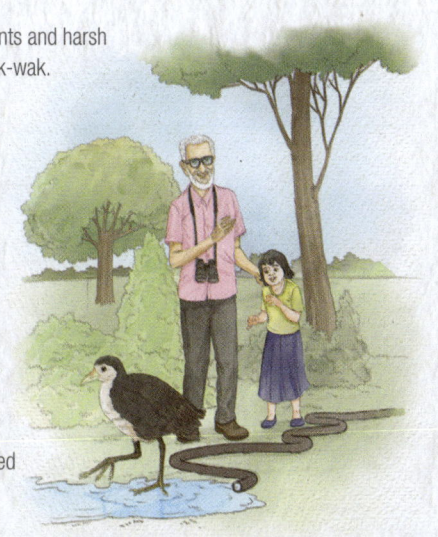

Jayantika Dayé

Black-winged Stilt

Scientific name: *Himantopus himantopus*   Size: *38 cm*
Hindi name: *Gaz Paon, Tinghur*
Sanskrit name: *Yashtik*

Description

In winter, in and around wetlands and water bodies, you will see this elegant, boldly pied, very long-legged bird with bright pink legs, giving it the very apt Hindi name of Gaz Paon – the bird with the legs that are 1 m long! As it flies, its bright legs stick out way behind its tail…an unmistakable identifier.

Habits

Black-winged Stilts are largely carnivorous, picking up all kinds of aquatic larvae, beetles, bugs, flies, crustaceans, tadpoles, worms, tiny fish and sometimes seeds. They prefer to search for their food in shallow water, using their eyesight, and sometimes probing in soft mud to see what emerges. Their stilt-like legs enable them to go in much deeper than other waders, so they often stand out among the group. They have a rather mincing walk, with long legs pulled backwards and out of the water, and then curled forward and extended to enter the water again.

They nest around April–June, and any intruder at a nesting site is greeted with loud cries and much aggression!

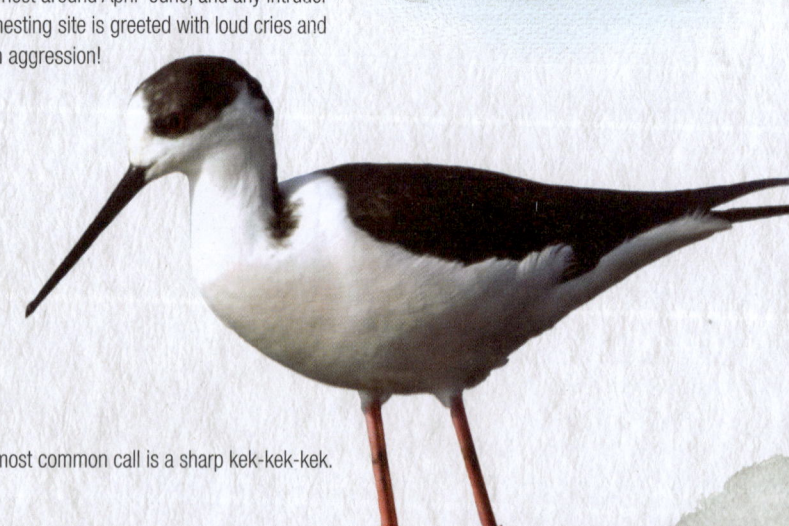

Call

The most common call is a sharp kek-kek-kek.

Indian Skimmer

Scientific name: *Rynchops albicollis* Size: *40 cm*
Hindi name: *Panchira, Dhruv, Jal Vardhani, Sharari*
Gujarati name: *Jal Hal*
Sanskrit name: *Jalavardhani*

Description

The sandbanks of Chambal River, a two-hour drive from the Keoladeo (Bharatpur) Bird Sanctuary… February, the start of the nesting month… and it's time for us to go for our annual sighting of the globally endangered Indian Skimmer. A short-legged, elongated, medium-sized black-and-white bird, with a most remarkable feature! Its large, heavy, downward-drooping red bill tipped with orange-yellow has the lower mandible significantly longer than the upper! A dentist's nightmare!

Habits

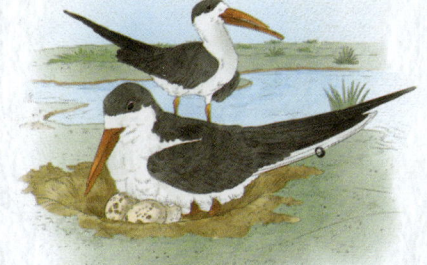

The Panchira is a winter visitor to the northwest of India, and also a resident in some parts of North and Central India. It is seen mainly on the sandbanks of large rivers, where it feeds on aquatic life that can be taken from the surface of the water, by using the longer lower mandible as a scoop and sieve, justifying its earlier name of Scissorbill! Small groups fly slowly across the surface of a slow-moving river, up and down, almost as if they were ploughing it, all the while surface-feeding small fish, shrimp and insects. It is quite comfortable feeding even nocturnally, if the days have been too hot or too windy.

During the breeding season of February–June, conservation groups work closely with the forest and water departments to ensure that water levels in critical nesting areas are maintained at a certain level, so that nests are not destroyed. They nest communally on the sandbanks, together with pratincoles and terns.

Call

A barking kyap-kyap call!

Mythology, Tales & Trivia

This is a globally endangered bird, with the global population estimated at only 6,000–10,000 birds and declining.

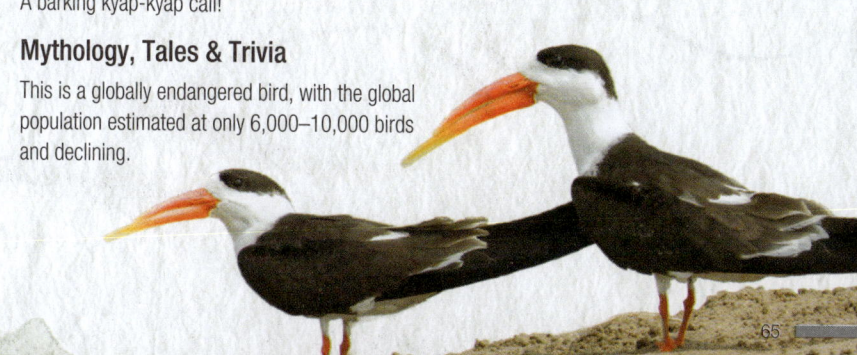

Jayantika Davé

Pied Avocet

Scientific name: *Recurvirostra avosetta*   Size: 43 cm
Hindi name: *Kusya Chaha*
Sanskrit name: *Kashikani*

Description
The hallmark of the tall and leggy Pied Avocet is its black head, three black curved bands on a white wing, and a distinctively upcurved black bill. A winter visitor, this is a very striking bird, seen around Delhi and towards the west of India…one of my personal favourites!

Habits
They mainly eat insects and crustaceans, and feed in shallow water or mud flats, scything their bills from side to side to catch their prey. The Pied Avocet feeds on its own or in small dispersed groups, but sometimes gets together in a compact group, and then the scything gets so frantic that they look as if they are practising ballet pirouettes!

Call
A sweet kluit…kluit, repeated continuously, which can be heard for long distances!

Mythology, Tales & Trivia
Interestingly, they have a crèche system where one or two adults volunteer to tend to up to 20 chicks.

The scientific name *Recurviostra* refers to the backwardly curving bill. The *avosetta* part of the name may refer to the black-and-white outfits of advocates.

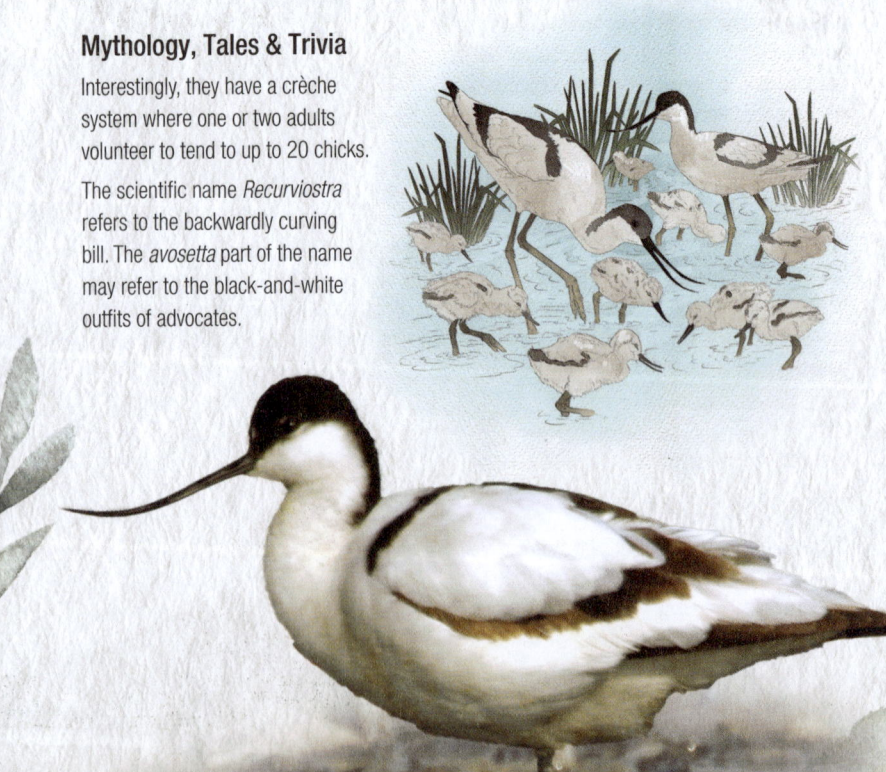

Lesser Florican

Scientific name: *Sypheotides indicus*   Size: *49 cm*
Hindi name: *Leekh, Chhota Charat/Charaz, Barsati/Kala Charaz or Tuqdar*
Sanskrit name: *Anjalikarn*

Description

This endangered, otherwise fairly nondescript bustard, in shades of brown, comes into its own in the breeding season – with the neck and stomach turning black, a white back collar and sides, and a crown of 5–6 elongated, spatulate, backward-curving feathers! Pretty stunning! A special visit to Velavadar in Gujarat, or Sonkhaliya, Rajasthan, during the breeding season is an absolute must-do!

Habits

The Leekh is an inhabitant of flat and open grasslands, scrublands, and can also be seen in cultivated fields of groundnuts and soybean. Its favourite foods are grass, seeds, berries, insects of all kinds, beetles, grasshoppers, lizards and frogs. The courtship display of the Lesser Florican is spectacular, and is best seen between July and September, closely linked to the monsoon. The male utters a harsh frog-like croak to draw attention to an explosive straight-up jump, at the top of which it then flutters its wings to descend slowly, and does it again…and again…and again!

Call

The Lesser Florican is a silent bird, only doing its harsh guttural croak during display, or a short whistle when disturbed!

Mythology, Tales & Trivia

One year we went to Velavadar, Gujarat, to see the breeding display. After searching for the Leekh for a long time, we were about to give up, and suddenly, walking down a raised bund between two fields, as if on a show ramp, struts this Lesser Florican in full breeding plumage. Having made sure all eyes were on it, it then proceeded to do the repeated squawk-jump-flutter…what a display!

The local name of Barsati is linked to its glorious breeding plumage, which comes into being only during the rains.

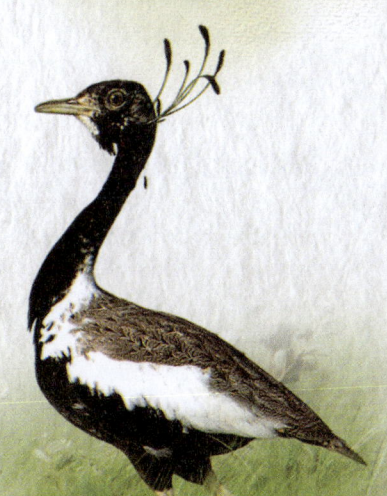

Jayantika Davé

Osprey

Scientific name: *Pandion haliaetus*   Size: 56 cm
Hindi name: *Machlimaar, Dhanesh, Banrao*
Sanskrit name: *Kurar*

Description

In winter, near large lakes, rivers or coastal waters all throughout India, the large dark-brown-black-and-white Osprey makes its appearance! It is easily recognizable due to its dramatic contrast colouring, and its very upright posture, with slightly open wings when at rest.

Habits

The Osprey's diet is primarily fish, and its talons and uplift abilities are so strong that it can pick fish weighing up to 2 kg directly from the water, using powerful wing strokes to lift this heavy load clear of the water! The Osprey has such sharp eyes that it can sight fish from 100 feet above water. It then hovers to ensure sight lock, and plunges feet first into the water to dig its talons into the fish and lift it into the air. The Machlimaar doesn't like to get too wet, so it typically fishes either in shallow water or focuses on surface-schooling fish.

The male Osprey usually mates for life, and has a dramatic courtship display, which involves showing off by flying in an undulating pattern over the nest area, while carrying a large fish, and doing its distinctive screaming call. Conservation efforts involve building tall nesting platforms, which are quickly adopted, and re-used, sometimes for up to 70 years!

Call

A loud screaming cry!

Mythology, Tales & Trivia

Since it mates for life, Chinese mythology uses the Osprey as a symbol of fidelity and harmony between husband and wife.

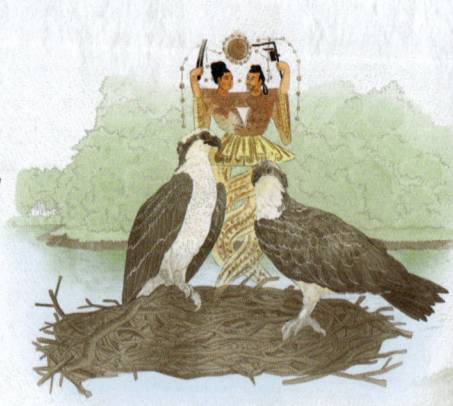

They have a reversible outer toe, allowing them to shift it to be a back toe, in turn enabling them to lift heavy fish with two talons in front and two at the back!

They can close their nostrils to keep water out!

Oriental Pied Hornbill

Scientific name: *Anthracoceros albirostris*   Size: 59 cm
Hindi name: *Dhanesh, Banrao*
Sanskrit name: *Matrinindak (generic for hornbills)*

Description

The striking black-and-white Oriental Pied Hornbill, with a bright-yellow ungainly casque over the bill, is quite a sight to see! These birds tend to move in groups, and are noisy, energetic feeders – impossible to miss if they have arrived on a nearby fruiting tree!

Habits

Resident in the Himalayan foothills and the eastern part of India, the striking Oriental Pied Hornbill inhabits evergreen and deciduous forests and plantations. Fruit trees are a big attraction, with worms, snails, lizards and small rats or small birds occasionally being taken to add variety!

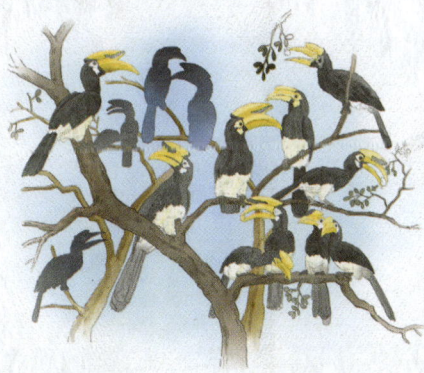

Once, when we were on a birding trip to Pangot in Uttarakhand, as the sun came up, we heard this loud noisy squawking and clamouring. We rushed out and saw that a fig tree, which was right next to our lodge, was full of a large group of the striking Banrao, giving us a great viewing! Another time, close to 40 of these birds were on a leafless fruiting tree – and what a sight they were, silhouetted against the blue sky!

The Dhanesh nests in natural cavities in trees, with 1–3 eggs being laid between February and April. The female enters the nest, and is sealed in by the mate, incubating the eggs for 25 to 27 days. It is no wonder, then, that when she emerges, she is a bedraggled sight, and the male too is lean and weary with his feeding duties!

Call

A cackling kek or kek-kek-kek.

Jayantika Davé

Black-crowned Night Heron

Scientific name: *Nycticorax nycticorax*   Size: *62 cm*
Hindi name: *Taal Bagla, Kokrai, Waak, Kwaak*
Sanskrit name: *Naktakronch, Chandravihangam, Koyishtha*

Description

Looking rather like an officious, stoop-shouldered, elderly judge, the stocky Black-crowned Night Heron with its black, grey and white robes, and long and white head plumes, is a dignified skulker on low trees at water edges. It is easy to identify due to its relatively short legs and heavy structure.

Habits

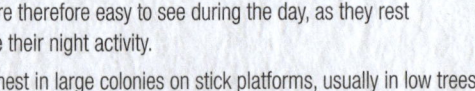

Night Herons, true to their name, are night or early morning hunters, thereby avoiding competition with other herons who are day feeders. As dusk falls, they set off to their feeding grounds in a steady stream, uttering a slow and steady 'kwark kwark' as they wing their way. Their diet is primarily fish and frogs, with the occasional aquatic insects, crustaceans and sometimes even small birds and mammals. They roost in large numbers, in low leafy trees around the water's edge, and are therefore easy to see during the day, as they rest before their night activity.

They nest in large colonies on stick platforms, usually in low trees.

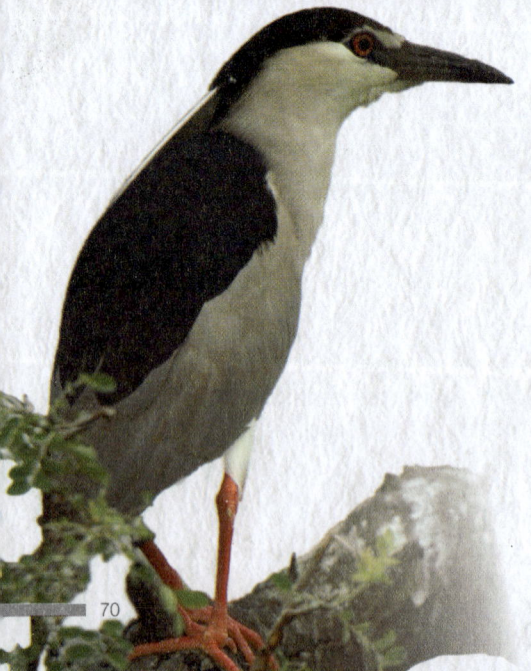

Call

A hoarse squat-squawk, seeming to describe their posture!

Mythology, Tales & Trivia

The scientific name *Nycticorax* is from the ancient Greek *nuktos* = night, referring to its nocturnal habits, and *korax* = raven, referring to its croaking call.

They are one of the few herons who use tools for feeding! They throw buoyant material into the water to attract fish close enough for them to strike.

Asian Openbill Stork

Scientific name: *Anastomus oscitans* Size: 68 cm
Hindi name: *Gungla, Ghungil, Ghonghila*
Sanskrit name: *Avabhanjan, Ghongak*

Description

The Asian Openbill Stork is a large stork with green-purple, glossed black wings, a black skull cap on an otherwise white-ish grey body, and a beak that somehow got warped and can't close in the middle! It soars high in small groups, and in the breeding season, its bright-red legs trailing behind are a lovely sight!

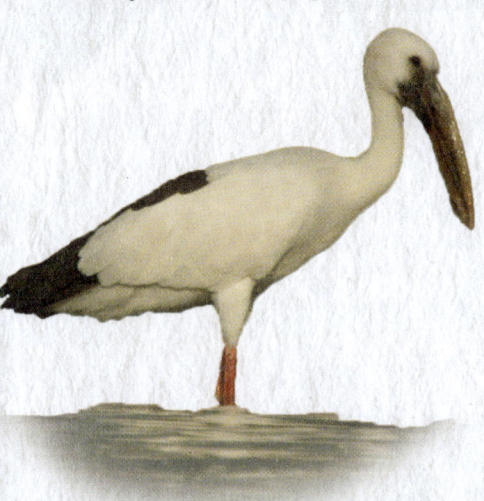

Habits

In the non-breeding season, the Gungla has a drab grey-and-black look, but in the breeding season it becomes almost unrecognizable, with the grey back turning into a bright white and the legs turning a bright orange pink! Their most distinctive feature is undoubtedly the beak, with an arched gap formed between the two mandibles, with the edges having very fine and small brush-like spikes, which help them to grip and crush snails better. Not a surprise then that T.C. Jerdon initially called them Shell Ibis. Their favourite feeding grounds are wetlands, where they pick up large molluscs, snakes and frogs.

Call

Like all storks, they are silent, except for a low honking call when greeting a partner arriving at the nest, and bill-clattering during breeding!

Mythology, Tales & Trivia

The scientific name *Anastomus* is from the ancient Greek word *anastomo*, meaning 'wide-opened mouth', and *oscitans*, from the Latin word meaning 'yawning'.

M. Krishnan shares an interesting story about the tradition of bird protection by villagers, which has been a practice in Vedanthangal. The villagers wanted a formal declaration of protection and in 1796, approached the then collector of Chinglepet, Mr L. Place, who announced it as a protected area. The villagers misplaced this declaration, and then had it re-stated in 1858 by George C. Tod, and again in 1936 by Mr A.H.A. Todd. Dedication and perseverance!

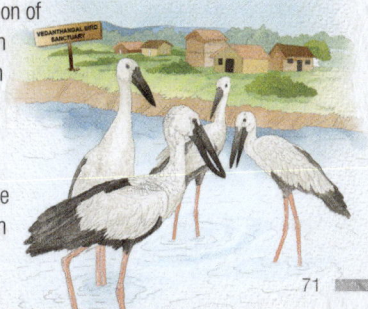

Jayantika Davé

Kalij Pheasant

Scientific name: *Lophura leucomelanos*   Size: *70 cm*
Hindi name: *Kaleej, Kukera*
Sanskrit name: *Kaalagyakukkat, Raktavartam*

Description

This elegant pheasant, dressed in glossy blue-black robes with white scaling, a bright-red bare skin mask around the eyes, and a lovely white or black crest, looks like the winning entrant to a masked ball! It is found in the forested hills of the Himalayas and the Northeast, in the vicinity of a stream, and usually best seen during early morning or at dusk. In our hill home, 6.00 a.m. in the morning, and soft chittering calls in the *gadera* (ravine) next to the house, mean that the local family of Kalij Pheasants has arrived! And as dusk draws near, they fly up into the utees (alder) trees at the lower edge of our property, to spend the night in safety.

Habits

Its favoured habitat is oak, sal, rhododendron or coniferous forests, with dense undergrowth and fine bamboo thickets. It is omnivorous, eating insects, small snakes, bamboo seeds, figs, forest roots, fern tips, acorns and other forest fruit and tender leaf tips. It forages in small family groups, with one or two males accompanied by a number of females. They are secretive and quiet in their movements. Oddly though, if one crosses a road or path, it is a good idea to wait quietly, as the whole flock will follow!

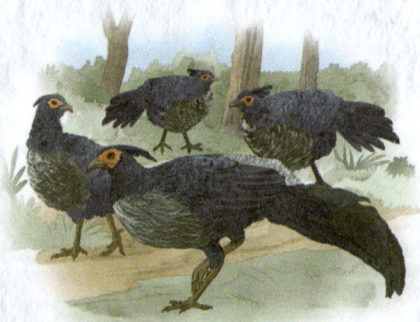

The male Kalij does a fierce-looking courting display – drawing itself up to its full height, extending its wings and rapidly vibrating them, making a drumming sound! Once, when my daughters were in our hill home around that time, the breeding activity was so intense that, at the lower edge of our property, while the girls were sitting there, the normally shy Kalij were hopping up and down into the rhododendrons, oblivious to the fact that human beings were sitting right there!

Call

Prefers to be silent, but gives soft chirruping calls while feeding, and a startled koorchi-koorchi, followed by a whistling klee-klee-klee call when forced to take flight!

Woolly-necked Stork

Scientific name: *Ciconia episcopus*   Size: 85 cm
Hindi name: *Haji Lak-lak*
Sanskrit name: *Shvet-kanth Mahabak*

Description
This black-and-white stork looks like it is always cold – with a black skull cap, and a heavy woollen fleece scarf around its neck! It is resident all over India, in areas that have wetlands and marshes. The feathers on the breast are longer, and shine with a coppery-purple sheen. Long red legs and a black bill complete the picture.

Habits
These birds were first described by a French naturalist in 1780, from a specimen collected from the Coromandel coast. Their preferred habitat is ploughed fields during the summer and monsoon, and freshwater wetlands in winter. They also forage alongside irrigation canals when water levels are low, looking for frogs, reptiles and insects, with a fair distance being covered with a steady gait.

They soar on thermals, with the typically outstretched neck of a stork, and can fly far. They are generally seen singly, in pairs, or in small family groups.

Call
Not very vocal, occasionally doing a two-tone whistle!

Mythology, Tales & Trivia
The genus name *Ciconia* refers to the Latin word for stork, and the *episcopus* is from the Latin for bishop, presumably from its skull cap.

Jayantika Davé

Great Hornbill

Scientific name: *Buceros bicornis*   Size: *100 cm*
Hindi name: *Raj Dhanesh, Banrao, Dhanesh*
Sanskrit name: *Khatvaang*

Description

The distinctive, noisy and large black-and-white Great Hornbill, with a heavy, casqued yellow beak, is seen around fruit-bearing trees in the forests of the Himalayas, the Northeast and the Western Ghats.

Habits

Its sheer size, huge casque and strong and heavy flapping flight punctuated with glides make it an unmistakable sight! The huge casque does not seem to have a primary purpose, but the bigger it is, the more desirable is the male! Males also casque-butt aerially during breeding season. They can be seen in groups, feeding on fruits, tossing them up into the air, and swallowing them whole in their gaping beak. Small mammals, birds and reptiles are also eaten.

The breeding season is a noisy time, with loud duets of 'kok' calls, which start with one call a second, and then rapidly deteriorate into a cacophony of sound! They nest on the tallest trees, with the nest in the hollow of a large tree trunk, where the female settles in, and the opening is then sealed with a plaster made of mud. The male is the devoted father, feeding the female, who meanwhile loses all her feathers. After the chicks have grown somewhat, the female will emerge to help with the feeding, and the chicks are clever enough to re-seal the nest opening.

Call

Noisy kok calls. Whistler amusingly describes their calls as 'the most extraordinary rattling roars, cacklings and bellows!'

Mythology, Tales & Trivia

They have lovely long eyelashes, and the male hornbill has a red iris, while the female has a blue-white one!

While roosting, they tip their neck back, lifting the beak up, to keep the heavy weight somewhat supported by the neck!

A Great Hornbill called William was the model for the logo of the Bombay Natural History Society.

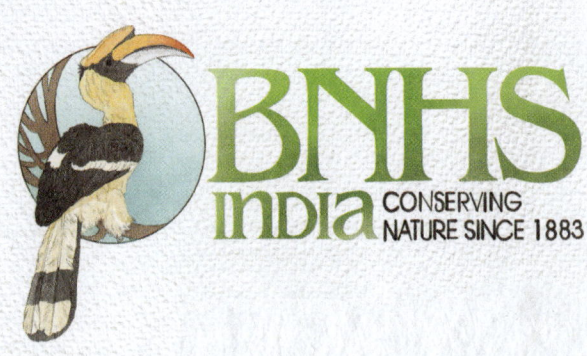

Tribal people, particularly in Northeast India, use the tail feathers for ceremonial head-dresses, and the casque and skull for festive decoration.

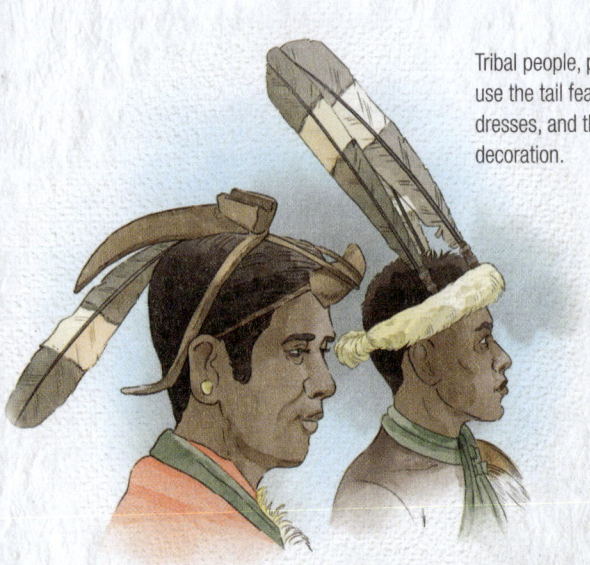

Jayantika Davé

Painted Stork

Scientific name: *Mycteria leucocephala*   Size: 95 cm
Hindi name: *Janghil, Dokh*
Sanskrit name: *Kaashtthasarangbak, Pinglakhag*

Description
The Painted Stork is a large black-and-white stork, with a bare yellow-orange head, a heavy and yellow downcurved beak, and with its shoulders and wings beautifully and delicately tinted with pink. They are a resident species, and are fairly common and easy to see in wetlands throughout India. In the monsoons, my parents and my children used to head to the Delhi Zoo for a picnic lunch because a colony of Painted Stork would always be there to start their nesting!

Habits
These storks feed in small groups in shallow wetlands and irrigated fields, and have a typical foraging action, sauntering sedately, submerging their open beaks in water, and sweeping the beak from side to side, snapping up any prey that they disturb. They also stir up the water with their feet to flush out other prey. Their favourite food is small fish, frogs, and even snakes. Strong fliers, they use late-morning thermals to look for good feeding grounds.

The Keoladeo Sanctuary in Bharatpur, Rajasthan, is a wonderful place to see them breeding – and the deafening clamour of the parent birds and the chicks can be heard for long distances! The conscientious parents protect the chicks from the mid-day heat, by standing in the nest with outstretched wings to shade the little ones. Feeding is through regurgitating the fish that they have caught.

Call
Like all storks, they are largely silent, though bill-clattering and some harsh croaking and moaning sounds are made!

Mythology, Tales & Trivia
Young chicks, when threatened, crumple to the bottom of the nest, pretending to be dead!

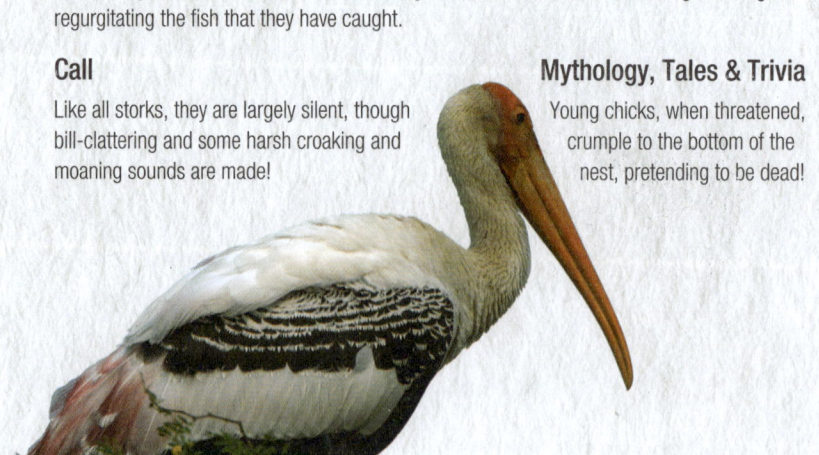

Black-necked Stork

Scientific name: *Ephippiorhynchus asiaticus* Size: 140 cm
Hindi name: *Loharjang, Loha Sarang*
Sanskrit name: *Sarangbak, Krishnagreev*

Description
In wet areas in the lowlands, look out for this gigantic, glossy, black-and-white stork, with striking bright red legs, smartly turned out for a military parade! It is not very widespread but is an unforgettable sight once you spot it!

Habits
The glossy bluish-black iridescent head of the adults, with the contrasting bright white back and bright red legs, are a sight to see! They are usually solitary in nature.

They are strongly territorial feeders, and ruthless too. In Bharatpur, I once saw one attack a hapless coot that happened to swim close enough. It was quite a frightening sight, to see it relentlessly jab the coot to death in shallow water, and then tear it apart and eat it.

They forage in natural and artificial wetland habitats, and their diet includes small waterbirds (coots, darters, grebes, jacana), fish, reptiles, frogs and invertebrates.

They have a beautiful courting dancing display, where the pair approaches each other beak to beak, extending their wings, fluttering their wing tips and clattering their bills.

Mythology, Tales & Trivia
Amongst the Mir Shikars, who are traditional bird hunters of Bihar, there was a ritual wherein a bridegroom-to-be had to capture a live Loha Sarang. Since the bird is a fierce fighter, this led to injuries and death. Thankfully this has now been stopped.

Call
Typically silent, other than bill-clattering and some hissing and groaning!

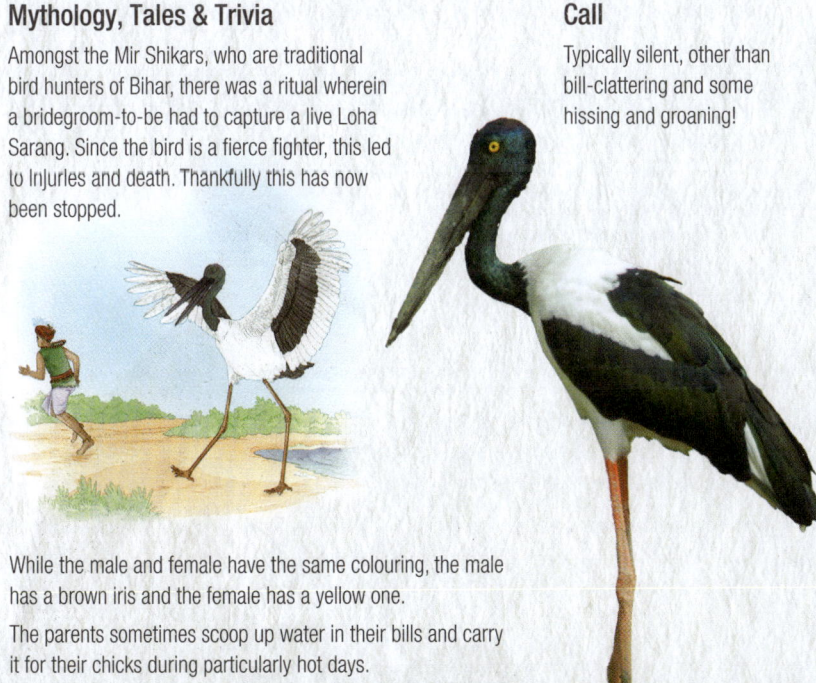

While the male and female have the same colouring, the male has a brown iris and the female has a yellow one.

The parents sometimes scoop up water in their bills and carry it for their chicks during particularly hot days.

Jayantika Davé

Adjutant Stork, Lesser & Greater

Scientific name: *Leptoptilos javanicus*   Size: *140 cm*
Hindi name: *Chota Garud, Chinjara, Chandana*
Gujarati name: *Nano Jamadar*
Sanskrit name: *Mahachanchubak, Deerghapaad*

Description

Dewar shares an amusing description of the Adjutant Stork, where he says that it looks from the back like an old hunchbacked man, with very thin legs, wearing a swallow-tail coat! It certainly is an 'old-man' stork – bald, wrinkled neck, stubble and a vulture-like ruff – a strange sight indeed! A winter visitor to parts of North India and the Northeast, it is not that common a sighting anymore. The Delhi Zoo often gets a number of them hanging out around the margins of the central lake.

A similar, though much larger, stork is the **Greater Adjutant**, which is distinguishable by its more prominent neck pouch and black marks on its face and neck…which are fancifully described as being similar to dried blood!

Habits

A distinctive feature of this stork is that unlike most storks, which fly with their necks outstretched, the Adjutant Stork flies with its neck tucked in, probably to better balance its very heavy bill.

A solitary or small group bird, the Lesser Adjutant is more commonly seen around wetlands, while the Greater Adjutant is seen around shallow or drying lakes and often at garbage dumps in the company of vultures, whose bare heads it seems to emulate. Favourite foods are fish, frogs, reptiles, rodents and scavenging.

They sit on the ground for long periods of time in a strange, folded-legs posture, often with outstretched wings to reduce their temperature.

Call

They lack vocal chords, and so are largely silent, with the only sounds being some aggressive hissing at the nest, and bill-clattering during breeding!

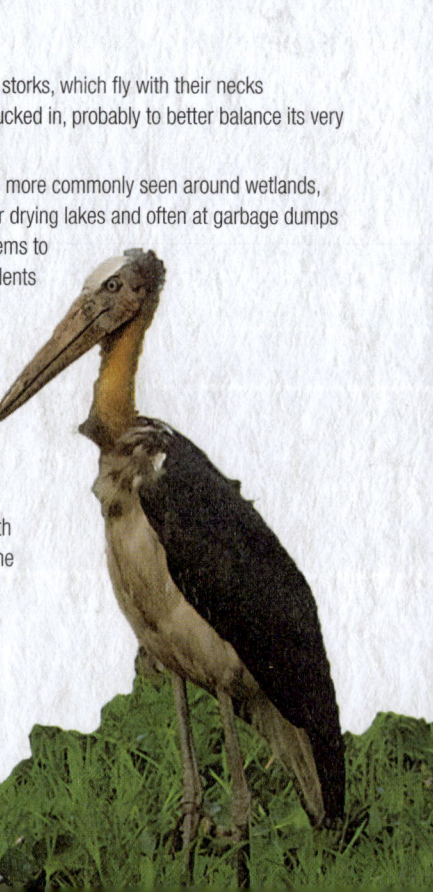

Mythology, Tales & Trivia

In the nineteenth century, Greater Adjutants were very common around Calcutta, and were valued as scavengers. The Calcutta Municipal Corporation therefore depicted them in their logo.

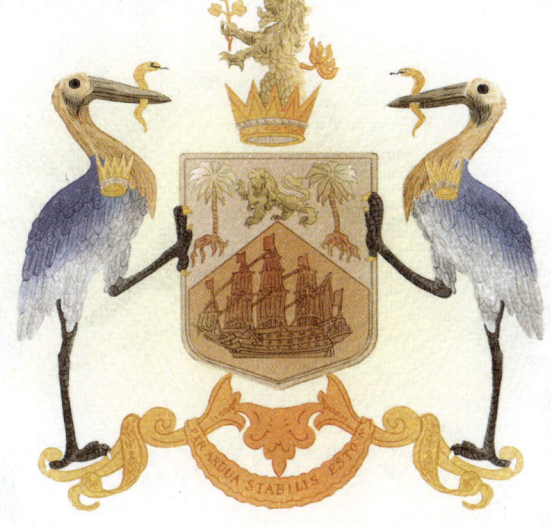

The Mughal Emperor Babur recorded a myth about a very precious 'snake stone' that existed inside the skull of the Adjutant Stork and was a magical antidote for snake bites.

The Adjutants have a stiff marching gait, from which they have got their name!

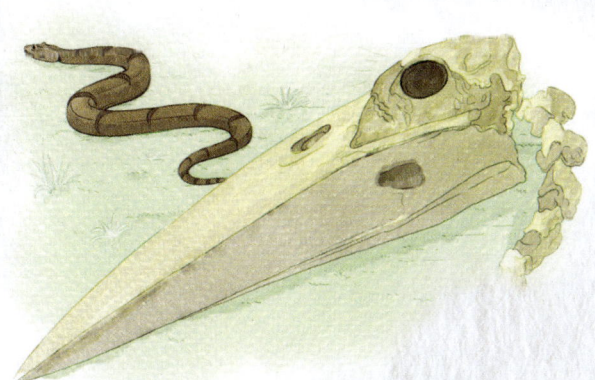

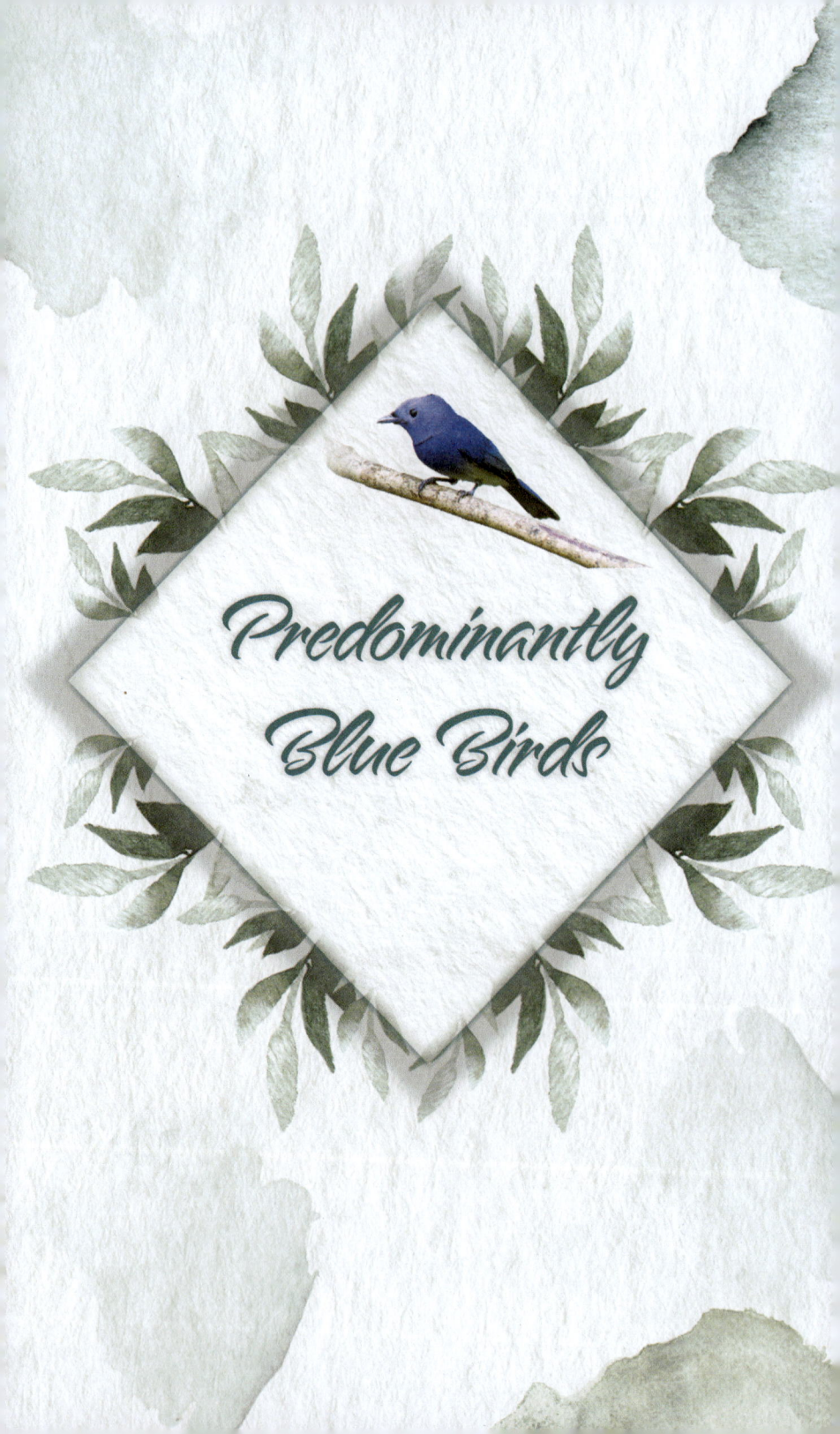

Each Little Bird That Sings

Indian Nuthatch

Scientific name: *Sitta cinnamoventris* Size: 12cm
Hindi name: *Siri, Katphoria*
Sanskrit name: *Pitta Raktodar Shilindhri, Kavak* (refers to the fact that when the bird is clinging to a tree trunk, it resembles a mushroom jutting out from a tree in a similar position)

Description

Creeping along the trunk of a tree, or the underside of a branch, is this little bird which looks and behaves like a woodpecker, but is not! It is the little Indian Nuthatch – a study in grey upperparts with deep chestnut undersides. The Indian Nuthatch is a bird of the lowlands, while a very similar bird is the **Chestnut-bellied Nuthatch**, which you will see only in the Himalayan foothills.

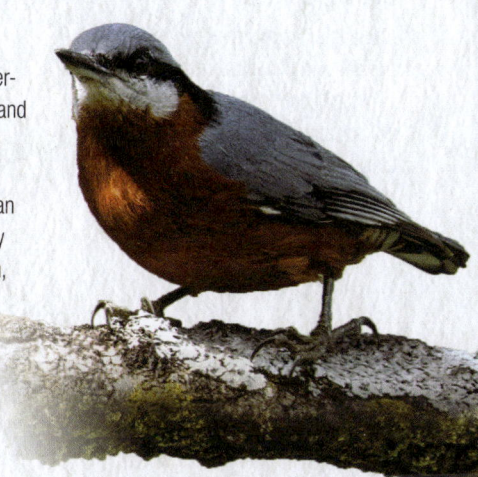

Habits

A variety of tree-dominated habitats are favoured, where the Siri forages for insects, seeds and nuts, running like a little mouse – upwards, downwards, sideways and backwards, amongst the trunk and larger branches, constantly cocking its head, and looking sideways to check for insects and interesting tid-bits. It has large claws, and so is very comfortable even travelling along the underside of branches.

Nuthatches either adopt a natural hole in a tree, or cut out a perfect round hole in the trunk or branch, making it smaller by sealing it off with mud mixed with the sticky fluid from some plants, so that other predators cannot enter.

Call

A melodious tsup, tsup or a soft sit-sit chatter!

Mythology, Tales & Trivia

In the Kandgalak Jataka tales, a woodpecker and a nuthatch were friends. One day, the woodpecker invited the nuthatch for lunch, and gave him lots of succulent worms. The nuthatch was so happy that he wanted to shift to the woodpecker's forest. The woodpecker warned him that he lived in a hardwood forest, and the nuthatch's bill would not be suitable for these trees. The nuthatch insisted, and the first time he tried to dig into the hard trunk, he broke his bill and died. The moral was, don't overestimate your abilities!

Jayantika Davé

Black-naped Monarch

Scientific name: *Hypothymus azurea*   Size: 16 cm
Hindi name: *Neel Mani*

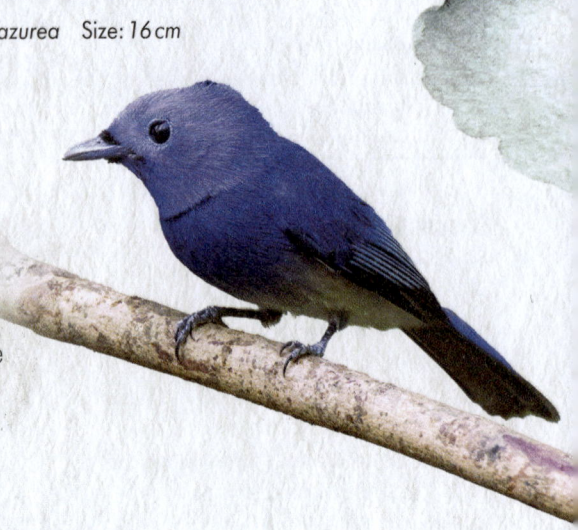

Description

A beautiful, widespread resident of forests and overgrown areas is this brilliant blue jewel! The Black-naped Monarch wears its black skull cap and black necklace proudly, on its azure-blue gown.

Habits

The Neel Mani is a typical flycatcher, always on the move, making aerial sorties from its perch, and capturing all kinds of flying insects. Its wings droop and its tail is cocked and spread out as it moves amidst the tree canopy, fluttering amongst the leaves to dislodge insects which are then quickly caught. Bamboo thickets and overgrown areas near a stream are an absolute favourite haunt.

Insects, butterflies, moths and grasshoppers are the primary diet.

Call

A high switch-witch and a three-noted pwee-pweepwee-pwee.

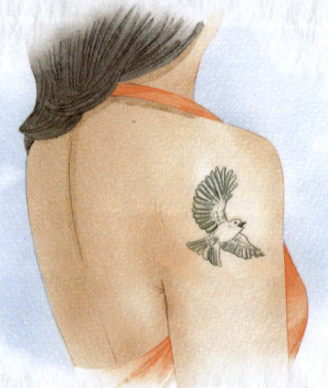

Mythology, Tales & Trivia

It is said that a flycatcher tattoo is a symbol of all the good things about flycatchers – energy, beauty and a quick wit, all in a tiny package!

Verditer Flycatcher

Scientific name: *Eumyias thalassinus* Size: 16 cm
Hindi name: *Nili Tik-tiki*

Description

In the forests of the Himalayas (1,200 m–3,000 m), a flash of distinctive copper-sulphate blue, and the active aerial sorties of a flycatcher, is a sure indicator that the sparrow-sized bird you are looking at is the Verditer Flycatcher. The blue is intense, with a thick, elongated dancer's black kajal line from around the eye to the base of the beak. Mackintosh shares that it used to fondly be called the Spring Flycatcher as it was the first brightly coloured flycatcher to appear after a cold winter!

Habits

The Nili Tik-tiki is not a shy bird, frequenting forested and cultivated areas, often near streams. It perches on bare branches above tree canopy height, and on electric wires, periodically launching forth after aerial prey, and usually returning to its original perch. Its primary food are bees, insects and ripe berries. An unusual habit is to flutter amongst the foliage to dislodge insects, which it then quickly picks up from the ground, doing a quick tail flick as it lands.

The nest is a beautiful open cup of green moss, grass and leaves, placed in creepers, under eaves or crevices in a tree or wall.

It nests outside the study in our hill home, so I can see the nest being painstakingly built up, with small beakfuls of moss brought in on each flight!

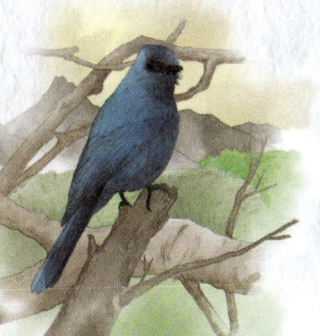

Call

A trilling call, pi-pi-pwee...pi-pi-pwee...pi-tititi-woo-pitititi-weyu, which comes tumbling down the scale, interspersed with a short, somewhat plaintive pseeut.

Mythology, Tales & Trivia

The birds get their beautiful colour not from actual pigment in the feathers, but from the feathers being structured in such a way that they scatter light and appear blue. A single feather found on the ground can therefore appear just grey.

Jayantika Davé

Common Kingfisher

Scientific name: *Alcedo atthis*   Size: 16 cm
Hindi name: *Chhota Kilkila, Chhota Machhrala*
Sanskrit name: *Manichak Matsyarank (Manichak = shining like a jewel or a flower)*

Description

The beautiful, small, sparrow-sized Common Kingfisher is anything but common! Look for this tiny brilliant spot of blue amongst the low overhanging branches of a lake or stream, and use your binoculars to appreciate its true beauty!

Habits

The Chhota Kilkila is found near clear, slow-flowing streams, or lakes with thick vegetation around the banks, and particularly enjoys spots where the bushes or low trees have overhanging branches falling close to the water. It is a very shy bird, and takes off with a characteristic whirr, revealing its bright blue back. The presence of these birds is a good indicator of the cleanliness of the water, and healthy ecosystems surrounding the banks and edges. Its main prey is fish, and the bird will position itself about 3–6 feet above the water for best success, scanning the water, and jerking its tail with a quiet 'chik chik' accompanying each jerk! On spotting a fish, the head bobbing will start to accurately gauge the distance, followed by a quick dive and capture. Back on the perch, the fish is held by the tail and beaten till dead, after which it will be swallowed head first. Shrimp and water insects are also eaten.

Call

The Common Kingfisher only calls in flight, and that call is a short sharp whistle like chee, repeated a few times!

Mythology, Tales & Trivia

Greek mythology talks about a young couple, Alcyone and Ceyx, who were very happy together. In jest, they called each other Zeus and Hera. This angered Zeus, who killed Ceyx with a thunderbolt. Alcyone, overcome with grief, killed herself too. Out of compassion, the gods changed them into 'halcyon' birds or Common Kingfishers, so that they could always relive their beautiful days together.

A kingfisher was said to be the first bird to fly from Noah's ark, and it received orange on its breast from the setting sun, and blue on its back from the sky.

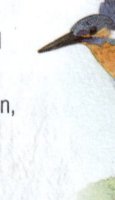
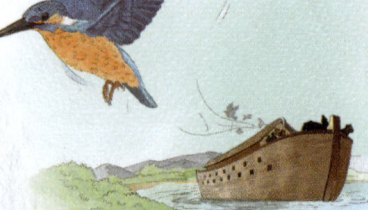

White-throated Kingfisher

Scientific name: *Halcyon smyrnensis*   Size: 28 cm
Hindi name: *Kilkila*
Sanskrit name: *Chandrakantha Matsyarank*

Description
A common sight on most roadsides, perched on wires or trees, is the large White-throated Kingfisher – bright blue and chestnut, with a heavy red bill and a conspicuous white bib. It is such a common sight now, and often nowhere near water, that I often wonder why it is called a kingfisher at all!

Habits
This Kilkila frequents a variety of habitats, often away from water, since its prey includes small rodents, reptiles, small birds, insects, caterpillars, squirrels, and of course everything that lives in water. So it is seen around habitation, in fields, around cultivation, and in forested areas that are not dense. It is not particular about its choice of the kind of water, and is seen around ponds, canals, dams, swamps, beaches and other water bodies. It has the typical kingfisher behaviour of waiting patiently on its perch, periodically bobbing its head and wagging its tail, before it spots its prey and takes it out with one dive. Prey is often battered on the ground before being carried up to its perch to be swallowed.

The males have a lovely courtship display of flicking open their wings and tail, and raising their bill high to display the startling white throat and front. Nest tunnels are made in mud banks, with both the parents flying into mud walls to make an indent to which they can cling, and which they then proceed to tunnel with their heavy beaks.

Call
The most typical call is a loud kiliililili as it flies!

Mythology, Tales & Trivia
This Kingfisher is the state bird of West Bengal.

In the 1800s, it was widely hunted for its bright feathers that were used to decorate women's hats.

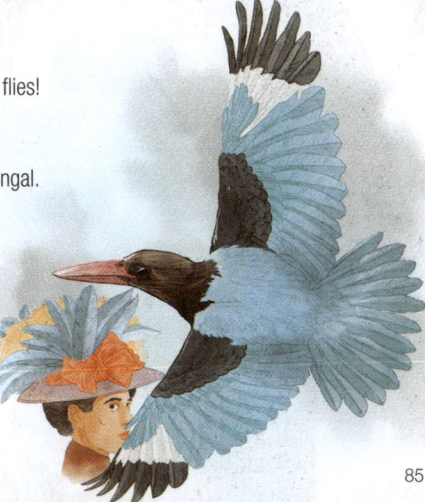

Jayantika Davé

Indian Roller

Scientific name: *Coracias benghalensis*   Size: 33 cm
Hindi name: *Neelkanth*
Sanskrit name: *Chaash*

Description
The beautiful, bright blue and pinkish-fawn Neelkanth is a stocky bird, which was called a Blue Jay when we were young, and is a lovely sight on wires along roadsides. Whistler puts it beautifully, and wistfully – 'To my last day in India I shall never lose the thrill that comes to me every time I see the sudden transformation of this dark lumpy bird into a flash of blue banded glory.'

Habits
The Indian Roller is a widespread resident in India, and is seen up to heights of 1,500 m. Its most common sightings are on wires alongside the road, in open countryside, near villages, fields and open forested areas. Insects, small lizards, snakes, frogs and mice are all part of its diet. It watches out for prey from an exposed perch and having sighted it, does a gentle glide to arrive next to it, grab it, and then beat it against the ground before swallowing it. The courtship is an acrobatic exhibitionist display of somersaults and nose dives, accompanied by many a harsh screaming call.

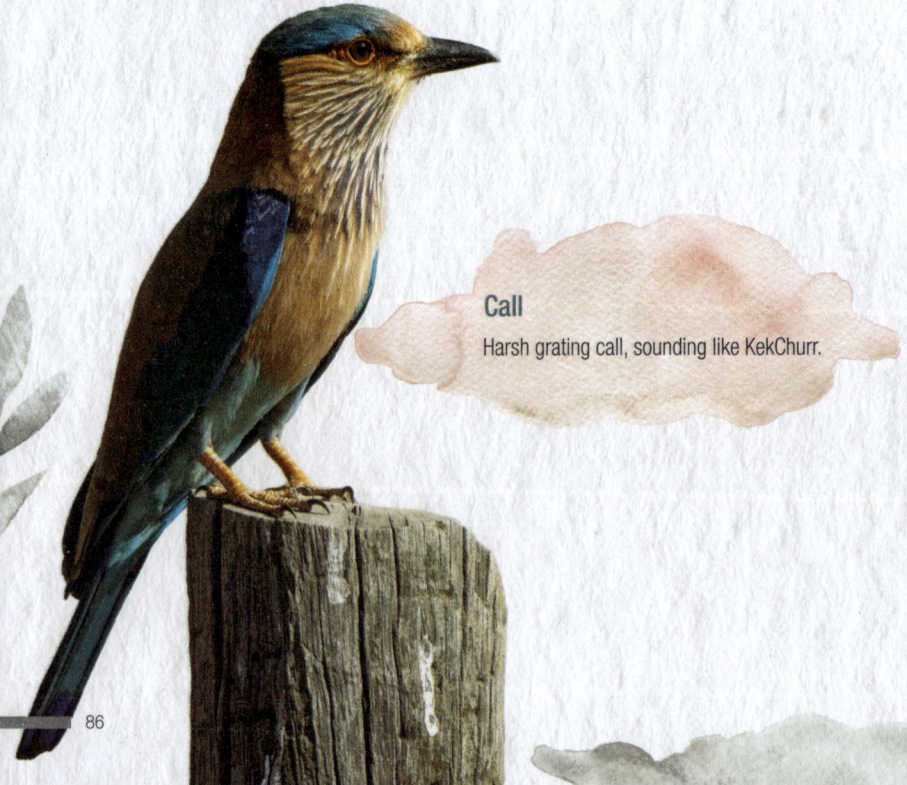

Call
Harsh grating call, sounding like KekChurr.

Mythology, Tales & Trivia

Thomas C. Jerdon in *The Birds of India* mentions that during Dussera and during the Durga-ji immersion ceremony, some rajas would ceremoniously liberate a Nilkanth to honour Shiva. Even when the image of Durga was immersed in the river, a Nilkanth used to be released.

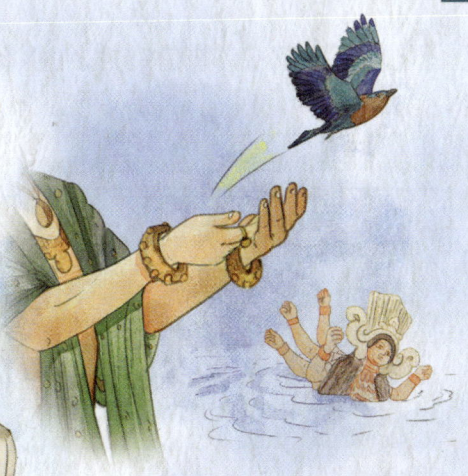

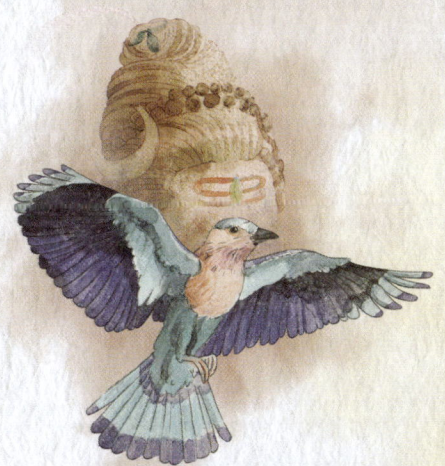

Legend also has it that it was called Milk-bird, because if a cow was giving only a little milk, a few of the Nilkanth feathers chopped up and fed to the cow would increase the milk production.

According to K.N. Davé, the Indian Roller has long been considered an auspicious bird, as it was one whose form Lord Shiva often chose to assume, and it therefore earned the colloquial names of Mahayogi and Neelkanth.

K.N. Davé notes how in the *Rig Veda* 10.97.13, there is a verse where the asthmatic cough of a patient is asked to leave the sufferer and go to the throat of the Roller, which anyway has a hoarse, guttural voice!

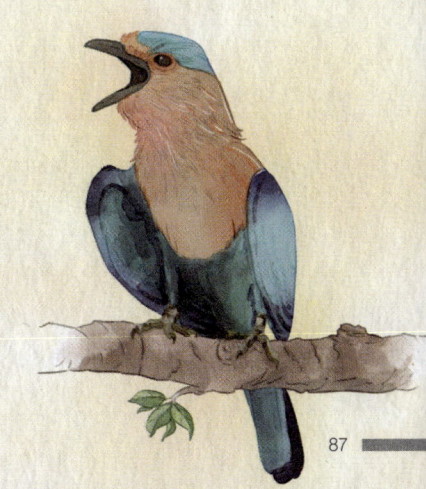

Jayantika Davé

Purple Swamp Hen

Scientific name: *Porphyrio porphyrio*   Size: *48 cm*
Hindi name: *Jamni Vanmurghi, Kharim, Khima*
Sanskrit name: *Jalranku, Manjul Datyooh*

Description

Marshy wetlands all over India are home to the plump, ungainly Purple Swamp Hen. The Jamni Vanmurghi is a lovely blue-purple in colour, with a distinctive red forehead shield descending to a red bill and bright red legs with long toes. The constant flicking of the tail reveals white flashes underneath. The blues on this bird truly blaze when the sun hits them, and the red contrasts make for a glorious picture!

Habits

The Jamni Vanmurghi appears in groups, feeding along vegetated water edges, amongst hyacinth and water reeds, while grunting and croaking all the time!
In Bharatpur one year, I remember seeing more than 500 birds on an open wetland, and as the sun rose, they changed from dark-grey blobs to this jewelled mass…one of those 'flash upon the inward eye' moments in times of solitude!

They have a quaint feeding system, pulling out aquatic tubers with their bills, and using their feet to convey the food to their bills. They also take fish, crustaceans, insects and other aquatic life.

According to Salim Ali, the male has a ludicrous courtship display, holding water weeds in his bill and bowing to the female with loud chuckles!

Call

Usually a constant series of grunts and groans, but with occasionally a long series of moaning calls!

Mythology, Tales & Trivia

According to Pliny the Elder, the Romans considered these to be noble birds, and kept them for decorative purposes in the gardens of large homes.

There are many descriptions in Sanskrit literature where the Purple Swamp Hen is described as moving among the beautiful blue lotus like a pretty little deer!

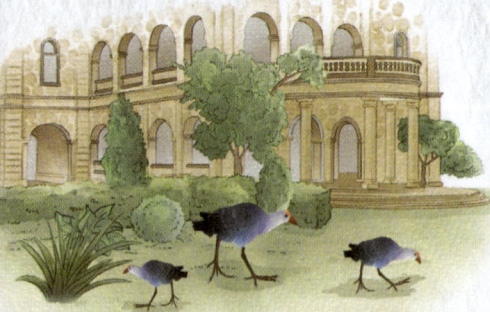

Red-billed Blue Magpie

Scientific name: *Urocissa erythrorhyncha*   Size: 66 cm
Hindi name: *Digdal*
Sanskrit name: *Poornakoot*

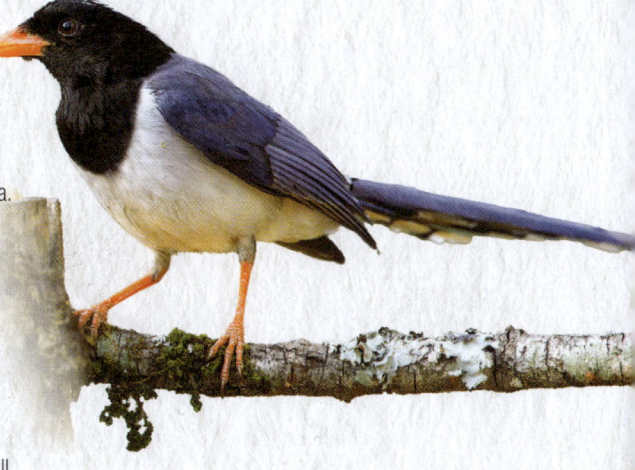

Description

This vivid, distinctive, large and noisy magpie is an unforgettable sight during a trip to the hills of North India. The Red-billed Blue Magpie is a lovely blue, touched with mauve, with a really long white-tipped graduated tail that dips gracefully downwards, and flutters gaily behind it when it flies! It is such a heart-lifting sight that when we were building our hill home, I always looked out for it on the drive up, and if I saw it, I treated it as a good-luck sign that we would make good progress on the construction! It is distinguished from the very similar **Yellow-billed Magpie** by its bright red bill.

Habits

It is happiest in forested surroundings, and not shy about appearing in gardens and terraces near forests. At our home, we put out fruit on our feeders, and that is a sure attractor! Their size and aggressive temperament makes sure that no other bird gets the first bite! While fruits seem to be a favourite, their diet also includes frogs, lizards, bird eggs and nestlings, small rodents, grubs and kitchen waste. They move in groups, and their loud calls draw attention to the movement, which tends to be at the tree-top level, with occasional descents to forage on forest floors. When they do descend to the ground, they hold their tails clear of the ground in a high arch!

Call

A harsh cha-chak, cha-chak, with a melodious loud whistle during flight!

Mythology, Tales & Trivia

According to K.N. Davé, an ancient Sanskrit name for the Blue Magpie is Durga, and comes from a description of the Goddess's complexion, said to have the colour of the light blue of the linseed flower. (Vasantaraja 4.21, 56-65; 11.2 & 5.)

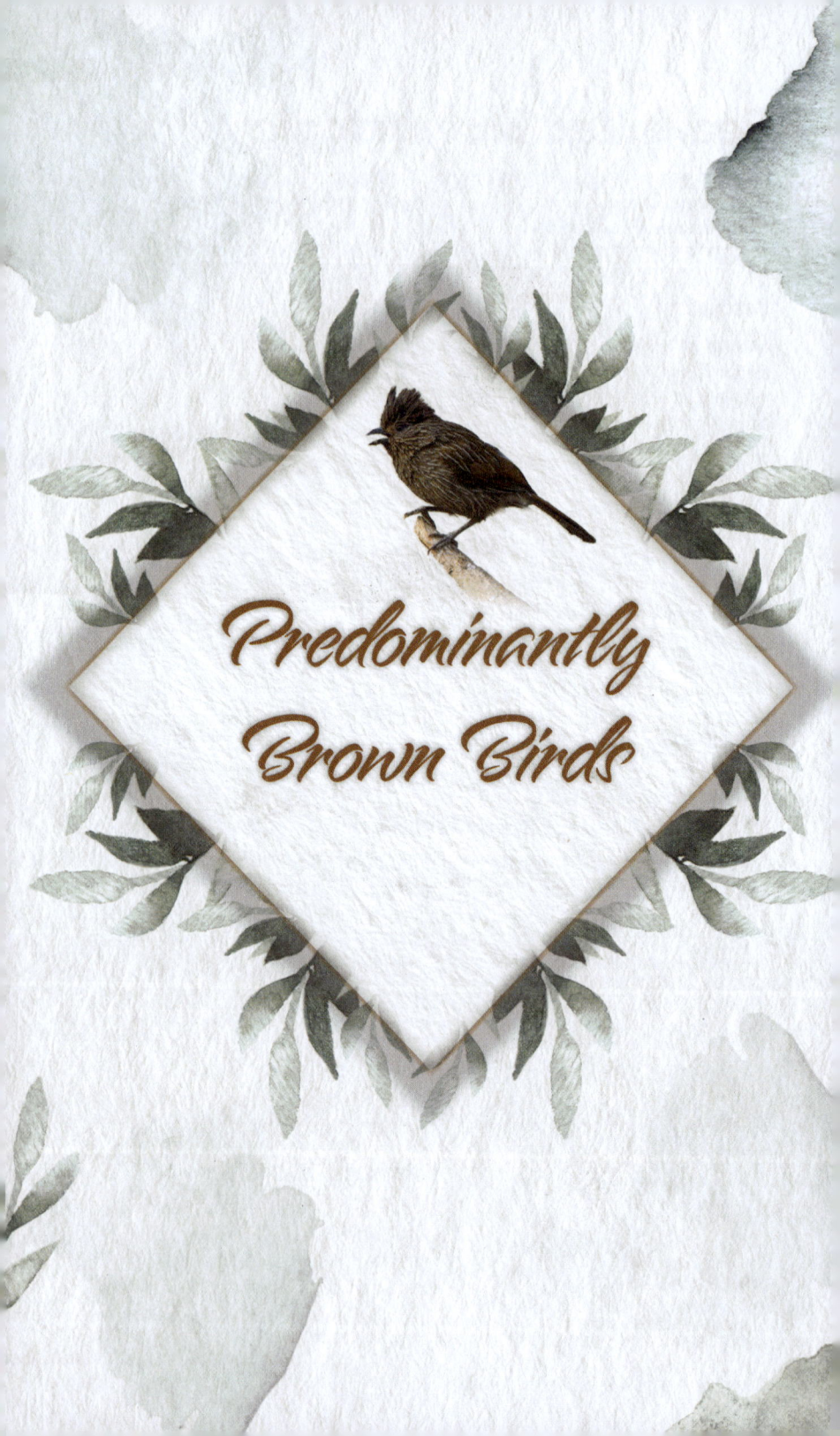

Scaly-breasted Munia

Scientific name: *Lonchura punctulate*   Size: *11 cm*
Hindi name: *Telia Munia*
Sanskrit name: *Paroshni*

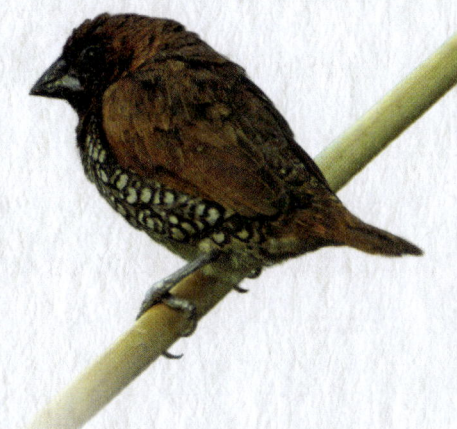

Description
A stalk of jowar seeds, or any other small seeds in a bowl in my balcony or garden, and these little brown beauties with beautifully scalloped undersides appear! They are quite comfortable with human presence and easily come quite close. The thick heavy bill is somewhat discordant with their otherwise slender, graceful bodies, but is a pointer to their seed-eating habit.

Habits
The Telia Munia is widely spread across India, and typically found in all kinds of grassy areas, shrub areas, cultivated fields, gardens and wastelands. Their favourite food is seeds of any kind, and it is a really pretty sight to see a small flock of them amongst tall waving grasses, climbing up the thin grass stem to get at the seeds on top. They are social by nature, and are often found in small to large flocks, sometimes together with other seed-eating birds, arriving and departing in an untidy, undulating flight mass!

The male has a lovely courtship act! He gets a thin stem of grass and drops it in front of the lady, and then gets to bowing and scraping, bending low, fluffing out his breast feathers, all the while bobbing up and down till she accepts him!

Call
A soft ti-tee repeated again and again, with sometimes a stronger kit-tee, kit-tee.

Mythology, Tales & Trivia
In Southeast Asia, trapped Munias used to be released during Buddhist religious festivals, with the releasing family earning merit for their release.

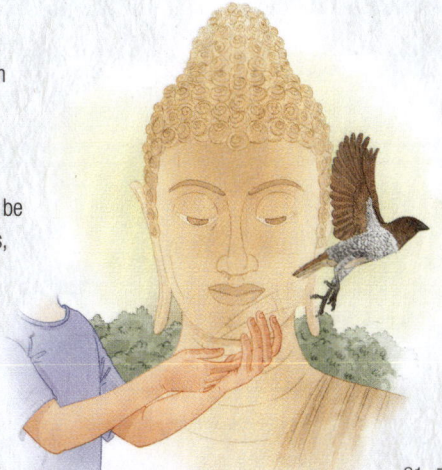

Jayantika Davé

Indian Silverbill

Scientific name: *Euodice malabarica*   Size: *11 cm*
Hindi name: *Charchara, Charga, Charakka, Pidda*
Sanskrit name: *Pirili*

Description

This pretty fawn-coloured little bird, with a silvery grey bill, is very Munia-like in appearance. Very comfortable around human habitation, it is a regular visitor to gardens and dry, scrubby open spaces. The Gujarati name of Shweth Kantth (or white throat) is an apt descriptor of the white underbelly.

Habits

A widespread resident, the Indian Silverbill occurs in the plains, and is also seen in the low foothills. Very gregarious in nature, it is seen in small and large flocks, usually in places where its favourite seeds can be found – the tops of tall grasses, and gleaning in cultivated fields of millets, both from the stalks and from the ground. Where suitable small grains are put out, whether in gardens or open scrubland parks, a flock of Charchara will always be around for an easy feed!

The male vigorously courts the female, offering her grass stems, and prostrating himself almost horizontally while puffing out belly feathers and jerking his head up and down!

Call

Single-noted calls, 'cheet, cheet', are made with sometimes a little song with a series of rising and falling notes!

Mythology, Tales & Trivia

It seems that one nest can also be shared by a number of females, and Hugh Whistler, in his *Popular Handbook of Indian Birds*, mentions that he has seen as many as 22 eggs in one nest!

The disproportionately large and untidy globular nest is sometimes used as a dormitory, with 6–8 birds using them just as resting places!

Ashy Prinia

Scientific name: *Prinia socialis* Size: 13 cm
Hindi name: *Kali Phutki*
Sanskrit name: *Parilika, Tuntuk*

Description

A lovely little resident is the Ashy Prinia, somewhat similar in build to the **Tailorbird** in terms of the small slender body and relatively long graded tail, but with completely different colouring. A rufous brown top with shades of grey on top, a distinctive red eye and a constant sideways wag of its long tail are the identifiers.

Habits

When you are out for a walk, a quick look in hedges, garden shrubs, tall grasses and all kinds of low overgrowth provides an easy sighting of the Kali Phutki. While they are not shy of humans, their general behaviour is to lie low and not attract attention. So they go about their business, alone or in pairs, foraging close to the ground for insects, spiders and flies, moving around inside bushes and on top of grasses. However, they will fly across your path, with a weak fluttering flight, and that will catch your eye! During breeding, all the colours get noticeably brighter, and the birds get really noisy, drawing attention to themselves! They are found up to 1,200 m in the Himalayas.

Pairs seem to have architectural style preferences for their nests – sometimes built as a bag woven from grass and stems, and wrapped around grassy stems; sometimes as a cup inside stitched leaves, like that of the Tailorbird; and sometimes stitched onto only one side of a large leaf!

Call

A most common call is a very cheerful jimmy-jimmy-jimmy accompanied by much sideways tail-wagging!

Jayantika Davé

Common Tailorbird

Scientific name: *Orthotomus sutorius*   Size: *13 cm*
Hindi name: *Darzi*
Sanskrit name: *Putini, Potiyak*

Description
A widespread resident, and a bird very easy to see in our gardens or balconies, is the Common Tailorbird. Look out for an olive-green-brown bird, with a long graded tail cocked at an absurdly high angle, and a smear of rufous on its forehead! And the best place to look will be around and under the low-hanging vegetation at the edge of your garden or balcony.

Habits
While the Darzi can be found up to 1,800 m in the Himalayan foothills, they are most often found in gardens, parks, villages and forest edges in lower altitudes. Their industrious search is for small insects, beetles, ants, flies and even small butterflies and moths. A sip of nectar is tempting, and they look really comical when they emerge from a deep trumpet flower, with a generous dusting of pollen all over their faces! A distinctive feature is the way their tail is carried — very high, and moving side to side constantly, almost as if it has come loose at the hinge!

We have been blessed by having a pair nest in our balcony every year, using the leaves of a philodendron creeper. The female is the Darzi, and the male a very willing and active helper. The Darzi chooses the few leaves that will make the outer shell, and pierces holes along their edges. The male then brings her cobwebs or other fibres, which she threads through these holes, pulling them closed to make a cone. This cone is then lined with a deep cup of webs, soft down or fine grass, and the eggs are laid.

Call
Throughout the day, their call of towit-towit-towit or pretty-pretty-pretty can be heard!

Mythology, Tales & Trivia
Jerdon tells of a Tailorbird that regularly watched the darzi stitching clothes in his verandah; as soon as he would leave his seat, the little bird would swoop down and pick up all the odd bits of thread to sew its nest!

Little Stint

Scientific name: *Calidris minuta*   Size: *14 cm*
Hindi name: *Chhota Panlowwa*
Sanskrit name: *Jalalobhin Jalrank*

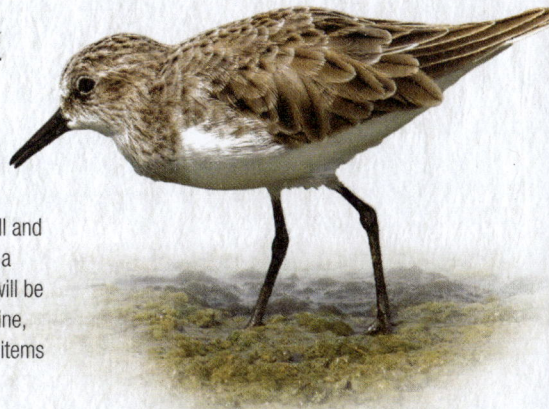

Description
In winter, the Little Stint makes its appearance across India flying in from Siberia and the tundras of Russia. Small and distinctively dark brown and white, it is a great lover of wet swampy areas, and will be seen pattering in and out of the water line, constantly moving and picking off food items from the surface.

Habits
The favourite haunts for the Chhota Panlowwa are the edges of water bodies of different kinds—rivers, coasts, lakes, mudflats and even seasonal water pools in flat areas like fields. The habitat provides its main diet of invertebrates, small beetles, water-bugs, ants, crustaceans, snails and even plant material. It has a characteristic feeding habit, pecking rapidly as it moves along, and then doing a quick run to grab at something that has just moved. It is usually seen in groups, as it is highly gregarious by nature. It is also happy to move amongst mixed groups of other waders, large and small. When disturbed, it takes off with a rapid flight, banking repeatedly, showing the upper side of one wing and then the underside – a beautiful blinking of black and white…black and white!

Call
Short sharp notes of pi-pi-pi.

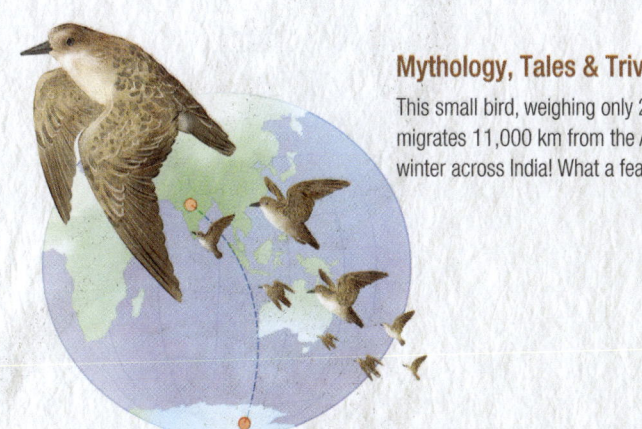

Mythology, Tales & Trivia
This small bird, weighing only 20 gm, migrates 11,000 km from the Arctic, to winter across India! What a feat!

Jayantika Davé

House Sparrow

Scientific name: *Passer domesticus*   Size: *15 cm*
Hindi name: *Gouriya*
Sanskrit name: *Ashvak*

Description
It is hard not to know the sprightly House Sparrow! It is around all our homes, in our balconies and in our gardens, unafraid of human presence, and lifting our spirits with its delightful cheerful chirping!

Habits
The Gouriya is a widespread resident, and true to its name 'domesticus', is the most comfortable around human habitation. It has a very varied diet of grain, seeds, insects, fruits and berries, as well as a host of household scraps. Primarily a ground feeder, it may perch on branches and twigs to reach fruit or seed heads. At the local grocer, it steals any and every kind of grain, pulling them out of little openings in sacks, and scattering them all over, making a big mess! It seems to be very particular about its appearance, and is often seen bathing – in water or mud, and then doing a lengthy preen, or wiping its bill repeatedly on the branch on which it is sitting.

Its nest is an untidy mess of grasses, scraps, feathers and fibres – really anything it can lay its beak on. It also takes very readily to nesting arrangements provided by us – a shoe box tied at a height, an earthenware pot with a hole, and cardboard or wooden nest boxes.

Call
A variety of cheeps!

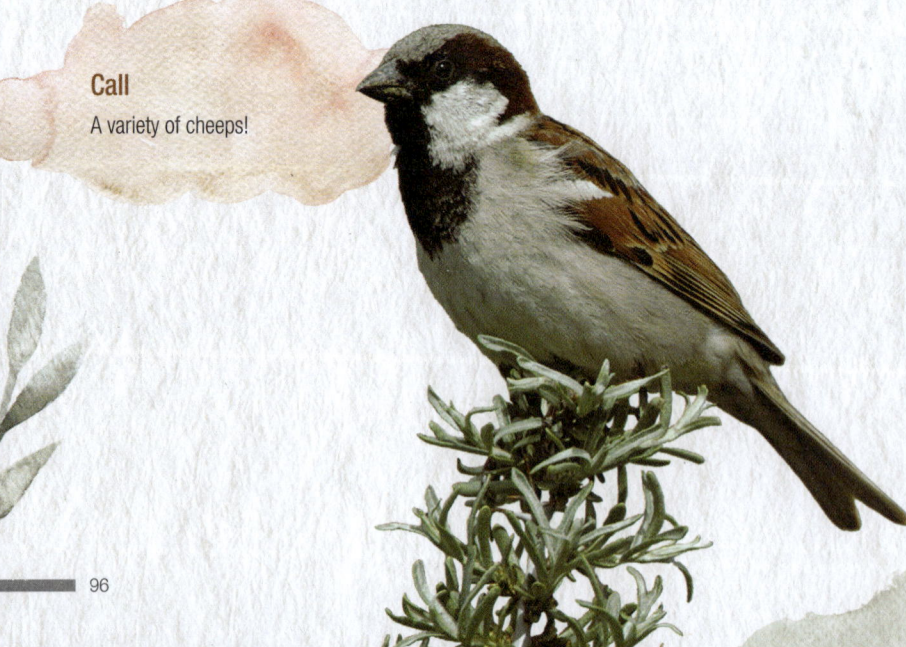

Mythology, Tales & Trivia

Just before the battle of Kurukshetra, elephants were used to clear the grounds of trees, and a sparrow's nest with four babies in it was knocked to the ground. The sparrow pleaded with Krishna to save her babies. Krishna said he did not interfere with the laws of nature, and did not promise anything, and only told her to stock her nest with food for three weeks. On the day of battle, Krishna lifted up Arjuna's bow and aimed at an elephant, knocking the brass bell from its neck. The battle lasted 18 days, and after it, as Krishna and Arjuna walked the fields littered with the dead, they came across an elephant bell. Arjuna lifted it, and there under it was the sparrow and her babies, all of them safe!

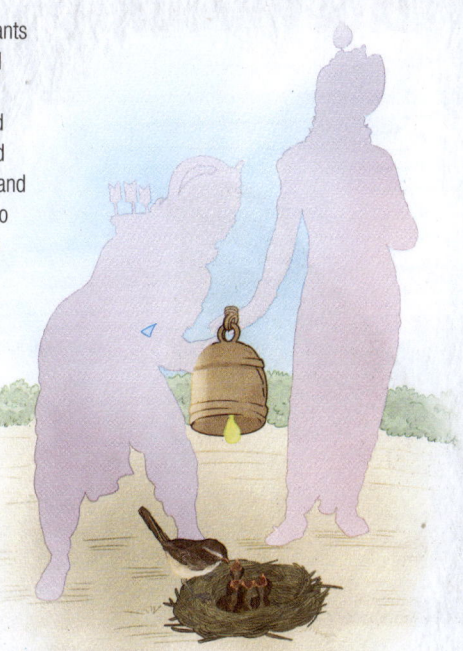

Our ancient texts used the name Ashvak or colt as a means of describing the similarity of behaviour between a sparrow and a frisky colt – active, handsome, carrying its neck and head high, flicking its tail, with an overall sprightly demeanour!

The dark bib of the male is a big draw for the ladies – the larger the bib size, the more the ladies are interested!

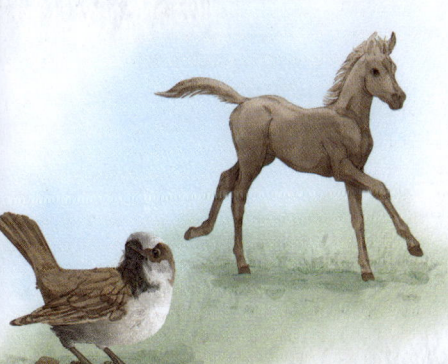

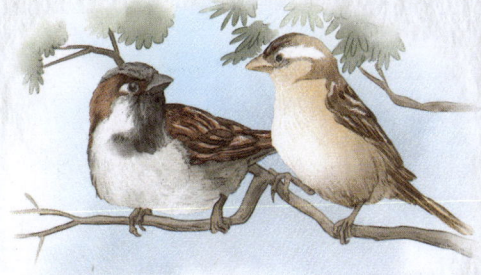

Jayantika Davé

Blue-throat

Scientific name: *Luscinia svecica* Size: *15 cm*
Hindi name: *Neelkanthi; Husaini Pidda*
Sanskrit name: *Chatika (generic)*

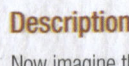

Description
Now imagine this…a medium-sized, upright brown bird with drooping wings, looking pretty unremarkable, till…it turns around! And what do you see?! A glorious blue bib, with a spot of rufous in the middle, and an outer edge of rufous too – truly a memorable sighting! So come winter, any walks we do in scrubland mean keeping a sharp eye out for the lovely Blue-throat!

Habits
A widespread winter visitor, it is not necessarily easy to see, because it tends to skulk and hide in thick vegetation around scrub, reedbeds and jheels. It is only when it decides to sing from the top of a rock or a branch that you get an easy sighting. Then the characteristic tail lift and jerk showing rufous sides, together with the blue bib, make the identification a certainty.
A quick short flight, a short run along the ground, interspersed with a quick stop and a tail fan, and it moves off again! It feeds by doing short quick runs, quickly collecting beetles, snails, flies, caterpillars, crickets, ants and other insects, including plant seeds or fruits.

Call
A harsh chack-chack-chack, or a trilling softer tree-tree-tree. During the breeding season, it is supposed to be an accomplished mimic of other birdsong!

Mythology, Tales & Trivia
In the Mahabharata, Bhima was bitten by a snake and would have died. A red-throated bird came and drank the venom and saved him, but itself began to die. The bulbuls then quickly arrived, and poured nectar into its throat and it revived. The mark left by the venom was the blue throat of the Blue-throat!

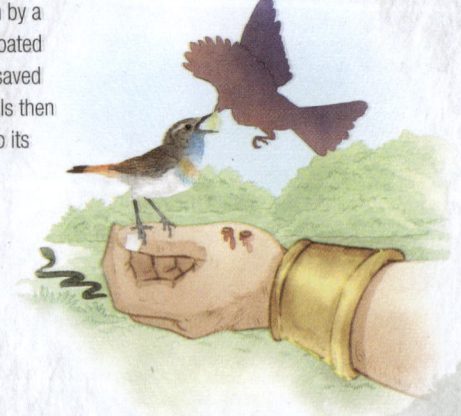

Each Little Bird That Sings

Paddyfield Pipit

Scientific name: *Anthus rufulus*   Size: *15 cm*
Hindi name: *Rugail, Charchari*
Sanskrit name: *Dhaan Tulika*

Description

When you are out walking in any grassy, arid, scrubland areas, you are most likely to see one of the Pipits. The most common one is the Paddyfield Pipit. A slim, longish, warm brown bird, with dark streaking, it moves quickly along the ground in a bobbing fashion, wagging its tail slowly and picking up seeds and insects as it goes along.

Habits

A widespread resident all across India, it is seen up to 1,000 m in the Himalayas, and sometimes even up to higher altitudes. A favourite habitat for the Dhaan Tulika is paddy fields, grassy areas, edges of woodlands and wetlands. It eats insects of all kinds, and also the seeds and green matter of grasses and weeds. The Charchari occurs alone or in pairs, and is usually quite reluctant to take to flight…taking off with a low, weak flight for a short distance, complaining bitterly with repeated soft plaintive notes, and settling down again quickly, to continue feeding.

The courtship flight is to fly up a short distance in a series of curves, singing all the while, and then do an abrupt fluttering descent. It is not particular about its nest site, and even a cattle footprint is deemed to be enough of a depression to hold its nest.

Call

In flight, it utters soft tseep-tseep notes, with the ground call being pipit-pipit.

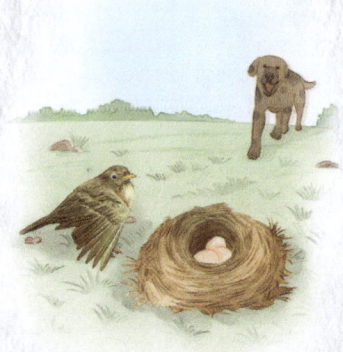

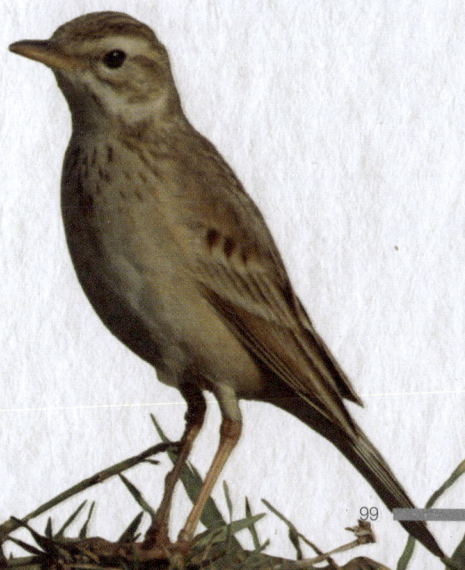

Mythology, Tales & Trivia

If the female is disturbed on the nest, she goes into the wounded bird decoy act, to try and draw the predator away from the nest!

Jayantika Davé

Baya Weaver

Scientific name: *Ploceus philippinus* Size: 15 cm
Hindi name: *Baya, Sonchiri*
Sanskrit name: *Peetmund kalvin*

Description

The Baya is a widespread resident across India, and in non-breeding plumage can be easily mistaken for a heavily marked sparrow. But all of us have seen and marvelled at the intricate bottle-shaped nests woven by the Baya, with often 50 to 200 nests in one tree! And with the rains, the Son Chiri comes into breeding plumage, flaming into an unmistakable bright yellow-and-brown beauty!

Habits

Grassland, scrubland and cultivated areas near water are the favourite habitats of the Baya, with the presence of trees being an essential requirement. They are only found up to 1,500 m in the Himalayas and are largely a lowland bird. Their primary diet is seeds of various kinds, as well as insects, flies, beetles, caterpillars, butterflies and small snails.

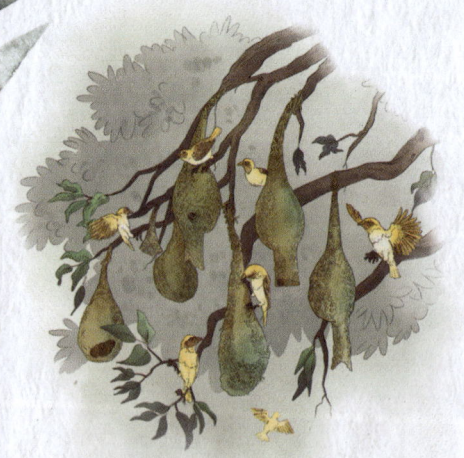

The building of the nest is an intricate process, with the males in full Son Chiri plumage doing the selection of site, tying a grass strand onto a branch, building an entrance porch and then proceeding to build an elongated nest chamber, with intricately woven sliced grass strips. Now is the time for the female to arrive for an inspection, and she really does rule the roost! She picks the home she likes, and agrees to the mate who was smart enough to build that particular home!

Call

A mix of twitters and whistles, with harsh 'chit' alarm calls!

Mythology, Tales & Trivia

Mackintosh tells of seeing these birds being trained to do tricks — such as firing a small toy cannon, and at the end of the trick, tipping up its head with a small nod as if to say, 'aha, what do you think of that?!'

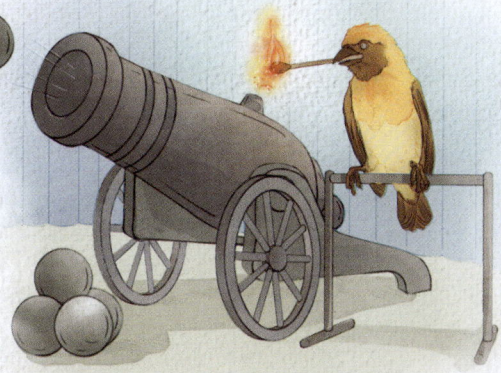

The legend goes that the male builds a small swing near the nest, so that he can sit near his mate while she is warming the eggs, and can swing and sing to her!

Another lovely story is that lumps of wet clay are placed in the nest, with fireflies on them, to light up the nest at night!

Jayantika Davé

Little Ringed Plover

Scientific name: *Charadrius dubius*   Size: 16 cm
Hindi name: *Zirrea, Merwa*
Sanskrit name: *Sarshapi Khanjanika*

Description

This little water-loving bird is a resident and a winter visitor across India. The Little Ringed Plover is very similar in size and behaviour to the **Kentish Plover**, but a quick differentiator is that the Little Ringed Plover always has a complete ring round the neck – black while breeding, or dark broken brown when not, but the ring is complete. In the Kentish Plover, the ring extends only to a little beyond the shoulders on both sides.

Habits

A widespread resident, the Zirrea can be seen up to 800 m in the Himalayas (even higher in the Nepalese area). It favours silt and sandy flats along slow-flowing fresh or salt water, or along the edges of artificial lakes and pools. Its diet comprises of insects and flies, spiders, shrimps and other invertebrates. It feeds in the typical Plover fashion of dainty small steps, and quick short runs ending with a bobbing jab at the food it finds. It is seen in small groups, as it is not as gregarious as some of the other Plovers. Its colouring blends in so well with sandy flats that the bird is not really visible till it does a sudden run to collect a tasty morsel. When threatened, it prefers to run and escape rather than fly, but when forced into flight, the sharply curved wings and strong low flight are a pretty sight!

The nest is just a little depression in the ground, sometimes left bare, and sometimes lined with some plants or stones, but always in the vicinity of water. It tries to lay its eggs near larger and more aggressive species, so that it gets natural protection from predators.

Call

Usually calls only during flight, with a soft, stretched-out complaining peeeyu.

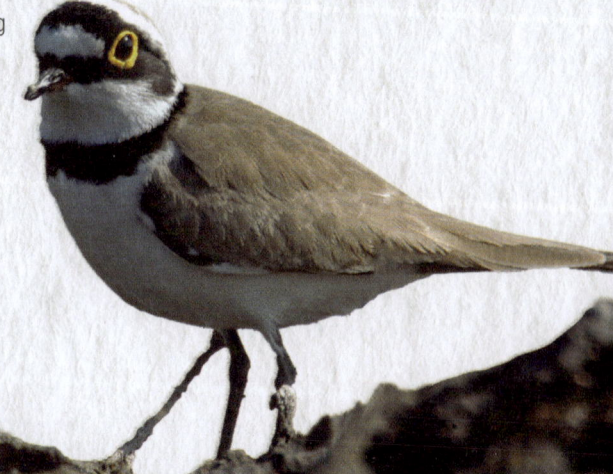

Oriental Skylark

Scientific name: *Alauda gulgula*   Size: 16 cm
Hindi name: *Bharat, Chandul*
Sanskrit name: *Bharadwaj*

Description

Our open grass and scrublands have a large population of the fairly nondescript Oriental Skylark – a warm brown all over, heavily streaked with black, and with a flattish crest. It blends so well with the background that it is not easy to see at first sight. So, stop a moment, allow your eyes to adjust to the brown lands around, and then you see it – this small active bird, moving around quickly with an upright stance, constantly singing and warbling to itself!

Habits

The Oriental Skylark is a widespread resident, and a winter visitor too. It frequents open lands that border cultivated areas, semi-desert, scrub, dry edges of marshes and coasts, and the edges of forest clearings. It can be found up to 4,000 m in the Himalayas. Its food is seeds and insects, and it forages constantly on the ground, alone and in pairs, and often in small flocks. When we are out walking in the Sultanpur flats, for example, these birds are present in large numbers, and as we come closer, they first prefer to squat and pretend that they don't exist! And if we continue to approach, they then flush out with a surprised chirrup and fly off, though only a small distance away.

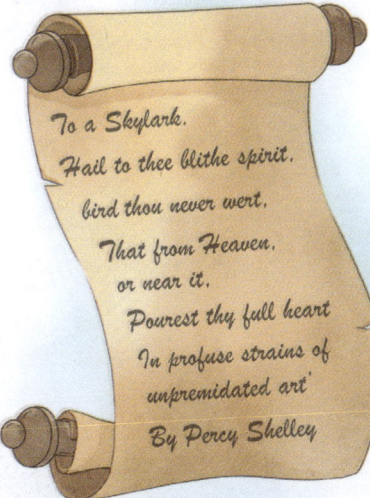

'To a Skylark.
Hail to thee blithe spirit,
bird thou never wert,
That from Heaven,
or near it,
Pourest thy full heart
In profuse strains of
unpremidated art'
By Percy Shelley

Call

The male sings a long quivering song, interspersed with warbling, twittering and whistling. It flies high up into the air, singing all the while, hovering on fluttering wings and continuing to sing, and then does a fluttering descent!

Jayantika Davé

Brown Rock Chat

Scientific name: *Oenanthe fusca*   Size: *17 cm*
Hindi name: *Matiya Shama*
Gujarati name: *Kalo Pathral Piddo*

Description
Around apartment buildings, rocky outcrops, and scrubby countryside in North India can be seen the bird I call 'The Sentinel' – the Brown Rock Chat. This dark, stocky, medium-sized bird sits quietly at a height in obscure corners, intently surveying everything that is around, all the while gently raising and spreading its tail and bobbing its head!

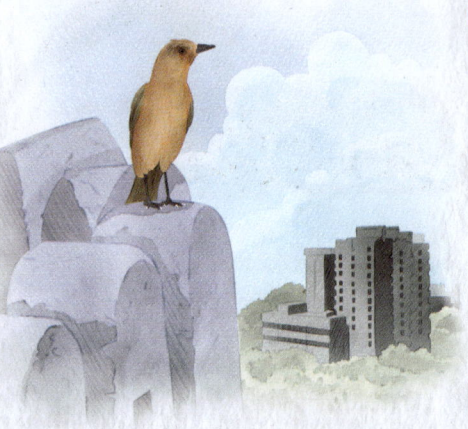

Habits
It loves stark habitats – old stone walls, forts, quarries, top-floor apartment balconies – positioning itself as this quiet dark statue, watchfully observing any movement. On our balcony, it is a shy bird that will quickly fly away at the sight of human presence. However, out in the countryside, we see it sitting on top of old stone walls, from where it does not frighten easily. In earlier times, writers like Hugh Whistler mention that it was unafraid of humans and often came into rooms even when there were people around…times have changed maybe? Favourite foods are insects, spiders, ants and beetles, which are typically picked off with a quick swoop.

Call
Fairly silent, bursting into a scolding tchuk-tchuk when alarmed, or a soft sweet whistle otherwise!

Bay-backed Shrike

Scientific name: *Lanius vittatus*   Size: *17 cm*
Hindi name: *Panchanag Latora, Chhota Latora*
Sanskrit name: *Latooshak*

Description
A very smart shrike with a grey head, a black forehead extending like a mask across its eyes, and a deep maroon-brown back – the Bay-backed Shrike is a widespread resident, and easily seen in dry open areas, along roadsides and in gardens.

Habits
We had a pair of Bay-backed Shrikes frequenting our large garden in Lodhi Estate, Delhi. My studying during the holidays would always be out in the garden, where I could observe the different birds that would go about their business every day. The Panchanag was very interesting to watch. It would perch on the top of a tall shrub or the exposed branch of a tree, launch itself after various winged prey and, having caught one, would immediately carry it into the bougainvillea creeper. I followed it one day, wondering what it was doing, and found that it would impale the insects on a large thorn of the creeper, and come back and eat them at will – its own personal larder! These shrikes feed mainly on insects and beetles, in flight or on the ground, occasionally also catching lizards or small mice. They are pugnacious by nature, and I have seen them driving away even the much larger drongo.

Call
Long rambling warbles, with the mimicking of many birdsongs mixed in it. Warning calls are a harsh churr-churr.

Mythology, Tales & Trivia
The male is a really good father, doing all the food-gathering to feed the nestlings, and passing it to the mother who stays close to the nestlings and feeds them.

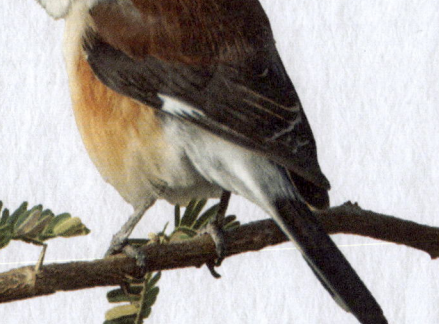

Jayantika Davé

Red-whiskered Bulbul

Scientific name: *Pycnonotus jocosus*   Size: 20 cm
Hindi name: *Kamera/Pahari Bulbul*
Sanskrit name: *Pushpvatansak* = *the red ear feathers of this bird, which looks as if it is wearing pretty floral ornaments in its ears*

Description

Of the bulbuls, the Red-whiskered Bulbul is my personal favourite – dapper, striking, glossy black head and tall perky crest, a slash of bright red on the cheek, and a red flash under the tail – an elegant beauty! It has a particularly cheerful 'pettigrew, kik-pettigrew' call which immediately lifts my spirits!

Habits

The Kamera Bulbul is a widespread resident across a lot of India, and found in a variety of habitats – from gardens to orchards to grasslands, and cultivation, and forest fringes and plantations. It is very comfortable around human habitation, and you are bound to see one as you look around green areas surrounding your home.

These bulbuls love fruit and nectar and treat that as their primary diet, while of course supplementing it with insects, spiders and kitchen waste. In our Empire Estate home, when the kachnar outside the balcony was in full bloom, our mornings would be brightened by their calls, as they loved the nectar and congregated on that tree! They are usually seen alone or in pairs, rarely in larger numbers.

The courting male assumes a begging posture, with tail spread, wings dropped low and quivering, and head bowed, all the while uttering soft calls.

Call

A cheerful 'pettigrew, kik-pettigrew' call!

White-eared Bulbul

Scientific name: *Pycnonotus leucotis*   Size: 20 cm
Hindi name: *Safed-kaan Bulbul*
Sanskrit name: *Shwet-karna Bulbul*

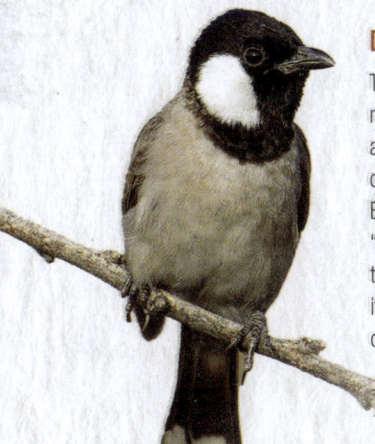

Description

This lovely medium-sized bulbul is a resident of the northwest parts of India. A typical-looking bulbul, with a dark black head, but virtually no crest, and a splash of sulphur-yellow under the tail. Whistler describes this Bulbul as a 'cheerful confiding individual, with a cheery "quick-a-drink-with-you" call — a familiar companion by the paths of man!' Always ready for a bit of fun — whether it is chasing a cloud of flying ants, or harrying a hapless owl or arriving at a table to pick up bread crumbs!

Habits

A lowlands bird of dry woodland, scrub, shrubbery, gardens and cultivated areas, the Safed-kaan Bulbul is a cheerful being, with a quick, repeated 'he-did he-did' call and many other cheerful bubblings in between. The fruit of the lantana and other shrubs are a favourite, as well as nectar and small invertebrates. It can be seen in pairs, or small groups, often descending to the ground to check for insects and seeds, and then flying back to its perch.

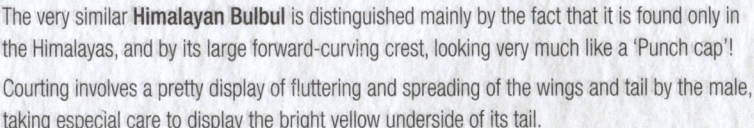

The very similar **Himalayan Bulbul** is distinguished mainly by the fact that it is found only in the Himalayas, and by its large forward-curving crest, looking very much like a 'Punch cap'!

Courting involves a pretty display of fluttering and spreading of the wings and tail by the male, taking especial care to display the bright yellow underside of its tail.

Call

'He-did, he-did' repeated a number of times, with pretty trills in the middle, likened to 'Quick-a-drink with you'!

Mythology, Tales & Trivia

Whistler mentions that in the wild state, the White-eared Bulbul hybridizes frequently with the Red-vented Bulbuls!

Jayantika Davé

Common Quail

Scientific name: *Coturnix coturnix*   Size: 20 cm
Hindi name: *Bater*
Sanskrit name: *Vartak, Garudayodhi*

Description

A widespread winter visitor to North and Central India, and resident in certain pockets across the country, is the Common Quail. This dainty, little, plump and almost tail-less Common Quail looks like the *chhota bhai* (younger brother) of the bigger Teetar or Grey Partridge. And M. Krishnan beautifully describes the babies as 'no bigger than a breakfast egg on red legs, and marvellously assured in deportment'!

Habits

The tiny Common Quail is a difficult bird to see, as it moves amongst vegetation, seeking every bit of cover that it can get, and if flushed, takes off in a low whirring flight, quickly lands and disappears immediately! It prefers open countryside, including cultivated areas and areas with low vegetation. Common Quails migrate in from the Western Palearctic region to India and Africa in winter. They can be seen up to 1,000 m and in some cases, there are sighting and breeding records in Ladakh and Bhutan. The Bater feeds off the seeds of grasses, weeds and small grains, and green vegetation including leaves, flowers and buds and flowers, as well as insect life, worms and molluscs.

Call

Its call of three short notes, likened to 'wet-mi-lips' or 'watwalak', is heard more often than the bird is seen. The call is repeated a few times in quick succession!

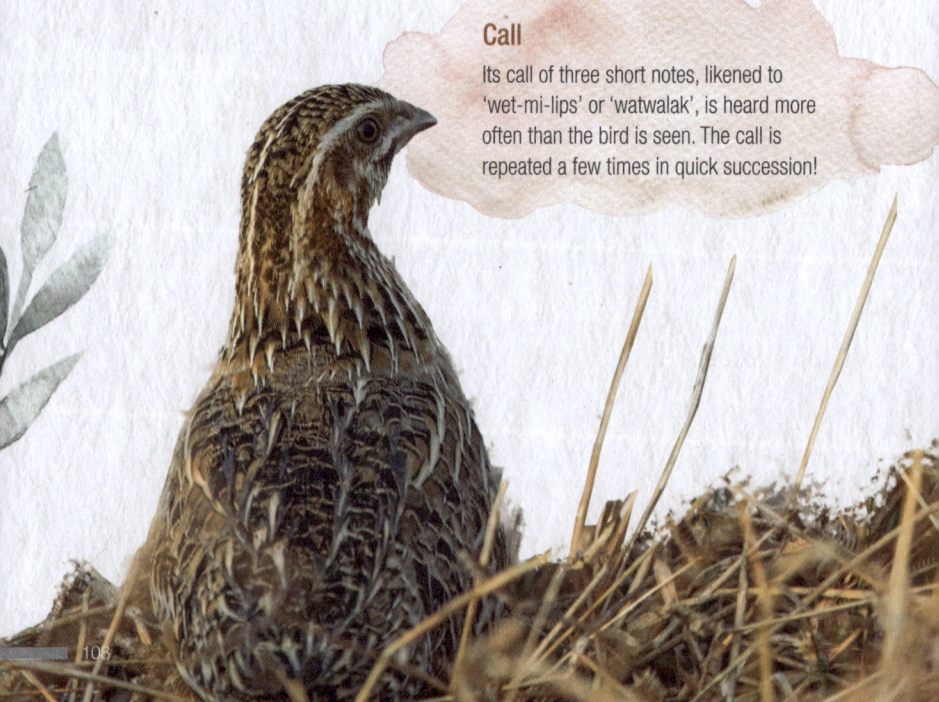

Mythology, Tales & Trivia

The Hitopadesha has a story about the Quail and the Crow, which lived together in a forest. Once, all the birds decided to go to the seashore to honour Lord Garuda, the king of all the birds, and the quail and the crow travelled together. On the way, there was a dairyman walking along with a pot of curds on his head. The crow kept swooping down and stealing the curds. When the dairy man saw his empty pot, he looked around for the culprit. The crow quickly flew away, but the quail was caught and punished. Moral – do not keep the company of villains and choose your friends carefully!

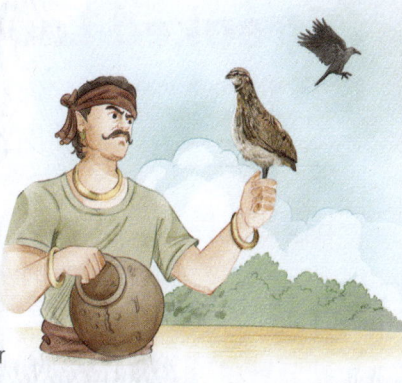

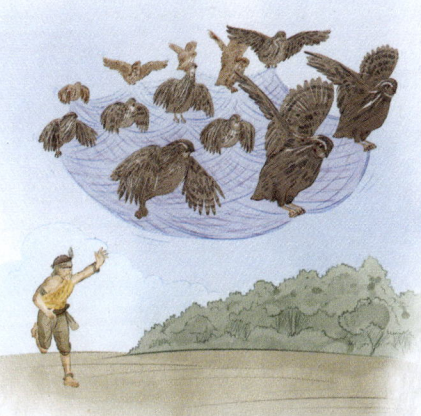

In the Jataka tales, a fowler learnt to imitate the call of the leader quail, and so managed to catch the whole flock. The leader quail was distraught, called the balance flock, and taught them that next time a net is thrown over them, they should put their heads through a hole each, and fly up with the nest, leave it on a thorn bush and escape from below. They did this very successfully. But one day, they began squabbling amongst themselves about who did more work while lifting the net, and in the process the fowler caught them all. United we stand, divided we fall.

Due to their pugnacious nature, they were kept as cage birds for fighting and betting, being then known as Garut Yodha.

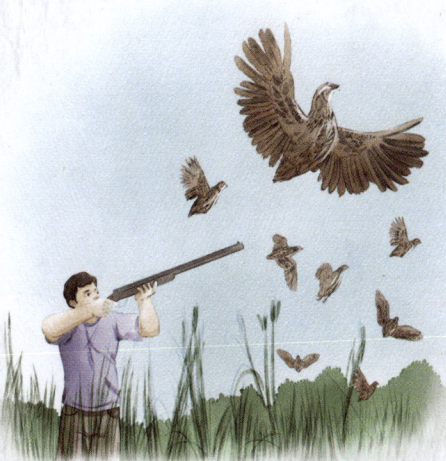

They were also hunted in large numbers, using call birds in cages mounted on poles, whose calls would cause the free birds to congregate in one area, from which the beaters would then cause them to fly to be shot for sport and for the table.

Jayantika Davé

Streaked Laughing Thrush

Scientific name: *Trochalopteron lineatum*   Size: 20 cm
Hindi name: *Goreeda*
Kash: *Sheen Pi-pi*

Description

This relatively small Laughing Thrush is a resident of the Himalayas. The Goreeda skulks through every bit of undergrowth it can find, and yet tantalisingly draws attention to itself with its lovely loud trilling call! As it emerges into the light, the chestnut earmuffs and black and white streaking on its brown and chestnut body become apparent. Hugh Whistler describes its habits humorously – 'occasionally it is inspired by ambition, and climbs out from the bushes into handy trees!'

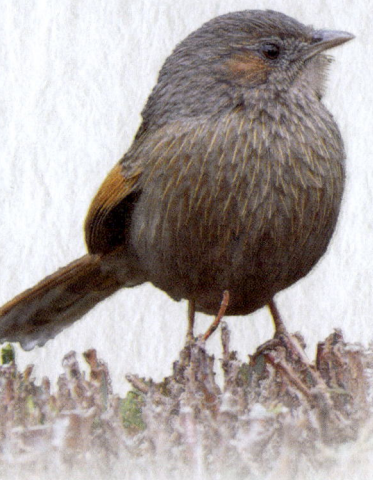

Habits

In our hill home, the first place where we see the Sheen Pi-pi is around the base of our stone pushta walls, from where it then moves on to hunt behind the ivy hanging from them, flying low and fearlessly across our veranda as we sit there, and finally arriving to steal food from our dog Buddy's bowl! The Streaked Laughing Thrush is a frequenter of bush lands, hill slopes, open forests, cultivated gardens, stone walls and also coniferous forests up to 3,000 m in the Himalayas, descending lower as it gets colder. Insects, spiders, moths, fruits, seeds and kitchen scraps are things it loves. These birds dribble from cover to cover with a broken weak flight interspersed with scuttles, as each bird overtakes the other.

Call

Loud chitters or a high-pitched whistling call, followed by a tsii-chu-tsii-chu call!

Mythology, Tales & Trivia

Hugh Whistler describes how a nesting pair of these birds tore apart the coir footmat outside his dining room, despite the fact that people kept moving in and out! The nest was easy to spot, with the brightly coloured fibres hanging out!

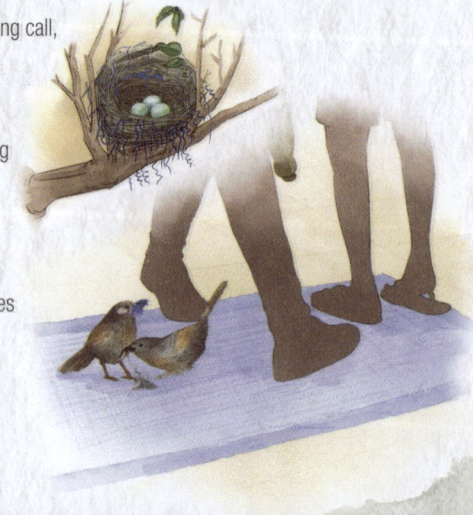

Common Sandpiper

Scientific name: *Actitis hypoleucos*   Size: 20 cm
Hindi name: *Jalrank*
Sanskrit name: *Bhatt, Ping*

Description

In winter, along the shores of water bodies across India, whether fresh or salt water, you are sure to see the smart, dark brown and white, medium-sized Common Sandpiper. As it moves along, it looks as if its body is jointed with springs, resulting in an incessant nodding of its head, and a continuous jerking of its tail up and down! While it has only a tiny tail, it wags it with great vigour, as if to prove to all watchers that it does indeed have a tail! A flash of a white wing bar as it takes flight, and you know it is the Jalrank you are seeing.

We have two other widespread Sandpiper winter visitors – the **Green Sandpiper**, which is darker and stockier, and the **Wood Sandpiper**, which has longer legs and a slimmer build. However, Sandpipers are difficult to differentiate for a beginner!

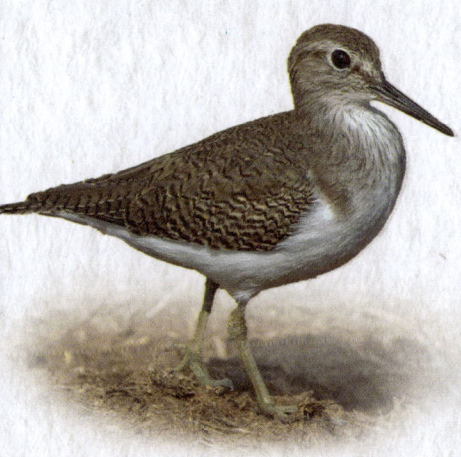

Habits

The Common Sandpiper arrives as early as August, and may stay on till May. Water body margins in winter, whether riverbanks, wetlands, small ponds, lakes or sheltered sea shores and even flooded rice fields, reservoirs or temporarily flooded grasslands will attract this visitor. It has been seen up to 4,000 m in the Himalayas and the Northeast hills.

The assiduous hunt is for insects, spiders, molluscs and crustaceans, with an opportune grabbing of small fish or frogs too. A bobbing scan, a quick run and a stab! It is usually a solitary bird, sometimes, though rarely, seen in small groups.

Call

Rapidly repeated set of 5 to 6 notes – tit-hidit-tit-hidit-tit-hidit or kitty-needie, kitty-needie.

Mythology, Tales & Trivia

The Common Sandpiper breeds across temperate and subtropical Europe, and can fly up to 4,000 km during its migration to India, Africa and Australia.

Called Sandpiper because they are largely found on sandy or wet soil, and have a plaintive, piping call.

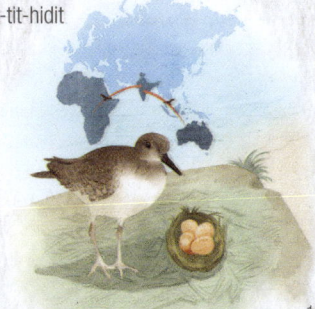

Jayantika Davé

Spotted Owlet

Scientific name: *Athene brama*   Size: *21 cm*
Hindi name: *Khakusat, Khusattia, Chugad*
Sanskrit name: *Shakuneya, Pingalika*

Description

This gorgeous little rounded spotted ball of fluff is one of our most common and widespread resident owls. For me, a trip to the Bharatpur Bird Sanctuary starts with a visit to the first bare tree near the entrance which has a number of round holes in it, and as the first rays of the sun strike this, out pop at least three of these lovely owls, basking in the sun – a painter's and photographer's delight!

Habits

The Spotted Owlet prefers relatively open forestation, and can be seen in open forests, gardens and parks and around habitation, fields and orchard groves. These birds are most active in the hour before sunrise and before dusk, and they emerge from their hole with much chittering and squeaking! They are also often seen on lamp posts and in gardens when the evening lights are on. One of the prettiest sights I have seen was in Bharatpur, where a whole family of seven of these owlet puff-balls used to emerge onto a completely bare tree at the inner entrance to the park, sit and sun themselves, while we marvelled! While sleeping, if it is disturbed, a puzzled round face will appear at the hole, asking you what you want…and if you don't answer, it will emerge further onto a branch, and begin its characteristic neck bob, full of curiosity and quite a bit of indignation! Its diet consists mainly of insects, with mice, small birds, frogs and lizards also being eaten.

Call

A loud screech of chiurr-chiurr-chiurr, interspersed with a cheevak, cheevak call!

Mythology, Tales & Trivia

Jerdon in *The Birds of India* writes that in earlier times, these little Owlets would be used by shikarees to catch other small birds. They would find an Owlet, tie it to on the ground near a small bush, and place branches around it, smeared with bird-lime. Other small birds, who hate owls, would then arrive to harass the poor owl, and get stuck to the bird-lime branches.

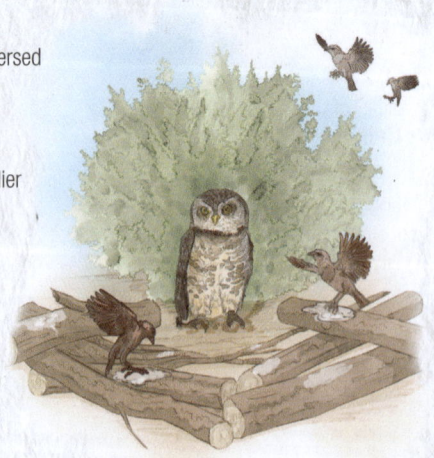

Each Little Bird That Sings

Brahminy Starling

Scientific name: *Sturnia pagodarum*   Size: 21 cm
Hindi name: *Brahmini Myna, Puhaia, Kalasir Myna*
Sanskrit name: *Shankara Shakunika*

Description

The Brahminy Starling is a lovely, very distinctive starling, with a long, black, wispy crest that gets blown about in the wind, green-blue eyes, and a soft rufous underside with a winged coat of grey! A widespread resident across India, it can sometimes be missed because it is not as common or as noisy as its other cousins.

Habits

It is found across India and up to 1,800 m in the hills, favouring open woodlands, forests, shrubs, scrub and areas around human habitation, particularly if there is some water around. Its main food are insects, the nectar of flowers and fruits and berries. It walks sedately along the ground picking up insects as it goes along, and does its nectaring and fruit hunting in the tree canopy. It is a communal rooster in medium-sized trees.

The nest is easy to see – a large, untidy, ugly structure of grass, leaves, papers and other discarded materials, lined with softer materials, and placed in the hole of a tree, often spilling out of it!

Call

A good songster, with a pleasant warbling song, and a variety of calls mimicking other birds too!

Mythology, Tales & Trivia

It is said to be a good mimic, learning the songs of other birds with ease.

The Brahminy part of the name is said to have come from the Brahminical *choti* or long hair on its head, and the 'pagodarum' from its frequenting of pagodas and temples in South India.

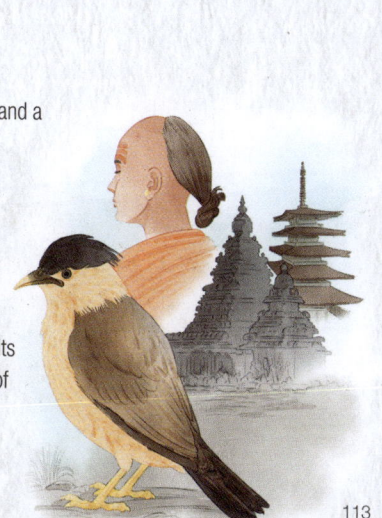

113

Jayantika Davé

Common Babbler

Scientific name: *Turdoides caudata* Size: 23 cm
Hindi name: *Chilchil, Dumri*
Sanskrit name: *Gram-haholika*

Description

Unlike its name, the Common Babbler is actually not a very common bird! It is a long, slim, brown bird, with strong dark streaking on the head and back, with a preference for skulking, and then running fast along the ground! When we are out for a walk in parks with trees and shrubbery at the fringes, this bird will often dart out from the undergrowth and quickly disappear on to the other side.

Habits

They enjoy mixed forests, gardens, orchards, dry stony areas and scrub jungles. These provide the ideal habitat for their diet of ants, beetles, grasshoppers and spiders. They also enjoy the berries of the lantana, and other seeds and grain, as well as some nectar, occasionally even stealing the eggs of small birds. They are reasonably gregarious, moving in small groups of about 6–7 birds, foraging along the ground with quick hops and trailing their tails behind, tipping over leaves and other litter, startling bugs that are hiding underneath. On being disturbed, they take off with a weak gliding flight, and the tail spread out, often looking like tiny pheasants! When agitated, 'the whole sisterhood combines to hurl invectives at the intruder, in a disorderly chorus,' as Salim Ali beautifully puts it.

The nest is a neat deep cup woven out of grasses, roots and twigs, and is often parasitized by the Common Hawk Cuckoo or the Jacobin Cuckoo.

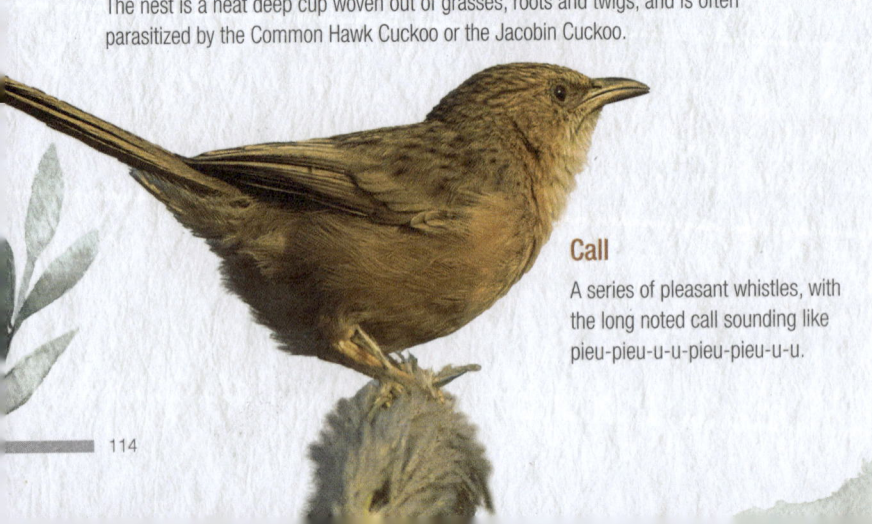

Call

A series of pleasant whistles, with the long noted call sounding like pieu-pieu-u-u-pieu-pieu-u-u.

Frogmouth, Sri Lanka

Scientific name: *Batrachostomus moniliger*   Size: 23 cm
Sanskrit name: *Dardur*

Description

This is truly an odd-looking bird – large head, big round eyes and a frog-mouthed appearance, with an exceptionally broad bill, with a very wide gape! It is not easy to see, as it is primarily nocturnal in its habits, and is found mainly in the Western Ghats in India down to Kerala, but is well worth the effort!

Habits

The Frogmouth has a strong preference for undisturbed forests, and roosts comfortably at 6–12 feet heights on shady branches, confident that its brown streaky colouring will camouflage it perfectly. These birds are most active at night, foraging for insects, moths and grasshoppers on branches, or picking them off the ground. They make short, quick flights through the trees, avoiding hopping or climbing through trees. We saw a pair in Thattekad where the male and female were snuggled close together, with eyes shut, pretending they could not see any of us.

Call

Harsh screeching calls, and some liquid chuckling calls!

Mythology, Tales & Trivia

When alarmed, they stretch their head and neck upwards, closing their eyes to slits, pointing their bills upwards, imitating a dead dry branch.

Once their chicks have hatched, the male removes the nest and throws it off the tree to hide any evidence of the nesting spot, as the same spot is often re-used.

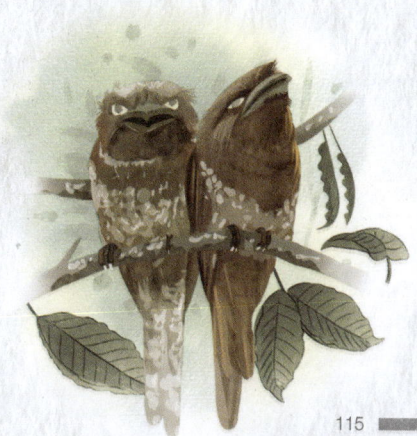

Jayantika Davé

Common Myna

Scientific name: *Acridotheres tristis*   Size: 25 cm
Hindi name: *Desi myna, Galgal*
Sanskrit name: *Kalehpriya, Chitranetra*

Description

The dapper, brilliantine-slicked, black-headed Common Myna is one of the most common birds around human habitation. As children, as we set off for school, we would look out for them, with the dictum that 'one for sorrow, two for joy' would dictate how our day would go! The pairs are well bonded, and you will see them strutting along together, indulging in soft conversation and stopping to neaten up each other's head feathers as a loving gesture!

Habits

The Desi Myna is a perky, self-confident, widespread resident across India, and found in large numbers around human habitation. An opportue ground-feeder, it is happy with grains, seeds, fruits, insects, nectar, birds' eggs, small animals and also kitchen scraps. In the fields, it will follow a plough to grab flushed insects, and will also sit on the backs of cattle to pick off their ticks. When they gather to roost in their hundreds, the noise is incredible!

Call

A scolding raadio-raadio-raadio, and a kok-kok-kok, accompanied by frenzied head-bobbing and frazzled plumage!

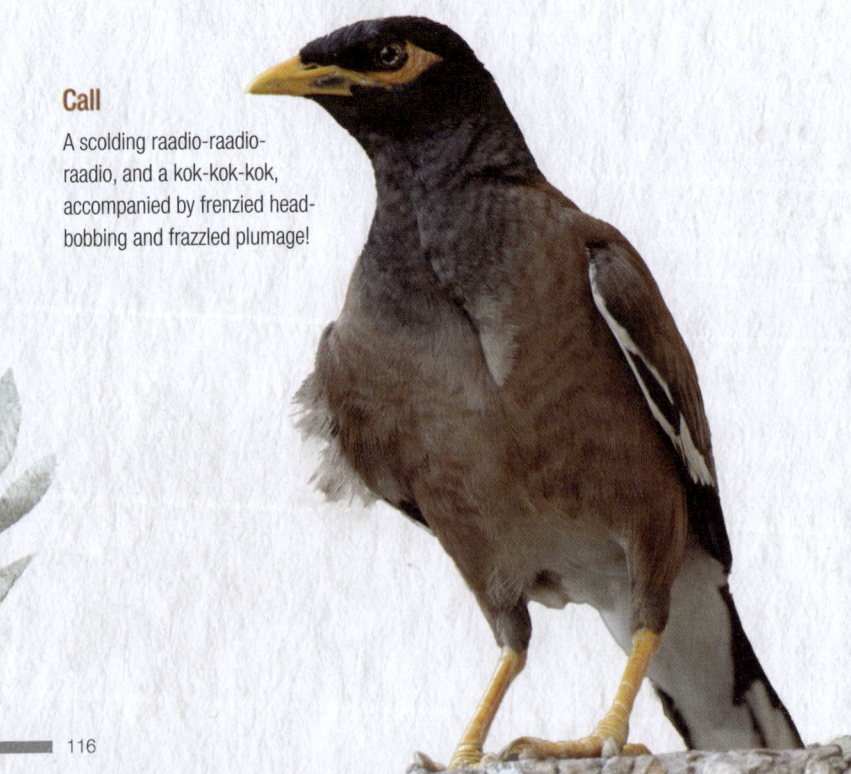

Mythology, Tales & Trivia

Once, in a forest, a myna tried to shelter in a tree where many crows were roosting. The crows threw the myna out, despite her pleadings. As the myna took shelter in another tree, a storm broke, with hail, thunder, lightning and rain. The myna found a hole in her tree, and was safe. The crows stayed where they were and many died. Ever since, the myna is deemed to be cleverer than crows, and mynas and crows are not friends.

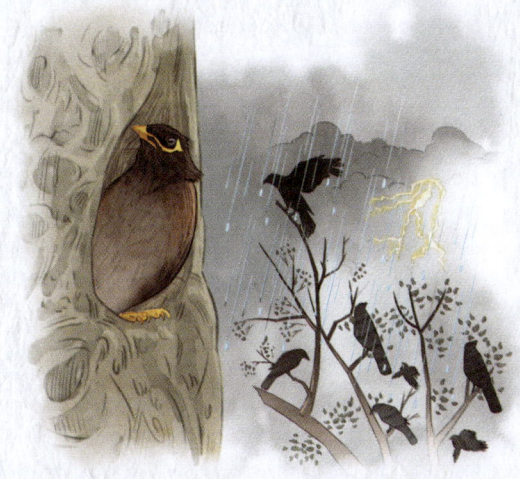

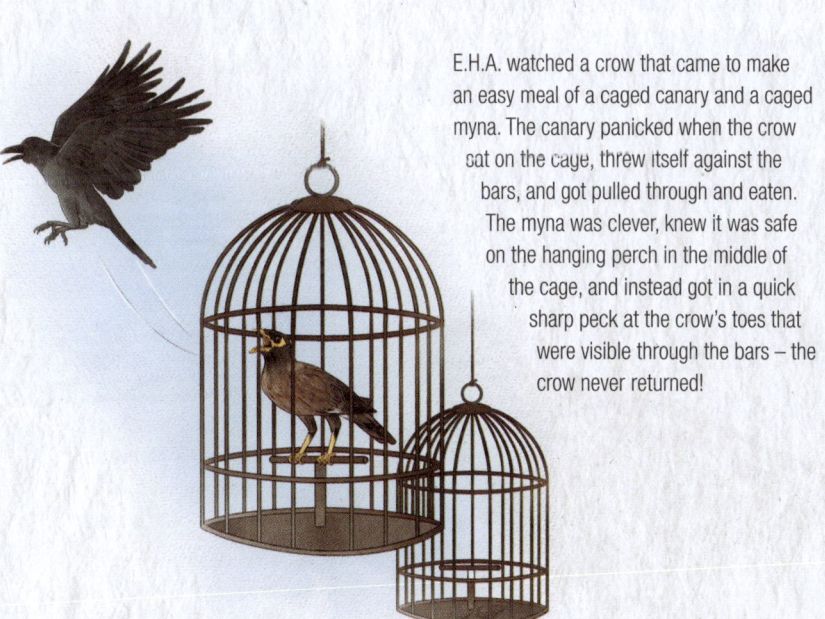

E.H.A. watched a crow that came to make an easy meal of a caged canary and a caged myna. The canary panicked when the crow sat on the cage, threw itself against the bars, and got pulled through and eaten. The myna was clever, knew it was safe on the hanging perch in the middle of the cage, and instead got in a quick sharp peck at the crow's toes that were visible through the bars – the crow never returned!

Jayantika Davé

Common Snipe

Scientific name: *Gallinago gallinago*   Size: 25 cm
Hindi name: *Chaha*
Sanskrit name: *Padankeer, Jalavartika*

Description
The Common Snipe is a rather badly put together plump, medium-sized bird – with disproportionately short legs, and an extra-long, very heavy beak! It appears throughout India in winter, and has a beautifully patterned back in dark brown and golden, with a prominent black eye stripe.

Habits
The Chaha is a shy bird, and hides in vegetation at the edges of wetlands, as it feeds on insects, earthworms, crustaceans and plant material. The large eye gives away its nocturnal nature, though it is seen during the day too. It has nerve cells at the end of its beak, which help to locate small worms! When alarmed, it takes off in a rapid zig-zag flight to confuse predators.

Call
When frightened, the Common Snipe utters a guttural 'escape, escape' or 'sni-ipe, sni-ipe' call!

Mythology, Tales & Trivia
From *The Book of Nature Myths:* Once, an Owl envied a Quail family which had many little ones, and asked the Quail for one of her babies. When the Quail refused, the Owl stole a baby at night, and disguised it by pulling on its beak till it became long. A little mole told the distraught mother Snipe what the Owl had done, and the Snipe went to the Owl nest and brought her baby back. But the others now laughed at him. Saddened, he went to live alone in the reeds, and since he liked the name Snipe, he adopted that!

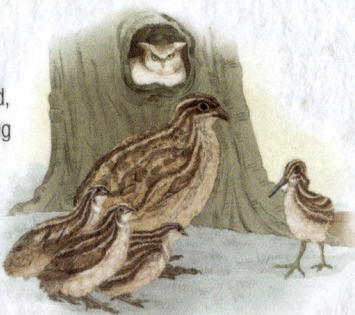

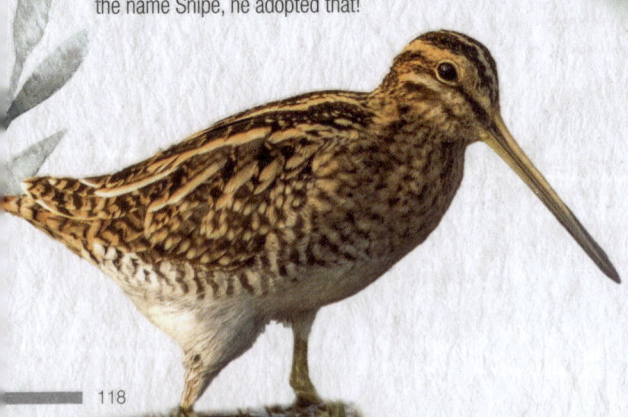

During courtship, the male rises high into the air and descends rapidly, changing the placement of its tail feathers to create an unusual drumming bleating sound. In many languages, therefore, the Common Snipe is known as the 'Flying Goat' or 'Heaven's Ram'!

Little Grebe
(Or Dabchick, as it was previously named)

Scientific name: *Tachybaptus ruficollis*   Size: 25 cm
Hindi name: *Pandubbi, Pantiri, Dubdubi*
Sanskrit name: *Vatrajul*

Description

The Little Grebe is a widespread resident of our open lakes and ponds all across India. Normally just a frumpy brown ball of fluff, in breeding plumage it gets rather gorgeous, with a bright rufous neck and a brilliant yellow patch at the base of its beak. It swims around busily, and then suddenly dives in and disappears, to surface a little distance away, while you are wondering where it went! This action gives rise to the very descriptive Hindi names!

Habits

The Pandubbi likes open water of any kind, and frequents lakes, canals, ponds and man-made reservoirs. Its diet consists of insects, water bugs, small crustaceans and small fish. While some food can be picked off the surface of the water, the majority of its food is got by diving down to at least 3–4 feet below the surface of the water, where it can stay submerged for up to 20 seconds as it tracks down its food. It is one of our most aquatic birds – almost never comes to land, and rarely flies any great distance.

The nest is a floating platform of water plants, and whenever the parent leaves the nest, it covers the eggs with a pad of weed, which continues to ferment in the sun and provides heat to help hatch the eggs.

Call

Loud and fast trilling call, with a wit-wit-wit as the alarm call!

Mythology, Tales & Trivia

A completely aquatic species, it is rarely, if ever, seen on land!

When it lands back in water after a flight, it catapults down onto its breast, which is well cushioned with fat and downy feathers!

In autumn, the wing feathers are shed, and it becomes almost flightless for a while!

Young Little Grebes are striped and can swim as soon as they are hatched.

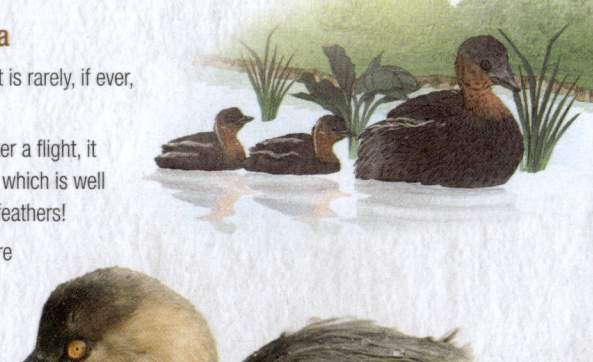

Jayantika Davé

Laughing Dove

Scientific name: *Spilopelia senegalensis*   Size: 27 cm
Hindi name: *Chhota Fakhta, Parki, Tortra Fakhta, Panduk*
Sanskrit name: *Kumkumdhoomra Kapot*

Description

This gentle vision in a dusky pinkish brown with blue-grey highlights is my favourite dove! Always revelling in the togetherness of pairs, the peaceful bobbing movement and the gentle cooing of the Laughing Dove bring with it a special serenity.

Habits

The Chhota Fakhta is found around gardens, human habitation and wooded areas where some water is to be found. They feed on fruits, seeds and grains, which are usually taken from where they have fallen on the ground, not normally from the plant itself.

My grandfather, Mr K.N. Davé, who was a great Sanskrit scholar and ornithologist, told me that if we cut out a piece of cardboard and placed it on a little bracket in our veranda, the Laughing Doves would build their nest on it. I didn't believe him, but did it nevertheless. Imagine my delight when very soon the doves began to arrive with their twigs. A nest was made, two white eggs were laid, and soon the babies arrived!

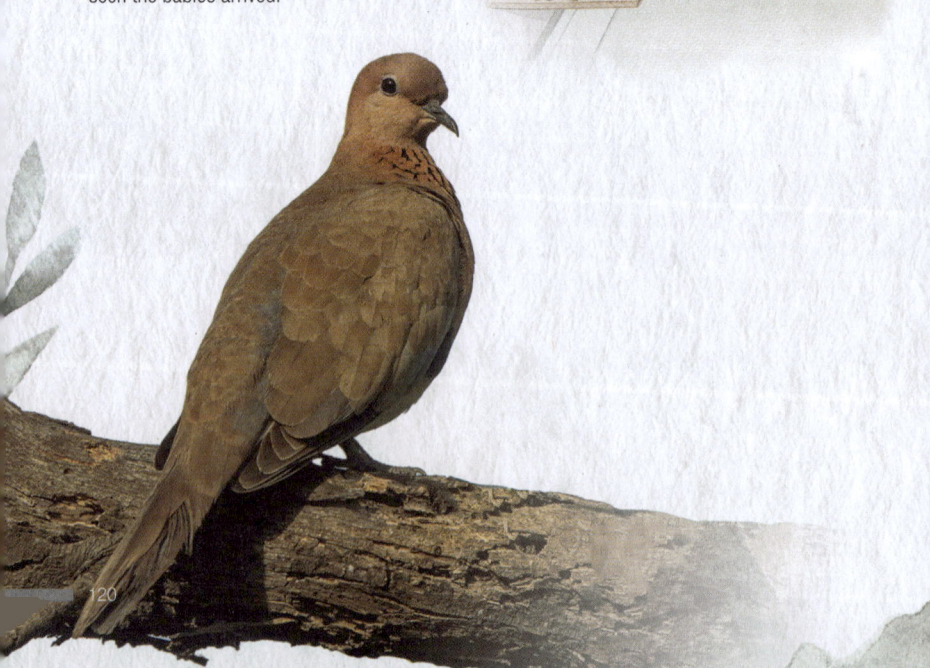

Call

A soft melodious coo-coorucoo-coo-coo-cu, repeated with gaps!

Mythology, Tales & Trivia

Legend has it that Tarakasur, an evil demon, had a boon from Lord Brahma that no one could kill him, except a son of Shiva. The Gods were afraid that Tarakasur would destroy the universe, and so persuaded Parvati to marry Shiva. When Shiva and Parvati were together, Agni the fire god took the form of a dove, and released their love as a drop into the Ganga, and the six-headed god Kartikeya was born, who went on to kill Tarakasur.

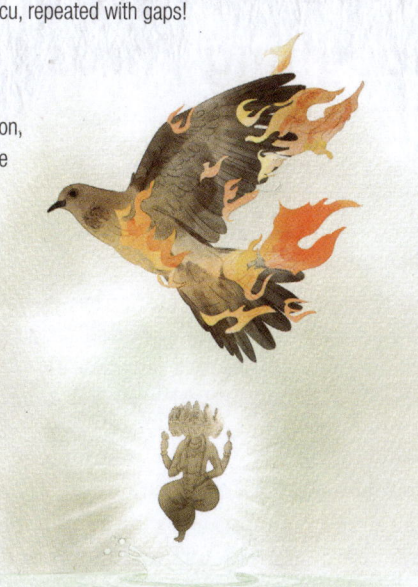

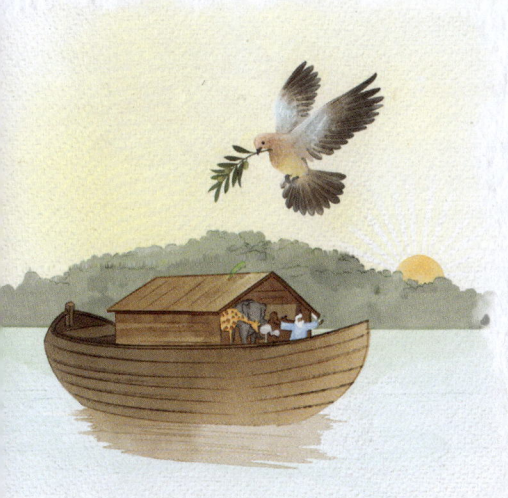

In the Old Testament, after the heavy floods, Noah sent the dove to look for land. It searched for seven days and finally returned with an olive branch. Ever since, a dove is considered to be a messenger of peace.

E.H.A. humorously describes their nest as 'composed of two short sticks and one long one'!

Jayantika Davé

White-throated Laughing Thrush

Scientific name: *Ianthocincla*   Size: 28 cm
Hindi name: *Safed kantthi*
Sanskrit name: *Kurubahuk (generic)*

Description

Eerie rustling in the forest, leaves being turned over with a soft 'the the', and then the burst into a discordant concert of noisy, wheezing, complaining calls! What adds to the ghostly air is the quiet glide of these birds through gloomy forests, with their newly laundered white bibs shining, and a curiously beautiful blue-grey iris.

Habits

The White-throated Laughing Thrush is a resident only of the Himalayas across to the Northeast, and is a lover of mixed forests of broad-leaved evergreens, conifers and deciduous trees. It is highly gregarious, always moving in small groups of at least 10–15 birds, staying above 1,200 m, and is also very comfortable in gardens with a lot of trees and bamboo groves. It hunts for insects, seeds and berries amongst the foliage, looks under cracks in the bark to find grubs, and often hops along the ground, cocking its head from side to side as it seeks out tasty morsels. These birds are a lovely sight, scrummaging busily on the forest floor, all the while keeping up a soft 'cheh cheh', chuckling and murmuring amongst themselves.

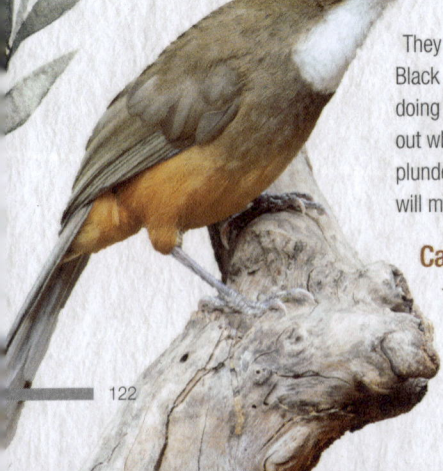

A hint of danger, and they take off with a loud complaining wheezy whistle. They have a particularly noiseless flight, looking almost eerie as they drift from one tree to another, their white bibs shining brightly!

They nest in bamboo clumps and trees. In our home, the Black Eagle knows the timing of this nesting, and starts doing sorties low above our bamboo clumps, checking out where the nests are being made, so that they can be plundered later. I sit and watch, praying that the eagle eyes will miss them!

Call

Thin wheezing plaintive call of tsweep, tsweeiu, chrr, chrr, with the flock constantly communicating with each other!

White-crested Laughing Thrush

Scientific name: *Garrulax leucolophus* Size: 28 cm
Hindi name: *Rawil-kahy, Safed Choti*
Sanskrit name: *Kurubahuk (generic)*

Description
A medium-sized, rich-brown-chestnut bird, with a startlingly white, raised spread-out crest, a white shirt-front, and a manic, loud laughing call! The White-crested Laughing Thrush – how could you possibly miss it! It is a resident, but only seen in our Himalayas, spreading across to the Northeast and wrapping around through to Bangladesh.

Habits
A flock of White-crested Laughing Thrushes are like a group of naughty, boisterous schoolboys, having just been let out of school, and now creating joyous mayhem with loud noisy bursts of laughter! A frequenter of broad-leaf, evergreen, deciduous and mixed forests, interspersed with bamboo, the Rawil-kahy is found between 1,000 m and 2,000 m. These birds move in medium-sized flocks, and you will hear them before you see them! The group forages for insects, spiders, beetles, seeds and berries, as also the nectar of flowers. They usually hunt towards the lower parts of trees, the tops of shrubs and on the ground, where they vigorously stab at the earth and toss aside clumps of leaves hoping to unearth an insect group. They are very alert, so that as soon as you are anywhere close, they burst into their loud laugh, making fun of you for trying to creep up on them!

Call
Prone to sudden outbursts of cackling laughter, with a lot of chatter in between, and then softer 'ow ow' notes being murmured as they hunt. Often one bird will burst into a mad laugh, with all the rest joining in, doubling over with merriment at the joke – truly a mad cacophony! Makes me laugh too, I must confess!

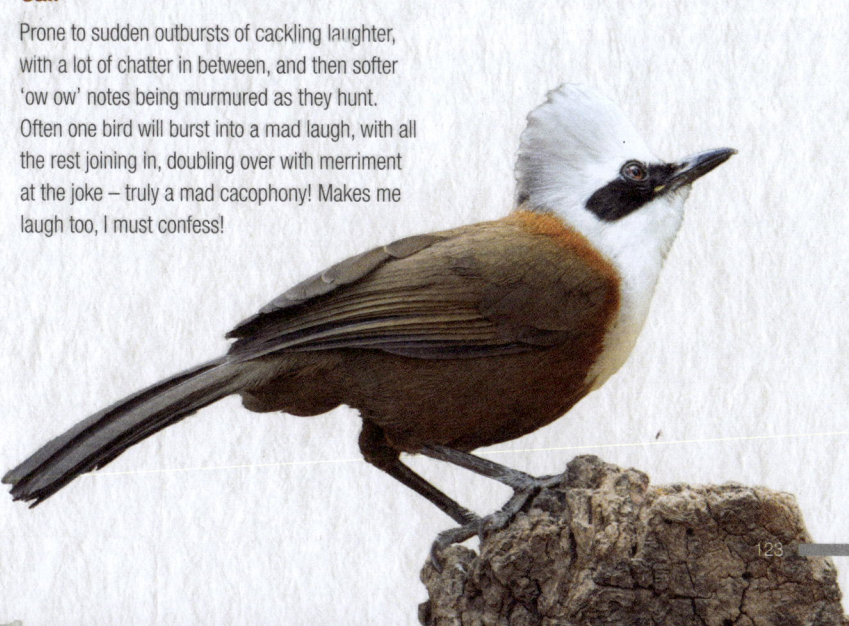

Jayantika Davé

Striated Laughing Thrush

Scientific name: *Grammatoptila striata*   Size: *28 cm*
Hindi name: *Bhiakura*
Sanskrit name: *Kurubahuk (generic)*

Description
I call this the Einstein bird! And when you see one, you will know why! A large, somewhat clumsy-looking brown bird, looking as if it is growing grey due to the fine white streaking, and with this crazy out-of-control mop of feathers on its crown, which it raises and spreads very often – truly looking like Mr Einstein himself!

Habits
Like a lot of the Laughing Thrushes, this is an inhabitant of the Himalayas and NE, frequenting broad-leaf evergreen and deciduous forests, and bamboo groves. While it is somewhat shy, it is still very visible in gardens with lots of trees and shrubbery, and around villages. Berries, seeds, insects, beetles and flowers and their nectar are favourite foods. I have rarely seen it on the ground, as it prefers to stay in the middle canopy of trees, flying into a tree from a safe place that has a thick shrubbery. It is found singly or in pairs, and even small flocks of 5–6 birds. A loud cheerful 'So Pleased to Meet You' call is a sign that you should be looking out for the Bhiakura!

Call
'So pleased to meet you!'

Common Redshank

Scientific name: *Tringa totanus* Size: *28 cm*
Hindi name: *Chhota Batan*

Description
A common winter visitor to most of India, particularly around the coastal areas or river banks and wetlands, is the brownish-grey Common Redshank, with a bright orange-red bill and bright orange-red 'shanks' or legs. A visit to a wetland will always yield a few sightings of these, so keep your eyes open for the orange-beak-orange-leg combination!

Habits
Wetlands, coastal areas, salt marshes and flooded grasslands and swamps are the favourite haunt of the Chhota Batan. All kinds of insects and spiders, molluscs and crustaceans are taken, including some small fish and tadpoles and worms. It wades briskly through the water, probing, jabbing, sweeping its bill as it wades, and moving in erratic dashes and spurts as it picks up its favourites. Usually in a small group, though spread out, sometimes alone or in pairs. It feeds in the day and even at night.

When we were young, Sundays were picnic Sundays, and Sultanpur was one of my Dad's favourite places to take us to. As we would approach near the park, there were small jheels along the road, and one of the first birds we would see would be the Common Redshank, which we would joyously point out!

Call
A nervous teeyu-hu-hu as it startles into flight, and a long-drawn tiyooo as it feeds!

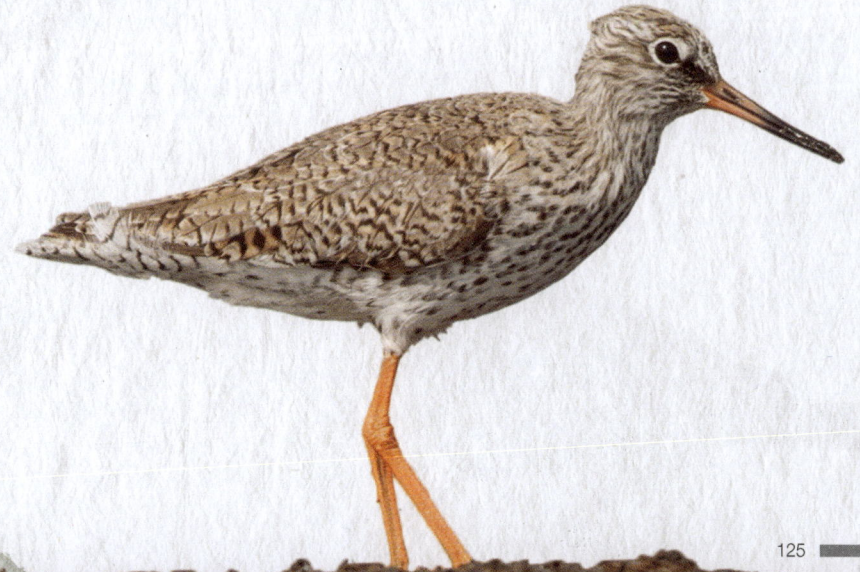

Jayantika Davé

Spotted Dove

Scientific name: *Streptopelia chinensis*   Size: 30 cm
Hindi name: *Chitroka Fakhta, Telia Ghuggu, Parki*
Sanskrit name: *Chitra Kapot*

Description

A medium-sized dove, with a pinkish-brown stomach, densely spotted wings and a black-and-white lace mantilla draped on its neck! Indeed, the Spotted Dove is a beauty! It is a widespread resident and can be seen in areas that have enough tree cover.

Habits

A lover of tree groves, whether in a forest or a park or at the edges of cultivated fields or gardens, the Chitrokha Fakhta is a resident across India, and can be seen in wilder areas as well as around human habitation up to 2,500 m in the Himalayas. A ground feeder, it forages for seeds and grains, and some green plant material and berries, as well as kitchen waste. It readily comes to grain feeders in homes where there is sufficient tree cover.

Spotted Doves have a lovely courtship display with the female strutting ahead, the male following, bowing and calling, with the spotted feathers of the neck fluffed out in an extravagant display! The male also sometimes flies up and comes floating down with wings spread out to land next to his lady love!

Call

Kuk-kroo-croo repeated a few times!

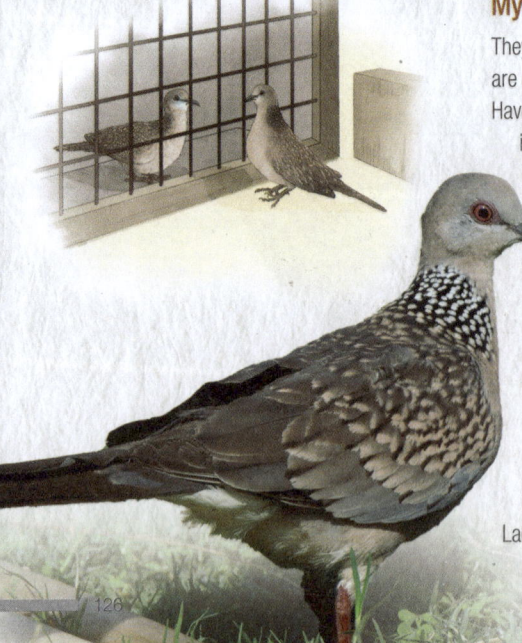

Mythology, Tales & Trivia

They tend to be seen in pairs, and the pairs are devoted to each other. One day in Glen Haven, our home in the hills, one of the pair inadvertently entered the house, and flew up to the skylight area, trying to get out again. The mate, in quiet desperation, paced on the terrace outside the skylight, not able to help, but unwilling to go away. This continued for the whole morning, till we were able to find a way to rescue the prisoner and release it! Truly touching!

A pretty name that pays tribute to the lovely spotted neck of this dove is Lace-necked Dove or Necklace Dove.

Eurasian Collared Dove

Scientific name: *Streptopelia decaocto*   Size: 32 cm
Hindi name: *Dhor Fakhta, Parki, Panduk, Gugi*
Sanskrit name: *Dhaval Kapot*

Description
Visible in parks, gardens and balconies in our cities is the lovely medium-sized Eurasian Collared Dove. It is larger than the more common Laughing Dove, and is a pinkish-grey fawn colour, with a distinct black collar around the back of its neck – hence its name!

Habits
Its diet is largely seed and grains, with some plants, berries and insects. It therefore tends to be seen around human habitation, though its original habitat is the drier scrub and small-tree areas of the country. It avoids dense forested areas, and is seen up to 2,500 m in the Himalayas. The Dhor Fakhta is a ground feeder, moving along with the stately dove gait, picking up little seeds and grains as it moves along. When it is not feeding, it perches on a tree or a pole, and preens…and preens!

During breeding season, a lovely little courtship dance plays out, with much 'koo-koo'-ing! The male puffs up its throat feathers, lowers its tail, and bows and scrapes, with the female reciprocating by ruffling up its feathers and lowering its beak to the ground.

Call
A melodious koo-koo-kook, or how-doo-do.

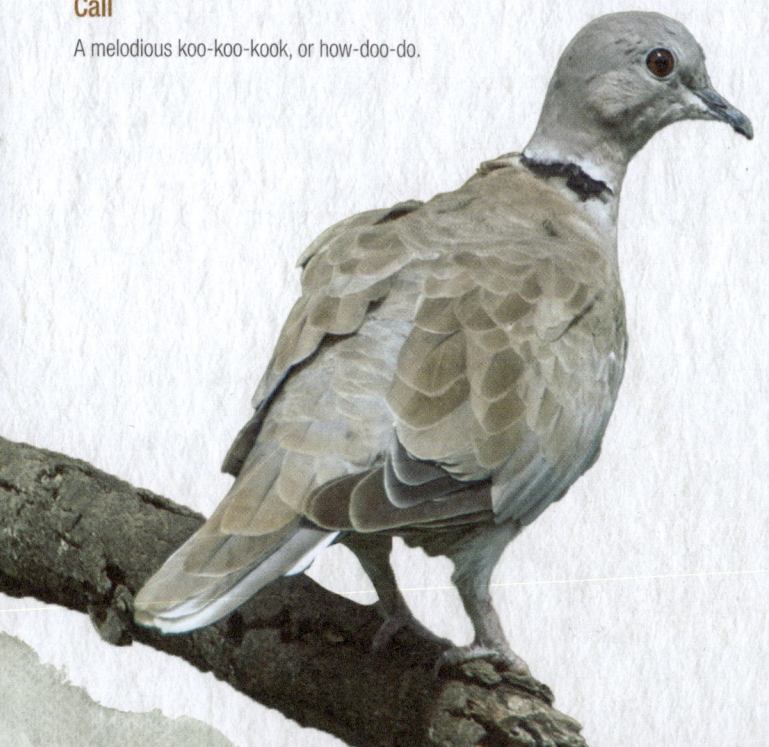

Jayantika Davé

Chestnut-bellied Sandgrouse

Scientific name: *Pterocles exustus*   Size: *32 cm*
Hindi name: *Bhat Teetar, Kuhar*
Sanskrit name: *Kakar*

Description

When we are birding in any of our desert parks or more arid areas, one of our 'must see' birds are the Sandgrouses, and of these, the Chestnut-bellied Sandgrouse is one that is a widespread resident across India. It is medium-sized, plump, short-legged, close to the ground in shades of light brown, fawn and gold, with a thin black necklace and a chestnut belly that is hard to see, as it is often hidden as it squats close to the ground.

Habits

Favourite habitats for the Bhat Teetar are deserts and semi-deserts, arid barren plains and thorny scrubland or fallow fields. It can be found up to 1,500 m. It feeds mainly on seeds, and sometimes insects and green material. It is most active during the early morning and late afternoon, tending to lie up under scrub during the hottest part of the day. Water is a necessity, and they come to drink in small flocks.

Once, when we were in the Little Rann, we were near a small pond just before dusk. The guide told us all to just wait and be still. And sure enough, flight after flight of the Chestnut-bellied Sandgrouse arrived to sit at the edge of the water and leisurely drink their fill of water, before winging their way to roost… Truly a memorable sight!

The nest is just a scrape in the ground, and 2–3 yellow grey eggs of a curiously elongated cylindrical shape are laid.

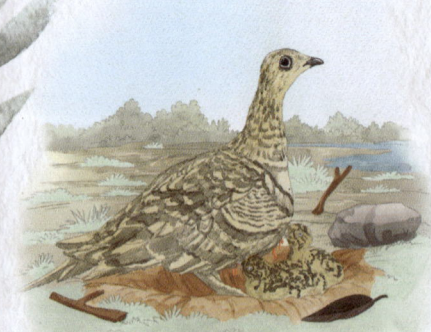

Call

In flight, a short 'whit!' followed by a hoarser kt-arrr. In flocks, they sometimes call continuously, sounding curiously duck-like, though softer!

Mythology, Tales & Trivia

The young are said to be given water by the male, who wets his front plumage with water, and then flies to the chicks so they can suck off this water!

Common Greenshank

Scientific name: *Tringa nebularia*   Size: *32 cm*
Hindi name: *Tantana, Timtima*
Sanskrit name: *Haritpad Jalrank*

Description
Pottering around the edges of our wetlands, marshes, lakes and ponds in winter is the medium-sized, long-legged, dark grey-brown Common Greenshank. As its name implies, it has green shanks or legs! In winter it is widespread across India.

Habits
The Tantana will be seen working its way steadily along and in shallow water, picking up insects, beetles, crustaceans and small fish. While it normally moves in a steady dignified way, occasionally it will dash and dart as something interesting catches its eye. Since it has an uptilted beak, it tends to pick up aquatic life from the surface of the water, rather than probe in the mud. It is quite comfortable being on its own, and mixes easily with other birds that feed in these habitats. It is easy to alarm, quickly taking fright and flying high up in a zig-zag way, all the time doing a 'thew-thew' alarm whistle! Foraging continues through the day and often nocturnally, with the bird taking advantage of marshy land of any kind – freshwater lakes, ponds, wetlands and flooded rice fields. While the green legs are often clearly visible, sometimes they get muddied up – so don't give up – take a closer look!

Call
A loud ringing too-too-too.

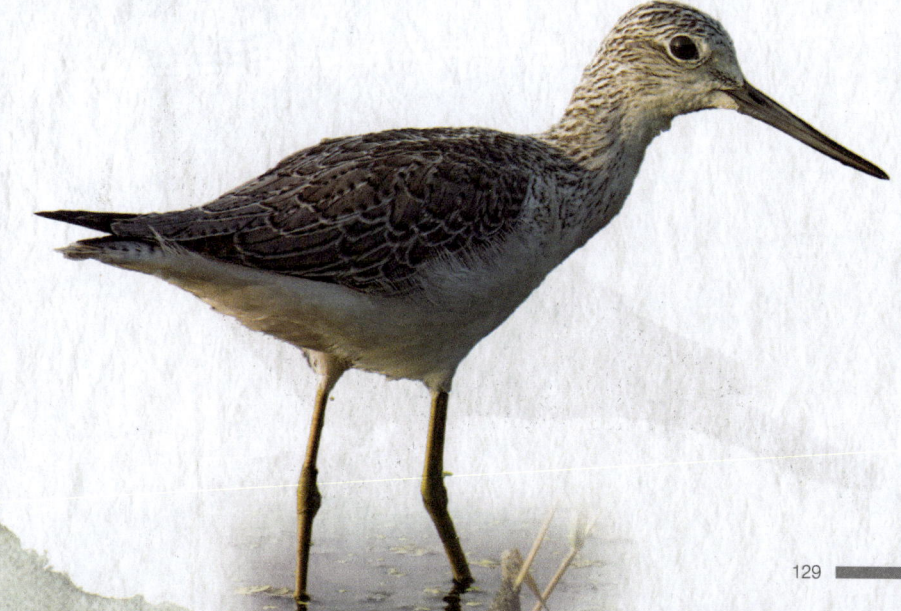

Jayantika Davé

Oriental Turtle Dove

Scientific name: *Streptopelia orientalis*   Size: 33 cm
Hindi name: *Kalstet Fakhta, Barko Fakhta, Ghugghu*

Description

The Oriental Turtle Dove is a plump, stocky dove, pinkish-brown grey, with the top part of its body being a rich chestnut-rufous-brown, with strong scale-like markings. Remember the song… 'On the second day of Christmas my true love gave to me, two turtle doves, and a partridge in a pear tree.'

Habits

It is widespread across India, being resident in some parts and a winter visitor in others. Equally comfortable in forests as well as glades and fields, it is found up to 2,500 m in the Himalayas. Seeds, grains and soft plant material are its main diet. In keeping with its plump, comfortable look is its call, which is deeper and more gruff than the other doves. It is not a gregarious dove, and is typically seen alone or in pairs.

The Ghugghu nests at different times in different parts of India. It does the typical dove nest thing – pulling together a few twigs, placing it in a shrub or a bamboo clump of a small tree, and calling it a nest!

Call

A gruff 'grrroo grroo cooo coooh'.

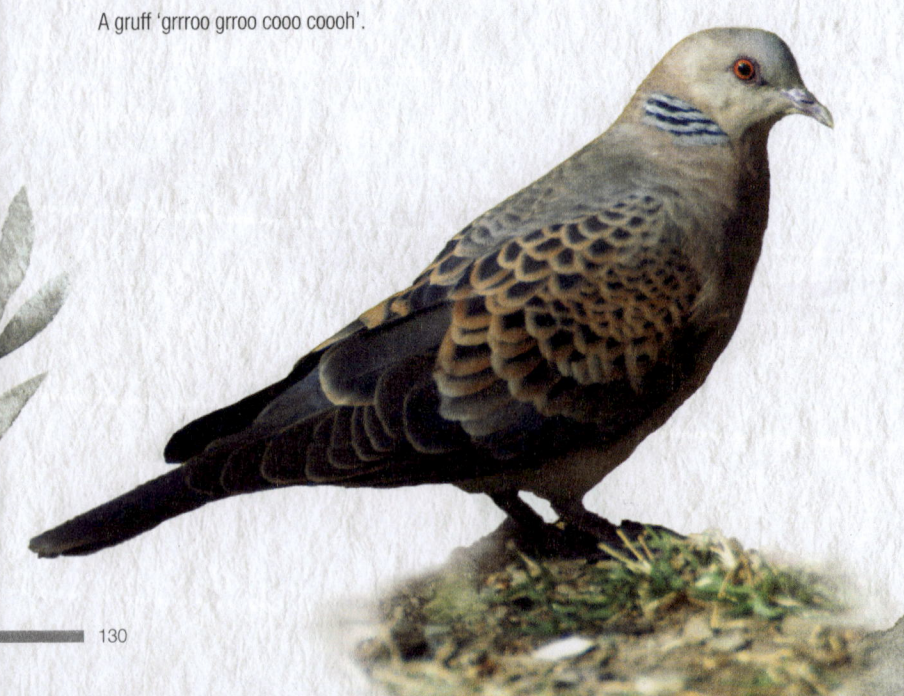

Red-wattled Lapwing

Scientific name: *Vanellus indicus* Size: 33 cm
Hindi name: *Titeeri, Titai, Titi, Titori*
Sanskrit name: *Tamramukh Tittibh, Andeerak*

Description

A tall and leggy, dark brown, black-and-white bird, striding confidently through an open park or garden, with a bright red beak and red eye shadow, and a strident demanding call of 'Did you do it… Did you do it?!' – and whether you did it or not, you are looking at the Red-wattled Lapwing!

A much-quieter cousin of the Red-wattled Lapwing is the **Yellow-wattled Lapwing**, which is a curious sight, though, with its fleshy yellow wattles starting below the eye, meeting above the beak, and then descending as two hanging lappets on each side! It is seen in drier open areas.

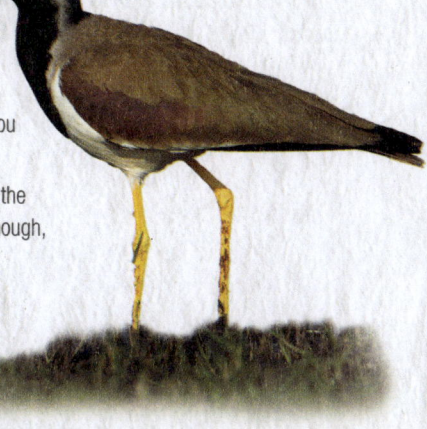

Habits

The Titeeri is a widespread resident across India, and favours open habitats of grasslands, cultivated lands, wastelands, parks and gardens. It moves along with a skittish, pattering gait, running in short spurts to pick up ants, bugs, beetles, grasshoppers and worms. An active noisy feeder, particularly at dawn, dusk and on moonlit nights! A ground dweller, it is never seen in the trees, even though it has a strong flight.

Once when I was walking in a park, I just avoided stepping onto their nest, carelessly placed in the middle of the park, the pair dive-bombing me and hurling the accusatory 'Did you do it'! There, under the shade of a tree, but otherwise out in the open, was this little hollow with three beautiful, stone-coloured, speckled eggs!

Call

A strident, ringing 'Did you do it… Did you do it!'

Mythology, Tales & Trivia

In earlier times, trained falcons would be unleashed to chase the Titeeri, since the Titeeri had a strong flight and endless aerial manoeuvres and therefore provided good sport for the watchers.

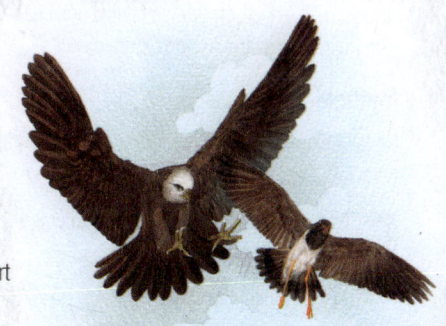

Jayantika Davé

Large-tailed Nightjar

Scientific name: *Caprimulgus macrurus*   Size: *33 cm*
Hindi name: *Dab Chiri, Chhipak*
Sanskrit name: *Naptrika, Chhippika*

Description

Come dusk, and the Himalayas and the Northeast of India resound with the loud chaunk-chaunk-chaunk calls of the Large-tailed Nightjar. It is a study in shades of brown and gold, though very difficult to see, as it emerges only at night. When you are out driving in these areas after dark, look out for them on the road or roadside, frozen in place by the light of your car, looking, as E.H.A. humorously puts it, like 'the heroine in a penny dreadful with large lustrous eyes'!

Habits

This nocturnal bird, originally called by many descriptive names like Eve-jar, Fern-owl or Night-hawk, prefers wooded habitats, forests, bamboo groves and other shrub areas, while also being found in the open countryside next to villages and cultivation. It has keen eyesight, and catches nocturnal flying insects of all kinds, making flycatcher-like sorties after its prey, with a silent glide, interspersed with a few leisurely wing flaps. The Dab Chiri is most active at dusk and before dawn, and the call continues through the night – very much a familiar sound of our hills and forests!

There are a number of Nightjar species in India, with very similar colouring, and they can mainly only be differentiated by their calls. But their habits are very similar.

Call

Moonlit nights ring out with the continuous chaunk-chaunk-chaunk – with most calling at dusk and before dawn!

Mythology, Tales & Trivia

Birds at the nest site will perform the broken-wing act to draw predators away from their eggs.

A Nightjar will always sit along the length of a branch, and not sideways like other birds.

Due to its wide gape, it was sometimes called 'Goatsucker', as it was assumed that it stole milk from goats and cows!

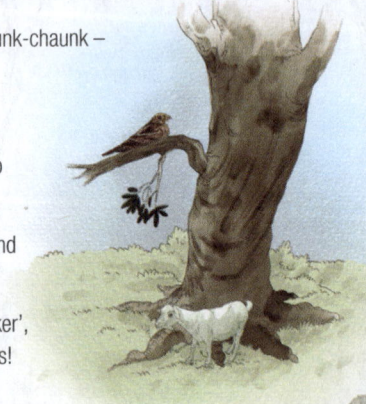

Grey Francolin

Scientific name: *Francolinus pondicerianus*   Size: *33 cm*
Hindi name: *Raam Teetar, Safed Teetar, Gora Teetar*
Sanskrit name: *Kapitrajal*

Description

The Grey Francolin or Teetar, as they are commonly known, are plump, upright brown, fawn-and-gold birds with pink legs, and are a quaint sight, as they waddle across a path, or along garden shrubbery. What draws the eye to them is their strident call resembling that of a seller of utensils – 'pateela-pateela-pateela', or the loud whirr of their wings when they take flight.

Habits

The Teetar is a widespread resident of India, and is a bird of open grasslands, parks, shrubby forest edges and areas where it can feed off village crops. It is also comfortable in man-made environs and so can often be seen in gardens, and even on golf courses! While seeds and grains are a favourite food, insects, small lizards, soft leaves and buds, fruits and berries are also enjoyed. We have enjoyed many a quiet evening sitting in a park along a golf course, watching a small group of Grey Francolin feeding, digging for roots and bulbs with their bills, and using their characteristic sideways kicking motion of the legs to clear away surface material so they can dig deeper. The pairs tend to stay with each other for life.

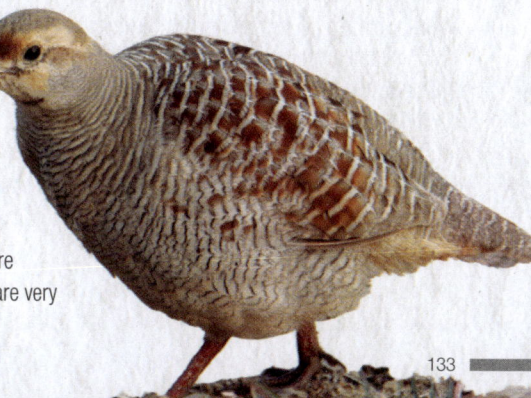

One of my best memories is watching a mother walk across the bottom of a long garden shrubbery, with a line of six balls of fluff following her!

Call

A start-up of a few chak-chak notes, followed by the loud ringing pateela-pateela-pateela or kateetar-kateetar-kateetar! It is most vocal during the early hours of morning and at dusk!

Mythology, Tales & Trivia

They become so tame that they follow their master around like a dog.

They were popular cage birds, and were kept for partridge fights as the males are very pugnacious.

Jayantika Davé

Barn Owl

Scientific name: *Tyto alba*   Size: 36 cm
Hindi name: *Kuraya, Karail, Buri Churi, Lakshmi Pecha*
Sanskrit name: *Chandrakolook, Shwaytokook*

Description

The Barn Owl is an endearing, striking, medium-sized owl, with a heart-shaped face, accented with a white facial ruff, and relatively light fawn-to-golden-brown feathers with spots.

The eerie unearthly call is well described by Thomas Grey in his 'Elegy Written in a Country Churchyard': 'The moping owl does to the moon complain / Of such, as wand'ring near her secret bow'r, / Molest her ancient solitary reign.'

Habits

The Karail is a widespread resident across most of India, and is a lover of open habitats, both rural and urban. It has modified its habits to be able to live amongst human habitation, often nesting in tall apartment complex buildings, and only emerging at night with its soft silent flight, to hunt for small rodents, bats, garden shrews, small birds and lizards in the gardens surrounding them.

On Diwali night last year, I looked towards my frosted-glass bathroom window, and there was a lovely big Barn Owl sitting on the ledge outside, swivelling its neck left and right in a Bharatnatyam dancer's motion, as it tried to look in!

Call

An eerie, unearthly, screeching cry giving rise to its earlier name of Screech Owl!

Mythology, Tales & Trivia

The Mahabharata has a story of the cat, the rat, the Chandrak owl and the mongoose. The cat is caught in the snare of a hunter, but the rat, the mongoose and the owl are free and are eyeing the rat for a meal. The rat makes a strategic alliance with the cat, hides under the cat's body till the mongoose and owl leave, and then cuts the net except for one strand, which he cuts only when the hunter approaches, as he cannot trust the cat to now not eat him, unless it is busy fleeing to protect its life! Clever rat!

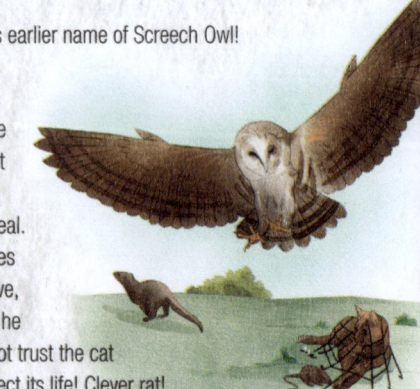

Owls hunt by sound too, and experiments have been done that prove that the Barn Owl has the best hearing in its species. The eerie unearthly call has given rise to some pejorative names for the Barn Owl—Buri Chiri in Hindi and Death Bird in Tamil.

Each Little Bird That Sings

Indian Thick-knee

Scientific name: *Burhinus indicus*   Size: 37 cm
Hindi name: *Karwanak, Barsiri*
Sanskrit name: *Giri Nakt Kurri*

Description

The earlier name for the Indian Thick-knee was the Stone Curlew, which is very descriptive of its habitat. This leggy, stocky bird with prominent and large yellow 'goggle' eyes, is very much an inhabitant of dry, arid and stony areas across India, sometimes even being seen in neglected parts of gardens and parks. It has an odd elegance and dignity in the way it carries itself; very upright, always watchful, and very sentinel-like.

Habits

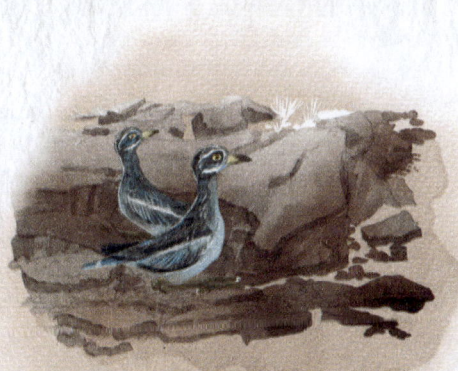

A widespread resident of India, usually found in the lowlands, and only up to about 1,000 m in low hills. It forages for insects, beetles, worms and sometimes seeds and grains. It is not very gregarious in nature, usually being seen in pairs, or small groups of up to five individuals, standing still, and then doing a sudden run with short quick steps to pick up an insect, with its neck retracted as if it is embarrassed to do this! Sandy stony banks of rivers or dry river beds are a good place to see them. Recently, we were returning from my brother's rewilding project in Corbett, and were riding back on a tractor on a dry stony river bed, and it was so lovely to see a single or a pair of Indian Thick-knees at almost every turn! It is active at night as evidenced by its exceptionally large eyes, and during the day, if alarmed, it squats close to the ground with its neck extended, and its colouring then helps it blend almost completely into the stony ground.

Call

Noisiest at dusk and at night, it utters a series of whistles, whi-whi-whit-whit, with each note getting louder and louder, sometimes prolonged as a plaintive and somewhat eerie whu-eet, whu-eet.

Jayantika Davé

Cinnamon Bittern

Scientific name: *Ixobrychus cinnamomeus*   Size: *38 cm*
Hindi name: *Laal-bagla*
Sanskrit name: *Jyotsnabak*

Description

As birders, finding a bird that is normally hard to see is always a particular thrill… And the Bitterns are really hard to see! So, when we sight this rich rufous-and-cinnamon beauty, there is much jumping for joy! The Laal-bagla is very similar in build to the Egrets but, unlike them, will hide out in tall grasses and reedbeds around wet areas.

Habits

The Cinnamon Bittern is a resident across India, and can be found in the dense reed-beds bordering our flooded fields, edges of wet marshy land, lakes, ponds, rivers – and anywhere with overgrown grasses and damp-loving shrubs. Its diet consists of frogs, insects, fish and other water-dwelling creatures. It is most active around dawn and dusk, and the rest of the time stays hunkered down on a low branch over the water. I have seen it, either startled out of hiding and bursting forth in a quick flight with a noisy kok-kok call, or, if lucky, sitting low near the water, head cocked, watching for prey below, which is then captured with a quick jab.

Breeding season coincides with the monsoons, around July–September. A small platform of sticks and reeds is made, lined with a little soft leafy matter, and placed on a clump of reeds or in a low tree or bush. About 3–5 white eggs are laid.

Call

A series of kwok-kwok-kwok most often heard at night or dawn, with a sharper kok-kok in alarm!

Mythology, Tales & Trivia

When alarmed, they tip their heads back and freeze, so that their silhouettes merge with the golden reeds and grasses amongst which they are hiding – quite a quaint sight! Salim Ali terms this as their 'on guard' habit!

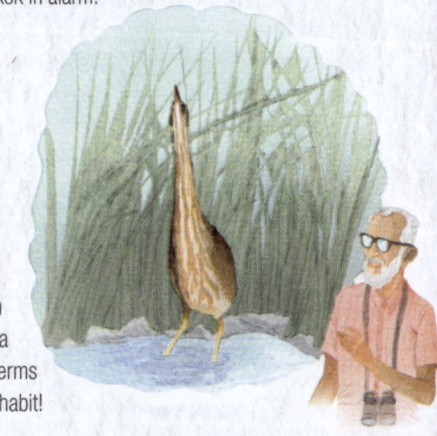

Sirkeer Malkoha

Scientific name: *Taccocua leschenaultii* Size: 42 cm
Hindi name: *Jangli Tota*
Sanskrit name: *Kairaat*

Description

This widespread resident of semi-arid thorny scrubland is not easy to see, as it is a ground skulker. What you are looking for is a bird that donned a brown cloak, a black mask and bright red lipstick, and headed for a masked ball!

Habits

I have seen the Sirkeer Malkoha in my walks in the Aravalli Forest Park in Gurgaon, when it emerged from its ground skulking to do some hunting in the branches of a really low thorny shrub… the sun came out just then, and lit up its 'party face' beautifully! The bright red beak has given rise to the Hindi name of Jangli Tota! It prefers to be in dry scrubby bush and forest, with lantana undergrowth, thick grass, thorny bushes and stony craggy hillsides as favourites.

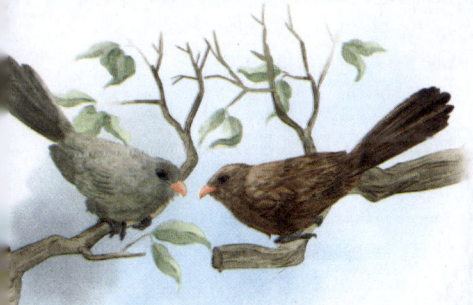

It is not usually seen above 1,000 m. It is a poor flier and, if disturbed, prefers to walk to the deepest part of the undergrowth, rather than fly some distance away. It has a curious run – doing a fast head-lowered dash, stopping to raise its head and body for a quick look, and then off it goes again! It is a ground feeder, and forages for berries, worms and caterpillars, large insects and lizards.

The breeding display has both the birds opening their beaks wide, bowing to each other, spreading out their long tails, all the while making these clicking sounds.

Call

A very silent bird, only very occasionally letting out a loud kek-kek-kerek.

Jayantika Davé

Peregrine Falcon

Scientific name: *Falco peregrinus*   Size: 42 cm
Hindi name: *Bhyri Baaz, Kohila, Shaheen, Safed Shaheen*
Sanskrit name: *Neelachhad Shyayn, Dhoomika, Mrigendra Chatak*

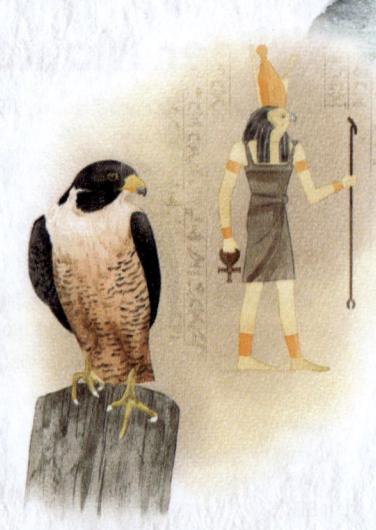

Description

This gorgeous medium-sized falcon is a resident in certain parts of India, as well as a winter visitor. So if you see a falcon with a light to dark grey top, and barred undersides that are rufous or white, look out for the identifier that distinguishes this from any other falcon, and that is the Horus-god-like black helmet extending down in a curve below the eyes!

Habits

The Safed Shaheen can be found in a variety of habitats, with a marked preference for being around water. On our visit to Chambal River, we scanned the underside of the large bridge that spans this river, and sure enough, there was a pair that had taken up residence on the thin ledge under the bridge, where they could not be seen easily. It is a fearless and accomplished hunter, chasing prey with great speed and agility, rising above the chosen one, and then hurtling down with great force, with wings almost closed, and talons digging into the prey to capture it, forcing it down onto land or water, from where it is then easily killed and eaten. Manageable prey is carried back up to the perch, whereas larger prey is dismembered, partially eaten on the ground, and the remains carried back to the perch.

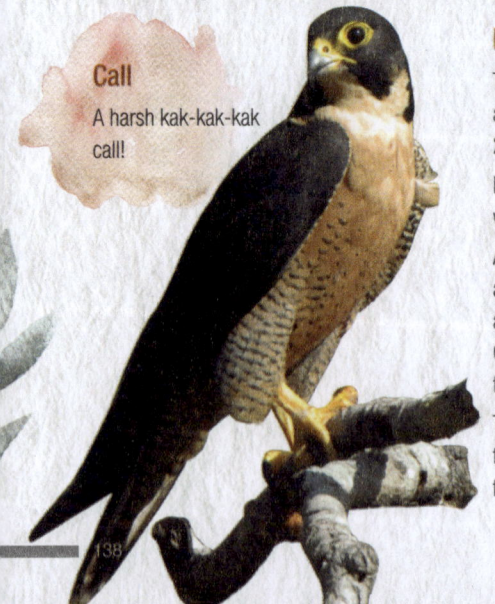

Call

A harsh kak-kak-kak call!

Mythology, Tales & Trivia

The name Peregrine means 'wanderer' and some Peregrines migrate up to 25,000 km annually!

It reaches speeds of up to 100 m per second when it is hurtling down to swoop on prey.

According to Jerdon, Indian Falcons are called Siah Chasm or black-eyed, as opposed to others which are called Goolab Chasm or light-eyed, referring to the Hawk family.

The Peregrine, or Bhyri as it was called, was trained for falconry and could be purchased for between Rs 2 and Rs 10 in 1840.

Indian Pond Heron

Scientific name: *Ardeola grayii*   Size: 44 cm
Hindi name: *Bagla, Andha Bagla, Chama Bagla, Khunch Bagla*
Sanskrit name: *Andh Bak*

Description

The dumpy brown bird that you see, with yellow beak and yellow legs, sitting with its neck tucked into its shoulders, unmoving for long periods of time, is the Indian Pond Heron. Come too close, and it will take off with a startlingly white flash of its wings and a harsh annoyed croak, and then your identification becomes a certainty! It was aptly called the Surprise Bird, because when it takes flight, the drab brown bird suddenly reveals its bright white wings!

Habits

The most preferred habitat for the Andha Bagla is shallow quiet waters overflowing from a main water source. It is however equally comfortable at the edges of lakes, marshes, small ponds, and particularly flooded rice fields, so much so that it used to earlier be called the Paddy-bird! A widespread resident across India, it has been found up to 2,000 m. The diet consists of aquatic insects, bugs and beetles, small fish, crabs, earthworms and other aquatic dwellers. It is a solitary feeder, but at good spots quite a few individuals will also join in, with patience being the main weapon! It sits hunched up in one spot, surveying what is happening around, often not even moving its head, and then a quick jab, and the morsel has been caught.

Call

A harsh, squawk wa-koo or kek-kek-kek call!

Mythology, Tales & Trivia

Its dingy colouring, and ability to stay still for many hours, has given it the characteristic of being invisible, and therefore the name Andha Bagla.

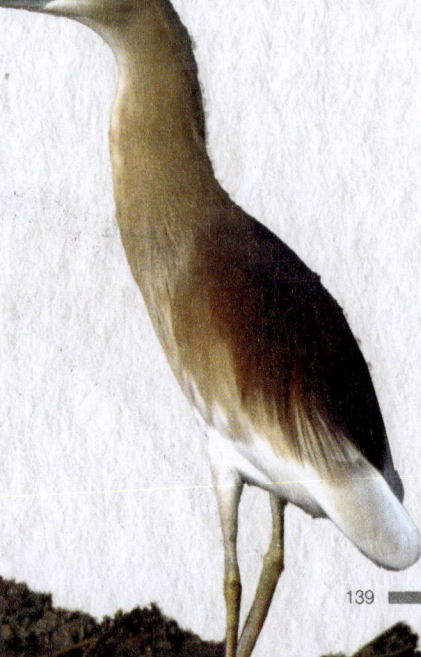

Jayantika Davé

Rufous Treepie

Scientific name: *Dendrocitta vagabunda*   Size: 48 cm
Hindi name: *Mutri*
Sanskrit name: *Koot Pakshi*
Bengali name: *Taka Chor, Handi Chacha*

Description

A smart dresser in shades of bright rufous-chestnut, black, grey and white, the Rufous Treepie draws attention to itself with its melodious ko-ki-la call, and its flight, which shows off its long, graded tail. A widespread resident, it can be seen anywhere where there are some tall flowering and fruiting trees.

Habits

Mainly arboreal, the Mutri is comfortable in a variety of habitats – open gardens and parks, villages and fields. They are very confiding birds; in Ranthambore for example, they have come and perched on our jeep, and even on our hats! While primarily a lowland bird, it can also be seen up to 2,000 m, though in the Himalayas it is replaced by the **Grey Treepie**, which is a very similar bird, with a lot more grey in it. A carnivorous feeder, it enjoys insects, beetles, snails, small birds and nestlings, small rats, bats, frogs and lizards, with figs, nectar and fruits for its sweet tooth! It is a dangerous predator at nesting time, and is constantly being chased away by other birds. At our feeder in Glen Haven, there is a feeding hierarchy based on aggressiveness – first the red-billed blue magpies, then the Treepies, then everything else. It appears in pairs or small family groups.

Call

Its most familiar call is the loud ko-ki-la, or goo-gi-lee, but it also has a variety of metallic harsh calls, and can do some mimicry too!

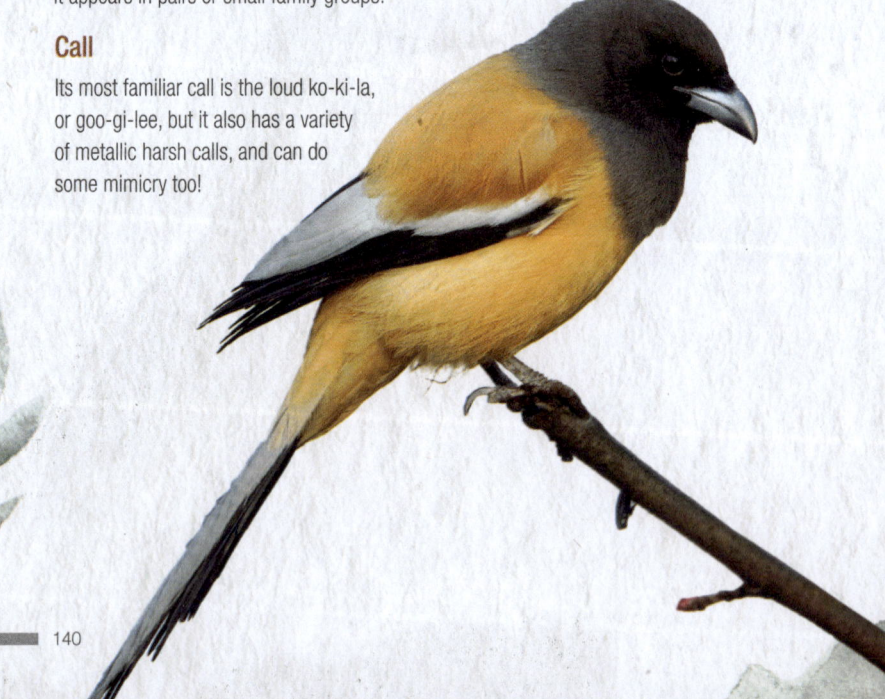

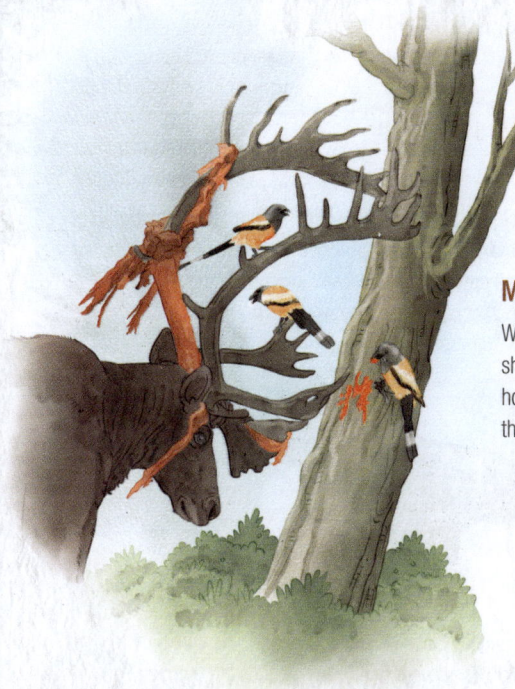

Mythology, Tales & Trivia

When deer, and particularly sambar, are shedding the velvet from their new set of horns, the Treepies pull off and consume these shreds.

Gourmet feeders! M. Krishnan once wrapped an omelette in cooked tomatoes, and stuck them on the thorns of a shrub. The treepie arrived, inspected the parcels, unwrapped them, and ate only the omlette inside!

The Bengali names seem to refer to their habit of stealing shiny things!

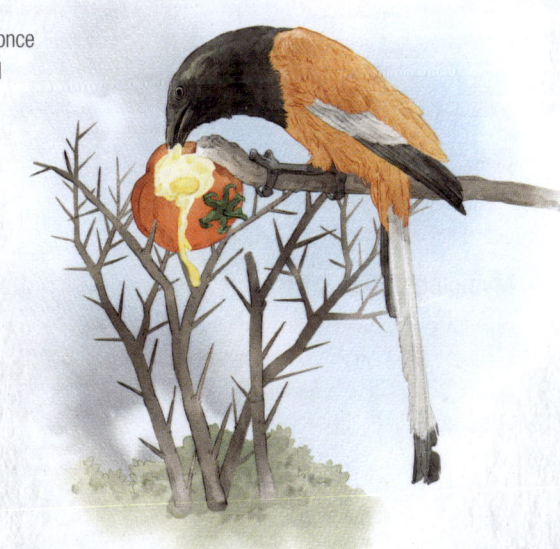

Jayantika Davé

Eurasian Marsh Harrier

Scientific name: *Circus aeruginosus*   Size: 48 cm
Hindi name: *Kutar, Kulesir, Safed Sira*
Sanskrit name: *Kucch Patri*

Description

A smart winter visitor to marshes and wetlands across India is this medium-sized raptor, in a colour combination of browns and chestnut, with a clear pale-coloured head. In winter, as we sit near a wetland looking at the wondrous combinations of wetland birds, and they suddenly rise in a frightened cloud of confusion, we only have to look up, and are sure to see the Eurasian Marsh Harrier that has appeared on a hunting mission!

Habits

The Marsh Harrier is a large, slim, long-winged Harrier that spends most of its time on the wing, carefully patrolling its chosen territory. The favourite hunting grounds of the Safed Sira are wetlands with reeds, marsh vegetation, lakes, rivers or reservoirs, or any similar habitat that would attract a wide variety of wetland birds and duck.

The Harriers have a typical V-shaped way of holding up their wings, and a measured flight low over the water, during which they can quickly grab small or medium-sized waterbirds from the surface, or in flight, as they arise in alarm. They also take small mammals, and sometimes fish, frogs and lizards too.

Call

A fairly silent bird, with a loud whee-ah call during the breeding season!

Mythology, Tales & Trivia

In earlier times, the Safed Sira had become adept at waiting around hunting parties, waiting to opportunistically grab a wounded duck before it could be picked up by the beaters.

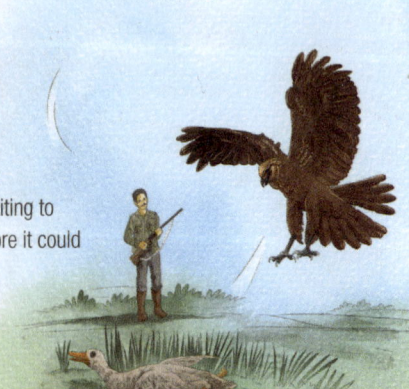

Each Little Bird That Sings

Eurasian Curlew

Scientific name: *Numenius arquata*   Size: 55 cm
Hindi name: *Goar Goungh, Bada Gulinda*
Sanskrit name: *Kukri Jalranka*

Description
A winter visit to our coastal areas is sure to throw up the Eurasian Curlew – a large whimsical bird, with an outsized, long, downcurved bill and a whitish centre parting on its head! It is patterned in shades of brown, overlaid with black markings, and will be seen in shallow coastal waters busily probing for edible aquatic life. It can be confused with the **Whimbrel**, which is smaller in size and with a similar, though smaller, beak.

Habits
I have had lovely sightings of this striking bird in Jamnagar in Gujarat, where there are large bays and estuaries, and as you sit and watch from the shore, flights of the Bada Gulinda come in and settle, making a striking sight. It is a winter visitor, and its favourite foods are small fish, all aquatic life, crabs, crustaceans and other amphibians, and on the shore, some seeds and berries too. It moves at a leisurely pace, deeply probing into the damp mud to unearth all its favourite foods.

Call
The call is a loud reverberating courlew-courlew-courlew, with sometimes a softer cui-cui-cui mixed in!

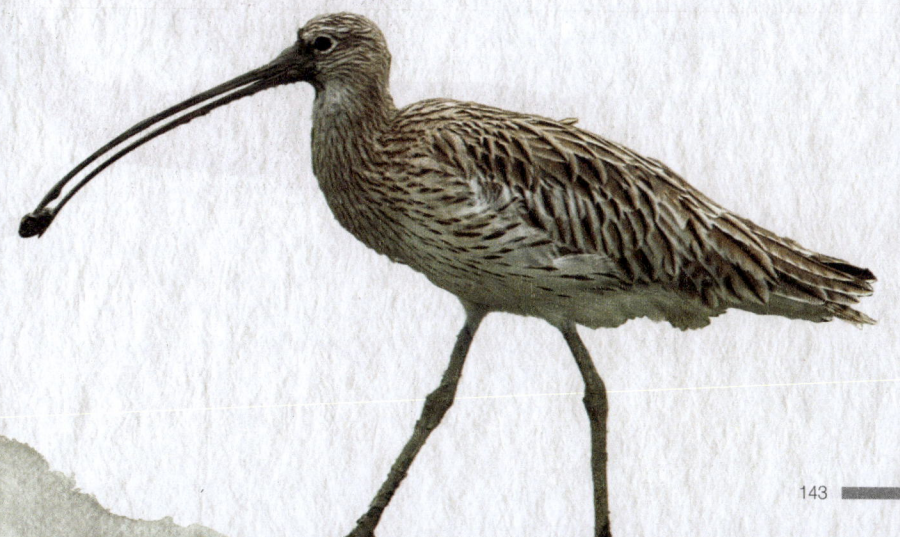

Jayantika Davé

Dusky Eagle Owl

Scientific name: *Bubo coromandus*   Size: 58 cm
Hindi name: *Jungli Ghughoo, Matiya Ghughoo*
Sanskrit name: *Mahakaushik, Mahapakshi*

Description

The striking grey-brown Dusky Eagle Owl is a sight not easily forgotten! A very large owl, with big upright ear-tufts, and large yellow eyes staring out at you from the foliage of a tall tree! You have to shake yourself to ask whether you are looking at a cat…or a bird!

Habits

The favourite haunts of the Jungli Ghughoo are forests of old thickly foliaged trees, interspersed with woodland, and generally near water of some kind. It is a bird of the plains, and is not seen above 250 m. The day is spent in sleepy naps, hunkered down on a branch and amongst a lot of leafy foliage. A couple of hours before dusk, it wakes up and begins to call in a leisurely way. Finally, from dusk to dawn, the hunting starts, with medium-sized birds like crows, pigeons and doves, and medium-sized mammals such as squirrels, hares and rats, as also reptiles and bird eggs, being taken. Its deep wo-wo-wo-oo-oo-oo call rings out as dusk falls, and is the perfect backdrop to the end of a satisfying day of birding!

It nests high up on an old leafy tree, and its chicks are a pretty sight – little balls of fluff peering over the edge of the nest, with those huge round eyes!

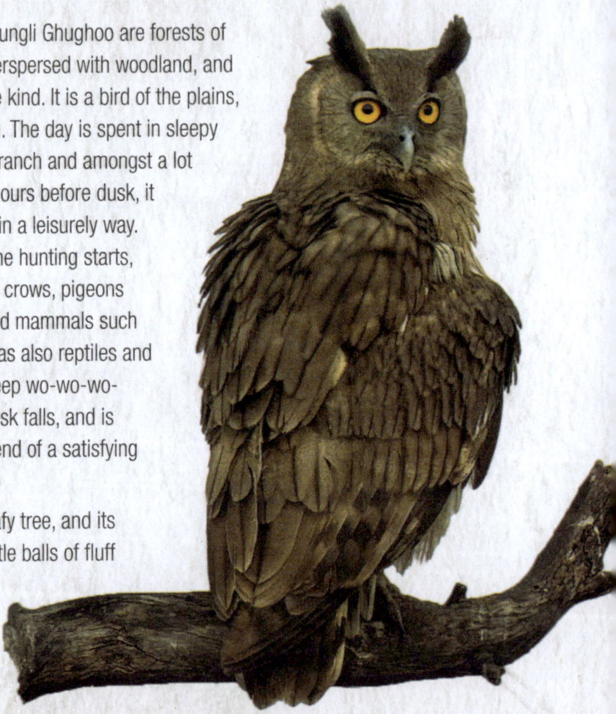

Call

A deep resounding wo-wo-wo-oo-oo-oo, which fades away with each note. The call is a deep mumbled hoo-hoo, and Stuart Baker says that when a pair was perched on his house roof at night, they sounded like two old men conversing in deep hoarse tones!

Mythology, Tales & Trivia

In the Mahabharata 1.2.296, Ashwathama works out a strategy of killing the Pandavas while they are asleep, after observing a horned owl attack sleeping crows at night.

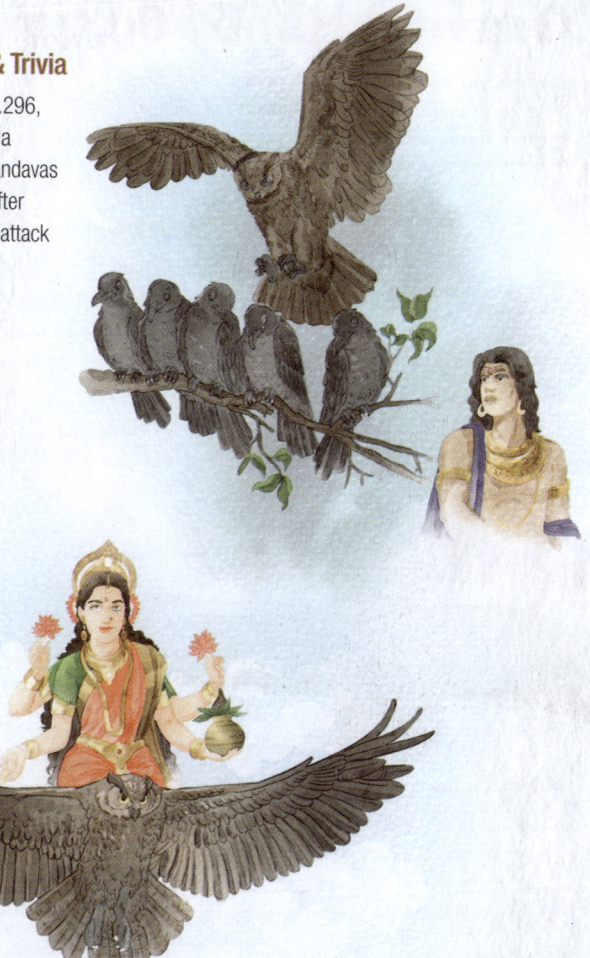

The Hindu goddess of wealth and prosperity, Goddess Lakshmi, is the consort of Lord Vishnu, and brings wealth while riding on or accompanied by an owl. Mythology seems to say that while Lakshmi brings wealth and prosperity, the owl is present to provide the wisdom to use it well, and not enter into strife.

Some of the larger owls have such large ear holes that you can easily see them, and they are large enough to put your thumb into them!

Stuart Baker observes that this owl is fearless, and he once saw one feasting on a big civet, which had all the marks of having been killed by the owl itself.

Jayantika Davé

Oriental Honey Buzzard

Scientific name: *Pernis ptilorhynchus*   Size: 58 cm
Hindi name: *Shahutela, Madkare*
Sanskrit name: *Madhuha*

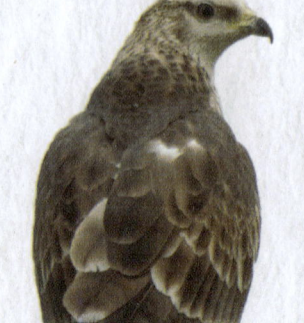

Description

The Oriental Honey Buzzard is one of the easier raptors to identify, since it has a relatively short, narrow neck, and a small, curiously flattened head, accented further by a flattened crest. Dark-brown scaled upper parts, with lighter brown barring on the underside, and a grey head complete the picture.

Habits

The Shahutela is a widespread resident across India, with a preferred habitat of broad-leaved trees, in dense or open wooded areas. It can be seen in the plains, as well as up to 2,000 m in North India. It has a very specialized dietary preference – no surprise – bees, their larvae, honeycombs and honey, seeking these out from honey bee nests on exposed branches or cliffs, and also within holes in trees. It also eats other insects and small mammals and birds.

Their breeding season is closely linked to the availability of bees.

Call

A high-pitched screaming whistling call, wheeeew, is occasionally uttered!

Mythology, Tales & Trivia

Since it feeds by preference on honey, its thinly feathered lores provide some protection.

Native observers say that they spread out their tails and make several passes over honeycombs to drive off the bees before they feed.

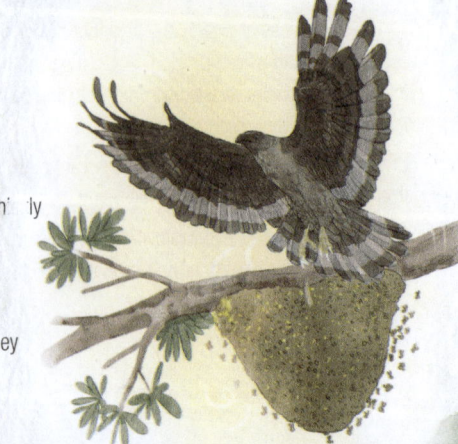

Glossy Ibis

Scientific name: *Plegadis falcinellus*   Size: 60 cm
Hindi name: *Kawari, Kowar, Chhota Baza*
Punjabi name: *Chamkila Buza*
Assamese name: *Jakmaki Akohi Bog*
Sanskrit name: *Pathrati*

Description

In winter, in flooded fields and marshes of western and southern parts of India, look out for what looks like a curlew having lost its way! This tall bird with a prominent downcurved bill looks predominantly dark brown, till it catches the sunlight – and wow! – the name 'glossy' takes on a new meaning – with metallic bronze, purple and green highlights coming to life! Some of the colloquial names – Chamkila Buza and Jakmaki Akohi Bog, all talk to the very fashionable highlights of this bird!

Habits

A frequenter of flooded fields, marshes, river edges and ponds, the Glossy Ibis feeds by probing into the wet marshy areas, and extracting insects, worms, grubs, grasshoppers, water beetles, molluscs, snails, frogs, lizards and fish, and even fresh rice grains. It moves along slowly and deliberately, probing repeatedly into the wet ground, and sometimes sweeping sideways to unearth its food. Foraging can be in small groups, or often in mixed flocks with other similar feeders.

It nests colonially with a variety of other ibis and heron species, building a large untidy nest in a small tree.

Call

A quiet ibis, with some croaking and grunting calls!

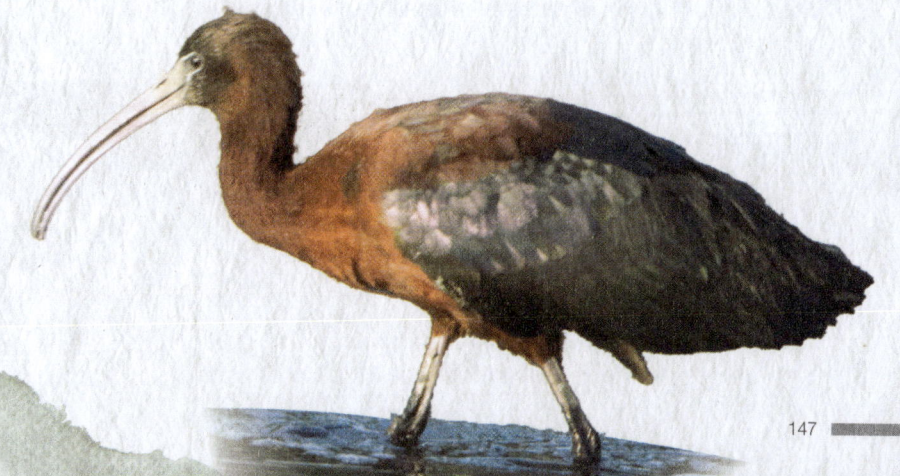

Jayantika Davé

Black Kite

Scientific name: *Milvus migrans*   Size: 62 cm
Hindi name: *Cheel*
Sanskrit name: *Shakuni*

Description

When we were in school, eating our sandwich on the school lawn, we would often hear a friend shout out 'Cheel Cheel!', warning us to hide our sandwich before it was grabbed out of our hands by this swift chestnut-brown robber with sharply angled wings and a forked tail! An ever-present raptor and a common sight in all our towns, villages and cities is the Black Kite. Even today, a lot of outdoor eating places will have strings or buntings stretched overhead to deter the aggressive swooping of the ever-hungry Black Kite.

Habits

The Black Kite is resident across all of India, and is very comfortable in all habitats, from human habitation to grasslands, semi-arid areas and light wooded areas, and can be seen very often around garbage dumps. The Cheel is more a bird of the lowlands, but can be seen up to 2,000 m. It forages at garbage dumps for any kind of scraps, is opportunistic in grabbing food from humans, and also hunts for live prey, like small rats, birds, bats, chicks, fish, lizards, worms and insects. It has a very agile flight, with adroit twists and turns using its sharply angled wings as rudders, flying high to survey the possibilities, followed by a spectacular dive to grab its food. And if the grab has been sighted by other Cheels, a mobbing party starts to try and steal the prize for themselves, accompanied by much screaming and jockeying!

Call

A musical drawn-out whistle like 'chee-ee-eel' repeated a few times, which is from where it gets its Hindi name!

Mythology, Tales & Trivia

In winter, Black Kites love to sun themselves against the warm stone walls of our school, resting for a long time, with their wings spread out like emblems on a flag!

Often the butt of teasing by crows, who seem to do this only to amuse themselves!

Eagles and kites usually remove hair and feathers from prey before eating. The balance are then vomited out as pellets.

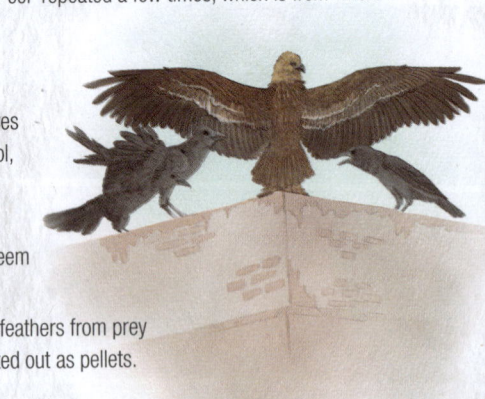

Crested Serpent Eagle

Scientific name: *Spilornis cheela*   Size: 65 cm
Hindi name: *Furj Baaj, Dogra Cheel*
Sanskrit name: *Garuda Farz Baaz*

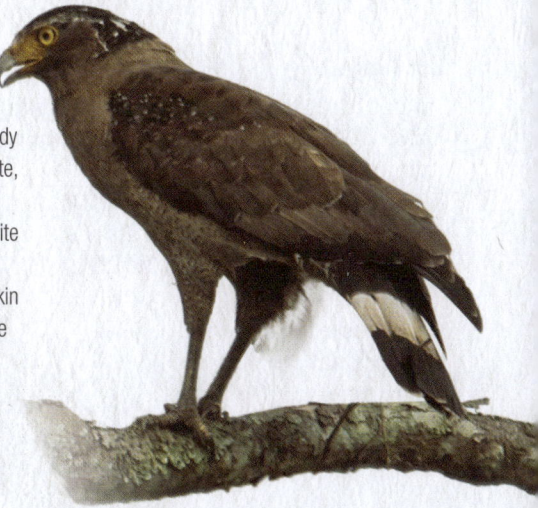

Description

The handsome Crested Serpent Eagle is a medium-to-large eagle, and is a study in shades of dark brown edged with white, to a lighter brown stomach with white barring, and a lying-down black-and-white crest, which is raised in excitement or when it flies in and lands! Yellow bare-skin spectacles around the eyes complete the compelling picture! When it flies, the striking black-and-white patterning along the edges of the wings is an unmistakable identifier.

Habits

A widespread resident across India, the Furj Baaj hunts in a variety of fairly open forested areas, remote or bordering cultivated areas, but with a preference for well-wooded, well-watered country. We have usually seen this bird in teak or sal or mixed forests, often up to 2,000 m, where it draws attention to itself by its noisy 'kuk-kuk-how-queeear' call! Its favourite prey is reptiles, particularly snakes – hence the name! It perches for a long time, remaining motionless and scanning for prey, which, once found, is quickly picked off the ground or a tree, and then either eaten on the ground itself, or carried back to its perch.

Courtship is an elaborate process, with the pair soaring together, and on landing, the male postures with wings raised, and head and tail raised, all accompanied by noisy calls.

Call

A loud and penetrating, though plaintive, whistling call, sounding like kuk-kuk-how-queeear.

Mythology, Tales & Trivia

In the old days, shikaris would say that the Serpent Eagle had the figure of God's chakra under each wing, and that would prevent the snake from going forward and escaping.

Jayantika Davé

Indian Spotted Eagle

Scientific name: *Clanga hastata*   Size: 65 cm
Hindi name: *Pahari Teesa*
Sanskrit name: *Jeevantak*

Description

The large Indian Spotted Eagle is a warm brown, with the feathers on its back having diffuse white tips, giving it its name. The spotting is sometimes not very visible, but a clear distinguisher is a very prominent yellow gape at the base of the beak, which is visible from afar, and extends to well behind the eye, giving it a wide-mouthed look! A similar, though larger, winter visitor is the **Greater Spotted Eagle**, which is overall a much richer darker brown, and where the spotting at the ends of the feathers is a very clear white, and so is much more distinct.

Habits

A resident across most of North and Central India, though not numerous. Favoured habitats are the lowlands with open forests, plains surrounded by groves of trees, wooded parks or cultivated areas dotted with trees. It is an adept flier, soaring very high and looking for prey, and then flying low over the tree tops as it spies interesting morsels, which it then speedily captures on the ground. Favourite prey is mammals, a variety of small birds, and lizards and snakes and frogs.

Call

A cackling laugh, sometimes interspersed with a few kleep-kleep yelping calls. Peter Simon Pallas describes the call as 'jeb jeb jeb'.

Mythology, Tales & Trivia

In raptors that hunt more agile prey, the female tends to be larger than the male. For more sluggish prey, the male tends to be larger.

Pallas' Fish Eagle

Scientific name: *Haliaeetus leucoryphus* Size: *80 cm*
Hindi name: *Machharang, Machhmanga, Dhenk, Patras*
Sanskrit name: *Puch Matsya Suparna, Kank Shyayn, Matsya Karur*

Description

Pallas' Fish Eagle is a large fishing eagle, which is a resident across large parts of Central and North India. The distinguishers are the size, the presence on a tree overlooking water, dark brown above, a whitish head, and a broad white band at the end of the tail, because of which it was earlier called the Ring-tailed Fish Eagle.

Another large resident fishing eagle is the dignified **Grey-headed Fish Eagle**, distinguished by its grey head and a chestnut inner jacket.

Habits

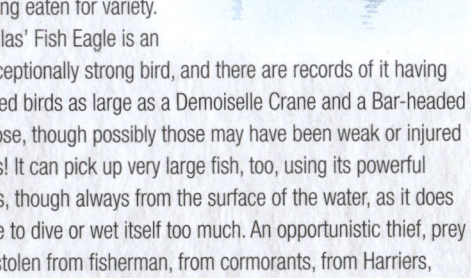

The statuesque Machharang frequents areas near lakes, rivers, ponds and wetlands, and can sometimes be found as high up as 5,000 m in Tibet. Its diet, as its name indicates, is mainly fish, with some rodents, frogs, reptiles, insects and even water birds being eaten for variety. Pallas' Fish Eagle is an exceptionally strong bird, and there are records of it having killed birds as large as a Demoiselle Crane and a Bar-headed Goose, though possibly those may have been weak or injured birds! It can pick up very large fish, too, using its powerful talons, though always from the surface of the water, as it does not like to dive or wet itself too much. An opportunistic thief, prey is also stolen from fisherman, from cormorants, from Harriers, sometimes from other hunters like an Osprey.

Call

The Machharang has a loud screaming call, rather like the grating creak of an unoiled cartwheel or wooden pulley of a village well!

Jayantika Davé

White-rumped Vulture

Scientific name: *Gyps bengalensis*   Size: 80 cm
Hindi name: *Giddh*
Sanskrit name: *Shitikarsha*

Description

Any cross-country road trip in my childhood was full of sightings of the huge, humped-up, naked head and necked White-rumped Vultures, fighting and squabbling over the carcass of a goat, cow or buffalo…a heaving mass of widespread wings, hissing and spitting, and heavy undercarriage landings with an ungainly run forward! A fascinating sight! Regrettably, their numbers have dropped significantly, due to eating of carcasses treated by the veterinary drug diclofenac…but the good news is that there is a slow comeback with the banning of diclofenac, and meloxicam being introduced as an alternate.

Habits

The Giddh is a great lover of open countryside near towns, villages and cities, sometimes going up to 1,500 m in the Himalayas. Large numbers tend to be seen near garbage dumps, or slaughterhouses, or near villages where there is a lot of livestock. Its primary diet is the remains of livestock, which is located by soaring high, and using its keen eyesight to quickly detect a carcass.

Vultures feeding are best described by E.H.A. as 'funeral wakes of riotous and ghoulish glee. The gourmands jostle and bump against each other and chase each other round the board with long, ungainly hops and open wings.'

Roosting is communal – remember the collection of vultures in the cartoon Mowgli, where they all sat on a branch in a line, necks tucked in, asking each other, 'What do you want to do?'…'I don't know, what do you want to do?', accompanied by much hunching and wing flapping – a scene which afforded my children endless merriment as we all sat together and mimicked them…asking each other 'what do you want to do?'

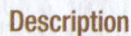

Call

A variety of grunts and hisses, with sometimes a burst of screeching when pushing another vulture away from a carcass!

Mythology, Tales & Trivia

Baby vultures are fed by the disgorging of lumps of meat, and crows will sit nearby, hoping for the proverbial 'slip between the cup and the lip'!

Each Little Bird That Sings

Great Indian Bustard

Scientific name: *Ardeotis nigriceps* Size: 90 cm
Hindi name: *Sohan, Gughunbher, Hukna, Sirailu, Gurain*
Sanskrit name: *Gonard, Gokshavedak, Gurukantth*

Description

The tall, stockily built Great Indian Bustard is globally endangered, and not easy to see. It is a resident of the dry, arid areas of India, but very sporadically present. Its favourite foods are the berries of ber, grains, shoots, and also insects, lizards and small rodents and snakes. A tall and heavy bird, the male is particularly striking with its flat-headed black cap and striking white neck.

Habits

We have seen it in the Great Rann of Kutch, as a lucky sighting…but what a sighting! We were driving around the Rann, and happened to see a pair landing some distance away. We started walking quietly, threading our way through the low, prickly ber fruit shrubs that are the favourite food of the Great Indian Bustard. As we climbed up out of a shallow ravine, there they were…not one, not two, but three…a pair and an almost full-grown baby! They hadn't seen us, and we watched them for a long time!

Breeding occurs throughout the year, and A.O. Hume writes a beautiful description of the Great Bustard male in courtship…'out goes the whole throat down to the breast…and the lower throat bag gets bigger and bigger, and larger and larger, till it looks to be within six inches of the ground…and looked at in front he seems to have a huge bag covered with feathers hanging down between his legs, which wobbles about as he struts here and there.' The nest is only a scrape in the ground, with 1–2 eggs being laid.

Call

A startled bark when alarmed, and a booming 'hrooom' when breeding!

Mythology, Tales & Trivia

The Sohan strangely sits down when it wants to drink, and doesn't drink standing up!

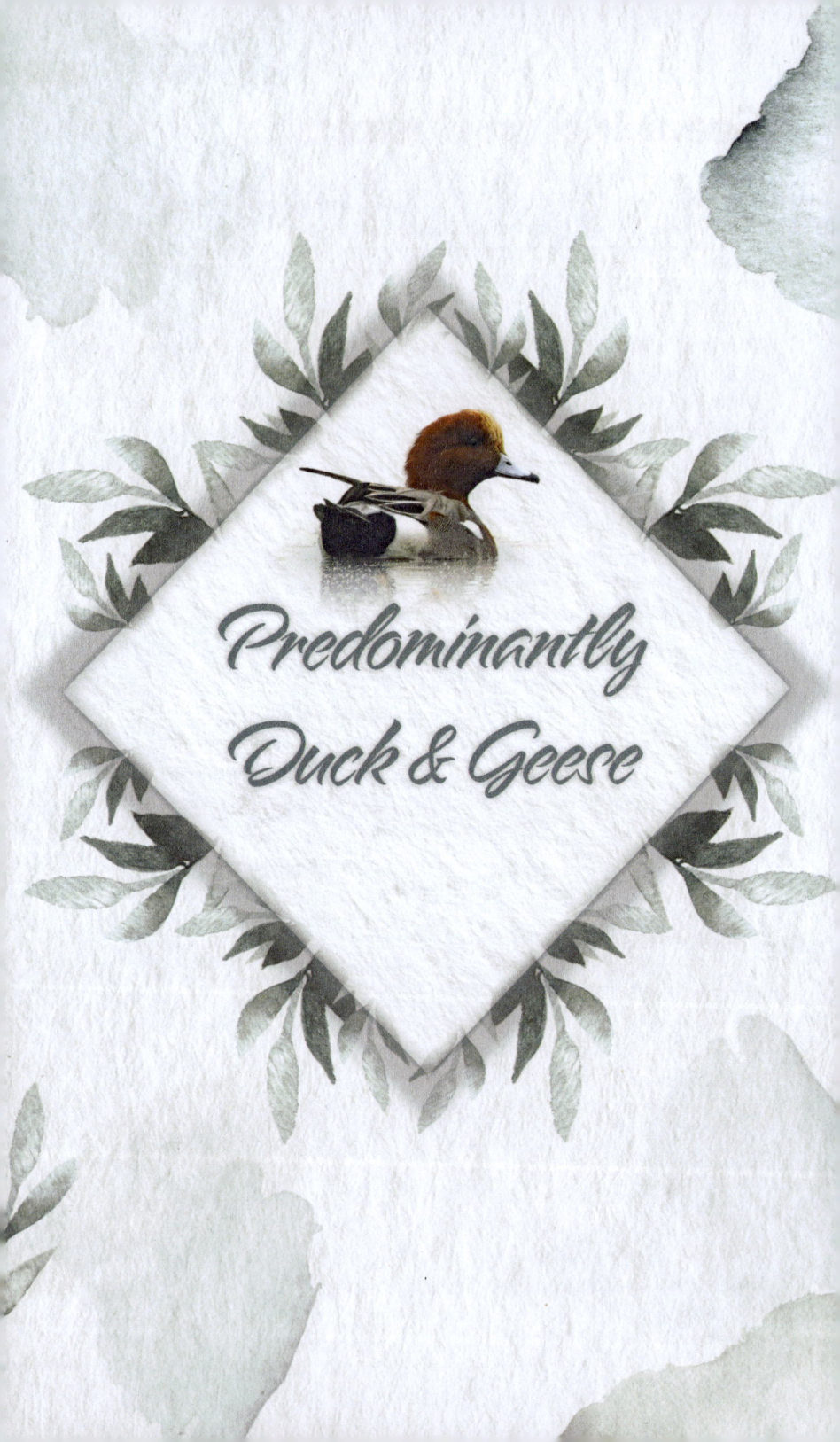

Cotton Pygmy Goose

Scientific name: *Nettapus coromandelianus*   Size: 34 cm
Hindi name: *Girja, Girria, Girri*
Sanskrit name: *Trinhans, Harithans, Ghargharak*

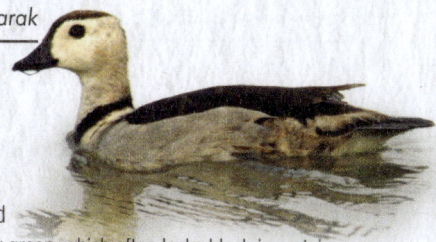

Description & Habits

One of the smallest of the ducks, the resident little Cotton Pygmy Goose, or Cotton Teal as it used to be called, is a small black-and-white duck with a black 'tilak' on its forehead turning into a cap, and a broad black necklace. The wings are actually a glossy dark green, which often looks black in certain light. More numerous in winter, they don't dive or upend, and are strong fliers. They have a loud, distinctive rattling call on the wing, sounding like 'fixed bayonets, fixed bayonets'! They used to be called the Cotton Teal due to the large amount of white in their feathers.

Common Teal

Scientific name: *Anas crecca*   Size: 36 cm
Hindi name: *Chhoti Murghabi*
Sanskrit name: *Rohinik Hansak*

Description & Habits

The Common Teal is one of our smaller ducks, but what a pretty sight it is when the sun falls on it! The iridescent green, broad eye stripe, chestnut head and yellow-outlined facial marking stand out clearly, while the yellow patch on the tail shows in all lights! A widespread winter visitor to our lakes and ponds, it is a dabbling, upending, gregarious duck that is seen in small flocks. The male is a deceptive Romeo, engaging in an elaborate courtship display but deserting the female as soon as she lays her eggs, moving on to greener pastures!

Garganey Duck

Scientific name: *Spatula querquedula*   Size: 39 cm
Hindi name: *Chaita*
Sanskrit name: *Saachi Hansak*

Description & Habits

One of the earliest ducks to arrive, and one of the latest to leave, is the Garganey Duck with its distinctive white eye-stripe that extends down the neck, and a feathered flow of shades of grey down the wings! It does surface feeding, with some dabbling, and becomes more visible once the other ducks have left.

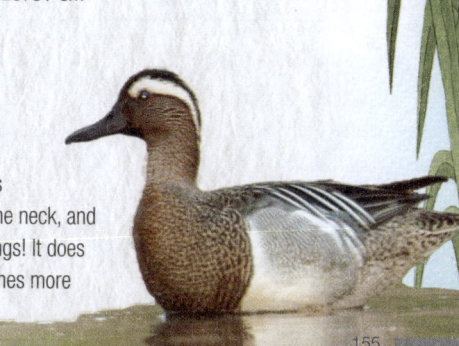

Jayantika Davé

Gadwall

Scientific name: *Mareca strepera*   Size: 41 cm
Hindi name: *Myla*
Sanskrit name: *Malin Hansak*

Description & Habits

Another easy to identify widespread winter visitor is the Gadwall, which is an indeterminate grey-brown above, but has this clear black triangular patch near the tail, which no other duck has! A slender black bill will confirm your identification. It feeds by upending, or dipping into the water, but not by diving. The only time it dives is when it is wounded and is looking to hide out from its attackers. It is highly gregarious and fairly abundant, and is a strong flier.

Lesser Whistling Duck

Scientific name: *Dendrocygna javanica*   Size: 42 cm
Hindi name: *Seelhi*
Sanskrit name: *Prakhyat Sharali*

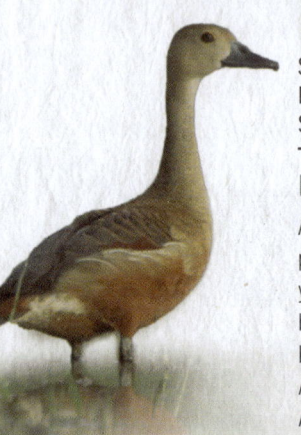

Description & Habits

As you wander near a water body of any kind, or a flooded field, preferably with vegetation and perhaps some submerged trees, keep your ears open for the sound of a flight of duck overhead, who will be having a non-stop whistling, murmuring conversation as they fly! Look up, and you will see a flock of Lesser Whistling Duck! A gregarious duck, it is normally found in groups of 30 or more. A somewhat similar-looking duck, though larger in size, is the **Fulvous Whistling Duck,** which is found mainly in Northeast India.

Common Pochard

Scientific name: *Aythya ferina*   Size: 44 cm
Hindi name: *Burar Nar, Lal Sir*
Sanskrit name: *Raktasheershak*

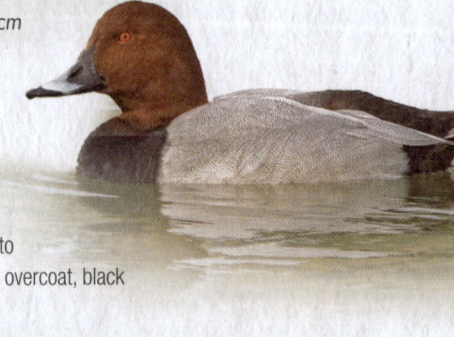

Description & Habits

The Common Pochard is a distinctive winter visitor to our larger lakes, ponds and rivers, and is a very gregarious duck. It is easy to distinguish from other ducks, with its pale-grey overcoat, black shirt-front and a lovely rufous chestnut head!

But now you see me, now you don't – because the Lal Sir is a bottom feeder, disappearing to depths of up to 7 feet at times to get a particularly tasty morsel!

Each Little Bird That Sings

Northern Shoveler

Scientific name: *Anas clypeata*   Size: 47 cm
Hindi name: *Tidari, Punana, Tokarwala, Girah*
Sanskrit name: *Khaathans*

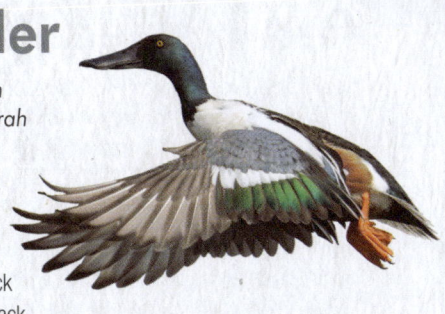

Description & Habits

This large duck is a winter visitor to most of India, and what catches the eye is the broad and flat thick bill…like a shovel! The head and neck can look black though it is actually an iridescent dark green in the right light, and the black back and clearly white chest and neck give it a very pied appearance. The toothed bill facilitates capturing of small crustaceans from the surface. Birds sometimes group together to swim in tight circles, to create a whirlpool effect that brings food to the surface!

Wigeon

Scientific name: *Anas penelope*   Size: 48 cm
Hindi name: *Piyasan, Patari, Pharia, Chhota Lalsir*
Sanskrit name: *Priyashan Hansak*

Description & Habits

The Wigeon is a very Common Pochard-like duck, pale grey above, with a chestnut head…but…and here's the identifier…as it turns to face you, you see the beautiful golden 'tilak' running from the base of the beak all the way to the top of the head – an anointed duck! A surface feeder on shallow lakes, and a vegetation grazer along water bodies, it is gregarious, and appears in small flocks.

Northern Pintail

Scientific name: *Anas acuta*   Size: 53 cm
Hindi name: *Sand, Seenkh Par*
Sanskrit name: *Shaku Hans*

Description & Habits

The aptly named Pintail is a winter visitor, and is easily distinguished by its chocolate head, white neck stripe and, most importantly, the pointing-to-the-sky, pin-like long feathers in its tail! A gregarious duck, it forages in flocks, being most active at dusk and dawn. The Northern Pintail is a varied feeder, grazing on land, dabbling for food on the surface, upending in shallow waters, and sometimes even diving.

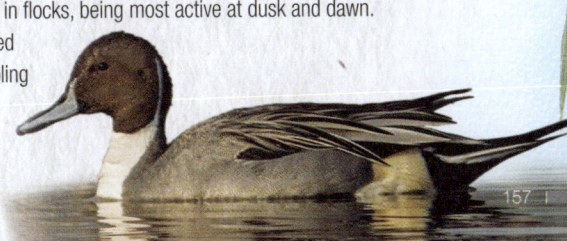

Jayantika Davé

Red-crested Pochard

Scientific name: *Netta rufina*   Size: 55 cm
Hindi name: *Laal Chonch, Laal Sir*
Sanskrit name: *Rakta Chood Majjika*

Description & Habits

In winter, one of our 'must see' ducks in the deeper lakes and ponds is the Red-crested Pochard. Early morning at a water body…the fog lifts…the sun comes up, and the first rays light up a flaming head, and a bright red beak – one of my 'flash upon the inward eye' moments of pure joy! The Laal Sir feeds by diving, and so frequents deeper, larger lakes and ponds.

Mallard

Scientific name: *Anas platyrhynchos*   Size: 58 cm
Hindi name: *Neelsira, Nir Rugi*
Sanskrit name: *Neelgriv Hansak*

Description & Habits

An unmistakable dandy is the Mallard – one of my favourite ducks! The glossy green head, bright yellow beak, white collar, and the jaunty, curled-tail feathers make it a duck that we always scan for in winter. The Neelsira is a surface feeder, and prefers shallow waters with enough vegetation to provide good cover. The Mallard has a small nail at the end of its beak that helps in efficiently catching and tearing off seeds or vegetation it wants to eat!

Indian Spot-billed Duck

Scientific name: *Anas poecilorhyncha*   Size: 60 cm
Hindi name: *Garm Pai, Gugral*
Sanskrit name: *Gharghar Hansak*

Description & Habits

The large Indian Spot-billed Duck is a widespread resident across India, and is found in all habitats – wild marshlands and ponds, and also the semi-wild ponds created in apartment complexes. We had one proud mother, with a host of chicks, who swam unconcernedly for some time in the main swimming pool of our apartment complex in Gurgaon! Scaled plumage in shades of brown and a distinctive yellow spot on the bill are the identifiers. It feeds mainly by dabbling and dipping into the water, sometimes upending itself to reach morsels from the muddy bottom.

Knob-billed Duck

Scientific name: *Sarkidiornis melanotos*   Size: 66 cm
Hindi name: *Nakta*
Sanskrit name: *Nandimukhi, Nasachhinna*

Description

The large, somewhat awkward-looking Knob-billed Duck was a favourite of my father, and he never failed to point it out to us! And it was hard to miss – a large glossy blue-black-and-white duck, with a curiously mottled head and a strange big fleshy knob on its beak! Only the male displays the knob, which reduces in size during the non-breeding season. The Nakta is a resident and can be seen across water bodies in large parts of India.

Habits

A vegetation feeder, it grazes or dabbles in the water, occasionally taking small fish and invertebrates. These ducks are reasonably gregarious, with a favourite habit of perching on low trees, but are never seen in very large numbers. Since they are not as semi-nocturnal as other ducks, they can easily be seen on water bodies across India.

The courting display is an interesting sight, with head-pumps, head-lifts as if drinking, together with bill-opening and hissing. The male can mate with up to five females, and vigorously defends them from other males.

Call

A very silent duck, except for a harsh croak or honk when surprised!

Mythology, Tales & Trivia

Sushruta had created a medical forceps named Nandimukh Yantra after the shape of the beak of this bird, with the comb being used as a curved grip, to pull out arrows embedded in soldiers during a war. The loop of the forceps would accommodate the thick part of the arrow, whereas the tip would grip the thin part and pull it out.

When wounded, it is said that it hides underwater by diving down, only exposing its beak to be able to breathe.

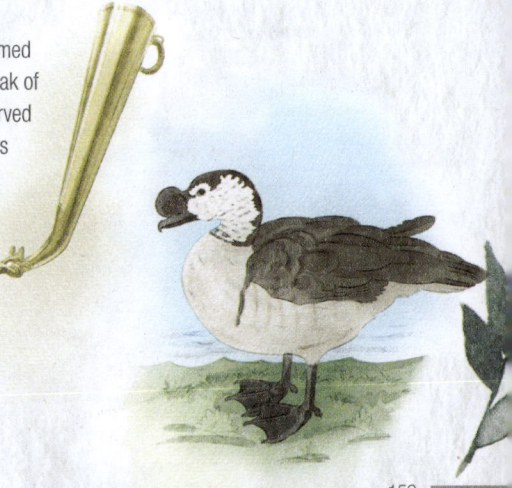

Jayantika Davé

Ruddy Shelduck

Scientific name: *Tadorna ferruginea*   Size: 67 cm
Hindi name: *Chakwa (M), Chakwi (F), Laal Surkhab*
Sanskrit name: *Chakrawak (from its call, which sounds like a squeaky wheel)*

Description

The Ruddy Shelduck is a large plump duck, in beautiful shades of gold, orange, rust, chestnut and white. They breed in Ladakh, and the parent birds have a fascinating practice! Each pair of birds has a number of beautifully striped chicks, and since they don't want to all be tied down with baby-sitting, one bird takes on the 'nursery' responsibilities for a number of parents, and keeps an eye on sometimes 20–40 chicks at a time!

Habits

A widespread winter visitor to large parts of India, the Chakrawak is a striking presence and is easy to identify on a water body due to its large size and bright colouration. It is very comfortable on land, grazing like a goose, and feeding on grasses, soft leaves and stems, aquatic life, small fish and grains and seeds. It is therefore often seen in fields, or dabbling for food at the bottom of shallow water or upending in deeper water. It is usually seen in pairs.

Call

Fairly noisy, calling both at day and night, with a loud, honking ah-honk, ah-honk call!

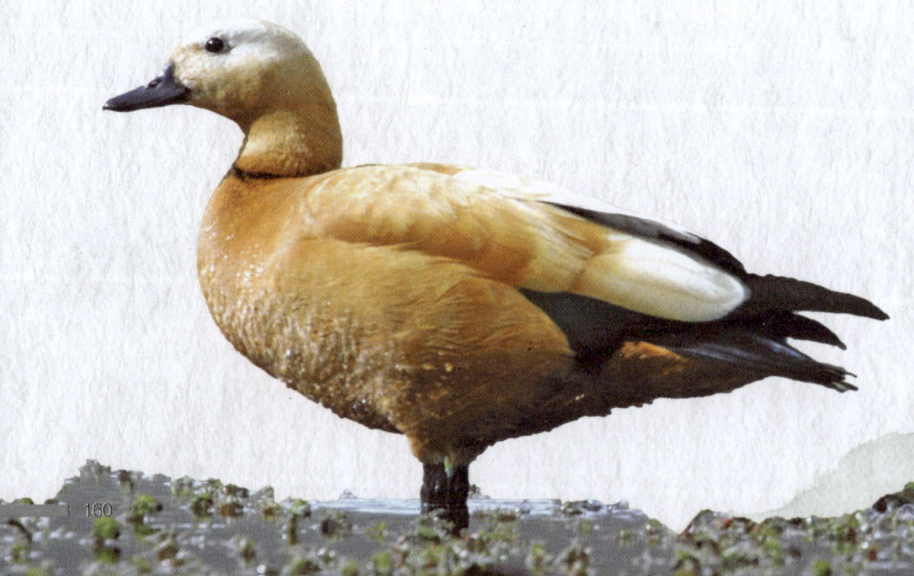

Each Little Bird That Sings

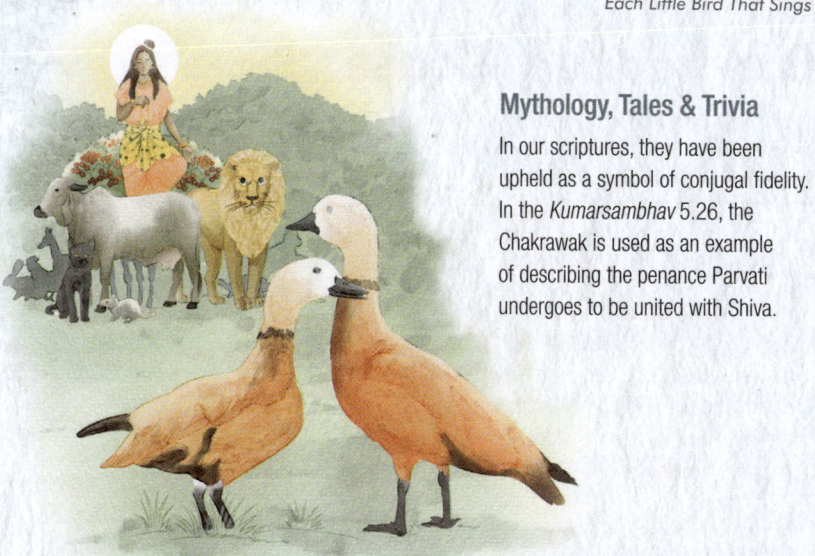

Mythology, Tales & Trivia

In our scriptures, they have been upheld as a symbol of conjugal fidelity. In the *Kumarsambhav* 5.26, the Chakrawak is used as an example of describing the penance Parvati undergoes to be united with Shiva.

In the Ramayana 5.16.30, Chakrawak are again referred to while describing the desolate condition of Sita in the garden of Ravana.

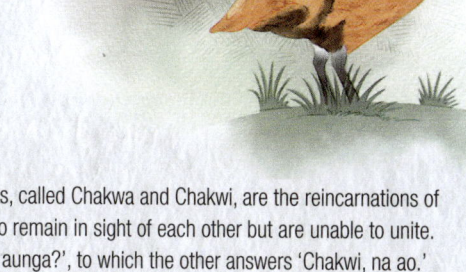

There is a legend that Ruddy Shelducks, called Chakwa and Chakwi, are the reincarnations of erring lovers who have been doomed to remain in sight of each other but are unable to unite. So the call is represented as 'Chakwa, aunga?', to which the other answers 'Chakwi, na ao.'

In Tibet, it is treated as a sacred bird, and so breeds with immunity.

Jayantika Davé

Bar-headed Goose

Scientific name: *Anser indicus*   Size: 74 cm
Hindi name: *Hans, Kareyee Hans, Raaj Hans, Birwa, Sawan*
Sanskrit name: *Kadamb Hans*

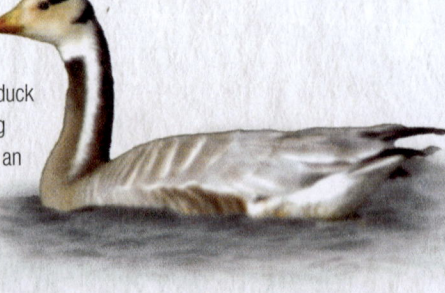

Description

Winter is the time for us to see a large variety of duck and geese, and the one we look forward to seeing every year is the Bar-headed Goose. Looking like an escaped convict, it is an unmistakable large grey goose, with a very white neck stripe, and two black bars across its head!

Habits

The Kadamb Hans breeds in Ladakh at 4,000 m–5,000 m, and is a widespread winter visitor to large parts of India, preferring lowland lakes, rivers and swampy marshes. It is primarily vegetarian, and feeds at night, grazing in grassland along the banks of rivers and lakes, or heading out into cultivated fields to eat young shoots or grain. Stems, soft parts of plants, berries, tubers and grains are what it enjoys, with sometimes aquatic insects and crustaceans for variety. The Bar-headed Goose rests up in large gaggles, and flies in the typical V formation, or in a straight line of geese, but never as just a muddled group.

It breeds in summer in Ladakh, with pairs of up to 100 birds nesting colonially, and re-using their nests each year.

Call

A slow, spaced-out, musical 'aang aang' in flight, which is a lovely sound as many members of the flight keep up the calling!

Mythology, Tales & Trivia

Bar-headed Geese can fly from the lowlands of India to the heights of Ladakh, reaching 4,000 m–5,000 m in 7–8 hours. They fly at a time of day when there are low winds, so that they can fly safely!

One winter, a dear friend, Nikhil Devasar, took us to check out the Basai wetlands, which have now been completely surrounded by tall buildings. As we walked in along the bund, imagine our joy when we saw this large group of maybe 100 Bar-headed Geese, with another large flock of Purple Swamphen feeding around them! What a sight!

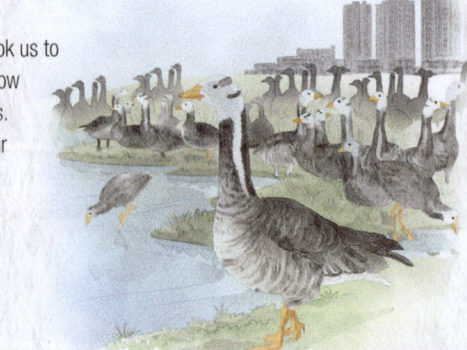

Greylag Goose

Scientific name: *Anser anser*   Size: 82 cm
Hindi name: *Hans, Kareyee Hans, Raaj Hans, Birwa, Sawan*
Sanskrit name: *Kadamb Hans*

Description
Winter in North and some parts of Central and West India marks the arrival of the large, stocky Greylag Goose. Unmistakable due to the combination of their thick pink bill and pink legs, they can be seen around our larger water bodies, flooded fields and rivers. Their deep, loud, honking 'ahnk ahnk' call draws us to look up and smile!

Habits
The Raaj Hans arrive in India in winter, choosing to land near water bodies ideally surrounded by fields, or even on large rivers. They are primarily vegetarians, eating seeds, grains, grass, stems and sprouts, and usually go out into the neighbouring fields to graze at dusk and through the night, returning to open water during the day. They are gregarious, with flocks of 30–50 or 100 birds being seen at a time.

The geese were a particular favourite of my father, and on Sundays, which was the only day that he was free, we would pack a picnic lunch and drive out to Sultanpur to camp on a quiet bank, and watch the flocks of both Greylag and Bar-headed geese!

Call
Noisy and communicative, with much cackling and honking aanhng-anhng-ung calls!

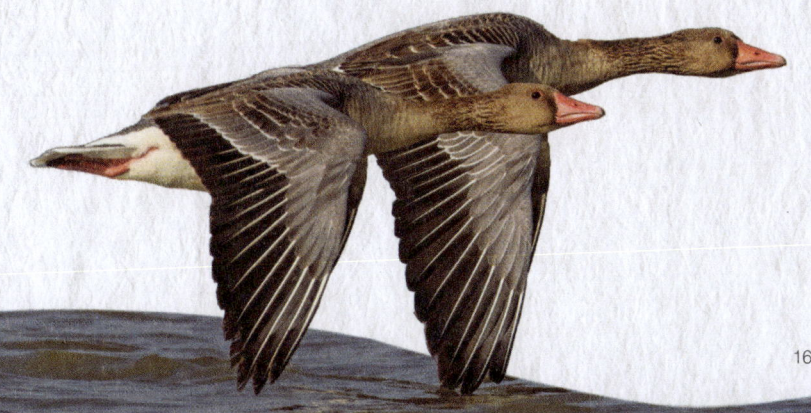

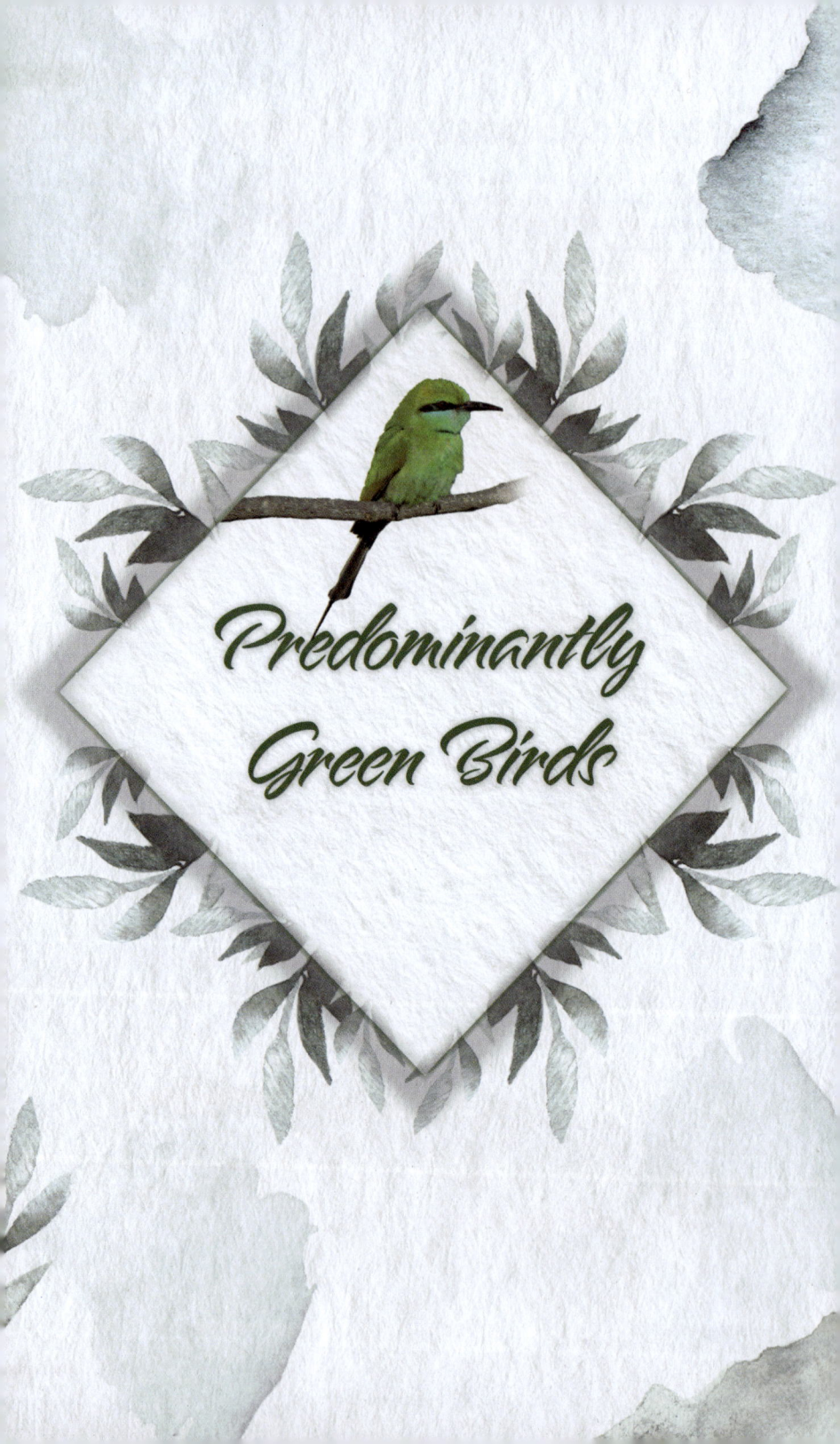

Each Little Bird That Sings

Coppersmith Barbet

Scientific name: *Psilopogon haemacephalus*   Size: 17 cm
Hindi name: *Kaathphora, Tambayat, Basanta Lisora, Chhota Basant*
Sanskrit name: *Dindimanvak*

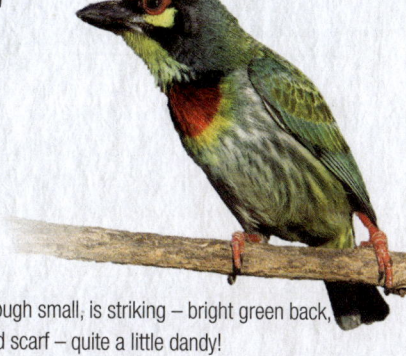

Description

The ventriloquist Coppersmith Barbet is a little beauty you would definitely have heard, if not seen, with the gentle took-took-took call from a fruiting tree, which seems to come from sometimes this side or that! This delightful barbet, though small, is striking – bright green back, red cap and throat, with bright yellow eye-glasses and scarf – quite a little dandy!

Habits

The Chhota Basant is a widespread resident across India, frequenting forests, gardens and orchards. Its main diet is fruit of all kinds, and if a peepal or badh is fruiting, you only have to stand there for a few minutes and a sighting is guaranteed! Guavas, mangoes, other berries, and small insects and crickets are also taken. On fruiting trees, up to 70 birds have been seen feeding together. At other times, it is solitary or in pairs. It is not normally seen above 1,500 m. The 'took-took-took' call rings out throughout the day, reminiscent of a coppersmith's hammer working on his metal vessel!

During breeding season, the male is an assiduous wooer – with throat puffs, tail flicks, singing and bowing! The nest is a neat round hole dug out in a tree, often on the underside of a branch, and is re-used.

Call

The took-took-took call is repeated many times through the day!

Mythology, Tales & Trivia

In our ancient scriptures, Sushruta and Charaka—given the regular beat of its call, accompanied by regular head movements to each side—gave it the name of Dindimanvak or small drummer boy; *dindi* = drum + *manvak* = small boy.

According to my grandfather K.N. Davé, the 'Hemkantarshu' has also been written about in the old scriptures of *Vayu Purana* and the *Manu Samhita*.

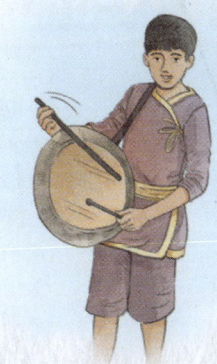

Jayantika Davé

Green Bee-eater

Scientific name: *Merops orientalis*   Size: *17 cm*
Hindi name: *Patringa*
Sanskrit name: *Pippak, Sharg*

Description

Electric wires in the countryside…the tops of tall trees in a garden…a bright green bird with a long graded tail, and a golden, bronzy brown head, and now you have an identification – the Green Bee-eater! And when the sunlight catches its head, Jerdon describes this beautifully as 'gold in the sun-beams!'

Another lovely summer visitor to large parts of North and Central India is the **Blue-tailed Bee-eater**, which then makes its way southward for winters in South India. A medium-sized bee-eater, with bright green above, a distinctive chestnut throat spreading to the sides, and a graded, distinctly blue tail.

Habits

A widespread resident, the Patringa is an inhabitant of arid wooded areas up to 2,000 m in India. It hunts for flies, bees, beetles and bugs from a perch on a wire, fence or small tree, and can also be seen perching on the backs of cattle, watching for insects that they flush! It has a very skilled aerial flight, with quick turns and twists, and a graceful gliding landing back onto its perch. It has small and rather weak feet, and so is incapable of walking or hopping on the ground, though every so often it descends to the ground for a vigorous mud bath. These birds are social roosters, with large numbers gathering to roost in one clump of trees.

The nest is a burrow dug into a mud bank at a low angle, ending in an egg chamber, with a very neatly cut circular entrance.

Call

A cheery tree-tree-tree constantly repeated!

Mythology, Tales & Trivia

In the Mahabharata, the war flag of the brave prince Abhimanyu was emblazoned with the figure of a bee-eater, symbolizing its habit of catching bees with a swift flight like an arrow (Mbh 7.23.89).

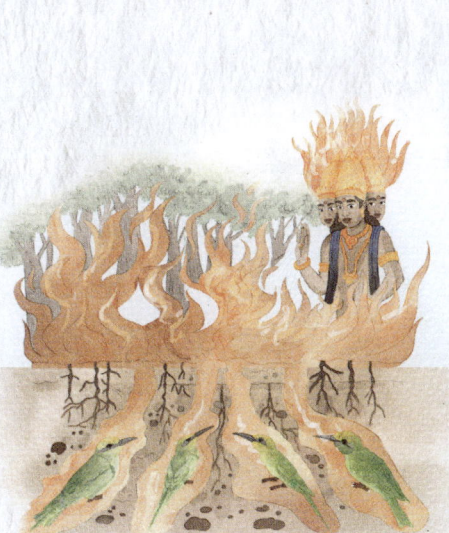

The Mahabharata has another story where the sage Mandapala assumed the form of a male bee-eater, and had four children, each of which, by their description, is one of the bee-eater species we find in India. He prayed to the god Agni for their safety, and left for the heavens. Many verses in the Mahabharata then depict how, when there was a forest fire, each of the four fledglings prayed to Agni *devata* to save them. Agni devata advised them to hide in their burrow in the ground, and the fire passed over them lightly. (Mbh.1.232.9,10)

Jayantika Davé

Golden-fronted Leafbird

Scientific name: *Chloropsis aurifrons* Size: *19 cm*
Hindi name: *Harewa, Sabz Harewa, Chhota Harrial, Chhota Harewa*
Sanskrit name: *Suvarna-bhal Patragupt*

Description

The Suvarna-bhal Patragupt – the Sanskrit name for this bird is so wonderfully descriptive! Golden forehead, the colour of leaves, and difficult to see in the foliage! One of our lovely residents, seen in the forests of the lower Himalayas and in the Ghats of the South.

Habits

The Harewa, or Green Bulbul as it was earlier called, is a lover of moist areas with forest canopies, broad-leaved, deciduous or evergreen, up to 1,200 m. The Golden-fronted Leafbird blends in so well with the leaves of trees that it doesn't catch the eye unless you are looking for it. It can be seen towards the tops of trees, taking fruit, nectar and different insects, some of which are even caught in flight in a fly-catcher fashion! It is an acrobatic feeder, and we have often seen it hanging upside down, or on its head with a tight grip on the branch, trying to reach inside flower throats to get to the nectar!

A hammock-like nest of thin twigs, grass, and cobwebs is hung between two branches.

Call

A variety of twitters and whistles, often with a lot of mimicry!

Mythology, Tales & Trivia

An accomplished mimic, the Harewa will mimic drongos, bulbuls, the White-breasted Kingfisher, and also migrants that have already departed, resulting in a lot of confusion amongst us birders!

They used to be very popular cage birds in the East and in Europe.

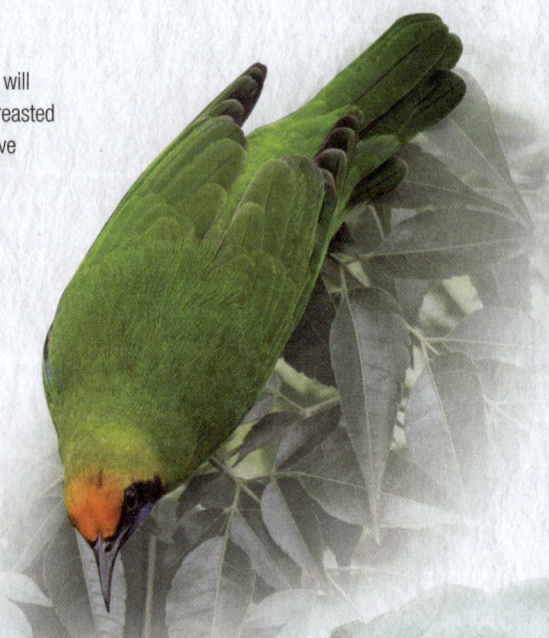

Brown-headed Barbet

Scientific name: *Psilopogon zeylanicus*   Size: 27 cm
Hindi name: *Bada Basanta, Katoor, Cumma*
UP name: *Kotur*
Sanskrit name: *Kutroo*

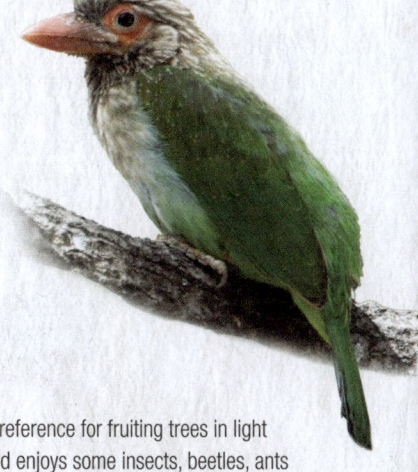

Description

When you are near a badh or peepul in fruiting season, be sure to look for this relatively large green barbet, with a largely brown head and breast and upper back, a striking patch of orange-yellow skin around its eyes, and a heavy orange-yellow bill.

The very similar **White-cheeked Barbet** is a resident of the Western Ghats, with the main difference being a significant white cheek and white dappling on its chest.

Habits

The Bada Basanta is a resident all across India, with a preference for fruiting trees in light forests, parks and gardens. It also takes some nectar and enjoys some insects, beetles, ants and termites. As summer warms up, the Brown-headed Barbet starts calling incessantly and with more fervour – kutrook-kutrook-kutrook…going on endlessly!

Call

The engine is warmed up with a harsh krr-rr-rr-rr-rr, which picks up speed, and then the kutrook-kutrook-kutrook calls burst out, being repeated endlessly, and often with other Brown-headed Barbets joining in, in a chorus!

Mythology, Tales & Trivia

The incessant kutrook-kutrook-kutrook call gives rise to the colloquial names.

I have a particular fondness for this bird, as through it I made a wonderfully interesting friend! One afternoon, Jasjit Mansingh and I were walking to the Delhi Gymkhana tennis courts for a game, and the kutrook calls started. She turned to me, and asked me… 'Now do you know what bird that is?' Without breaking my stride, I answered that it was the Brown-headed Barbet! She laughed joyously, gave me a hug, and said… 'Aha, a fellow birder!'…and that was the start of a lovely friendship!

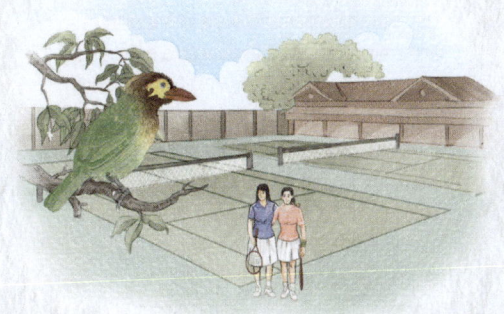

Jayantika Davé

Lesser Yellownape

Scientific name: *Picus chlorolophus*   Size: 27 cm
Hindi name: *Katphora*
Sanskrit name: *Darvaghat, Kashtthakukut*

Description

The Himalayas or the hills of South India, an old tree with cracked bark, a green woodpecker assiduously working the bark, with a flaming head the colour of mustard fields in bloom, and you can be sure that you are looking at either the Lesser or Greater Yellownapes. The Lesser Yellownape has some red in the crown too, while the **Greater Yellownape** has a more flamboyant yellow crest, and a streaked white throat, which is an easy distinguisher!

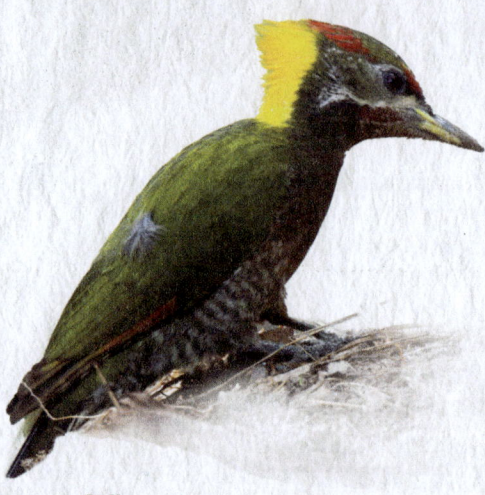

Habits

A lover of all kinds of forest, moist or dry, evergreen or deciduous, the Yellownape forages away busily on tree trunks, looking behind the bark for all kinds of beetle and larvae. It also enjoys berries and nectar, and during the Padam flowering season, it comes to a tree right next to our balcony to eat the gorgeous pink flowers! It has also started visiting our bird feeder, and is quite happy banging away with its powerful beak, enlarging the hole in the feeder till more bajra and rice come pouring down it, which it then speedily demolishes! It is usually a solitary bird, sometimes appearing in pairs.

Call

A loud drawn-out peeee-ui, also short chaks. Enjoys doing a drum-roll occasionally!

Mythology, Tales & Trivia

Once, my daughters, Vedika and Rushali, and a niece, Taarini, had climbed a hill behind the house, and were just sitting on the ground enjoying the breeze. From a tree right next to us, a Greater Yellownape dropped to the ground and started picking up some fallen fruit! And while our mouths were still open in amazement, another… and another…and another! We didn't move an inch…just feasted our eyes! One of my 'flash upon the inward eye' moments!

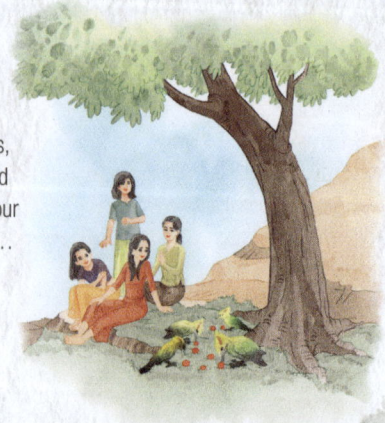

Great Barbet

Scientific name: *Psilopogon virens*   Size: *33 cm*
Hindi name: *Traiho*
Sanskrit name: *Pippal*

Description

So, it seems that God decided to experiment and see how many colours he could put on one barbet! The Great Barbet, which is our largest barbet, has a green body with a dark blue head, brown back, yellow streaks underneath, red under the tail, and a really large and heavy yellow bill!

Habits

A resident of our Himalayas, found up to 3,000 m, this noisy-flighted, purely arboreal bird comes to forests, orchards and gardens to pick figs, berries, flowers of rhododendron and wild pear, and a variety of insects. The incessant, endlessly repeated call of 'peeeao-peeeao' notes are what will draw your eye to look for this bird. In Glen Haven, we have a fruiting bush called tushar growing in the gaderas on the side and front of the house, and during fruiting season, there will be large numbers of the Traiho landing in the bush with a heavy swoosh, and then disappearing into it, plucking and eating the fruit whole.

The courtship is quite lovely, with tail-spreading and wagging, low head-bowing, and vociferous singing, often together in chorus!

Call

One bird will start with the resounding, melancholy peeeao-peeeao notes, and soon every other Great Barbet in the vicinity will join to form an endless chorus!

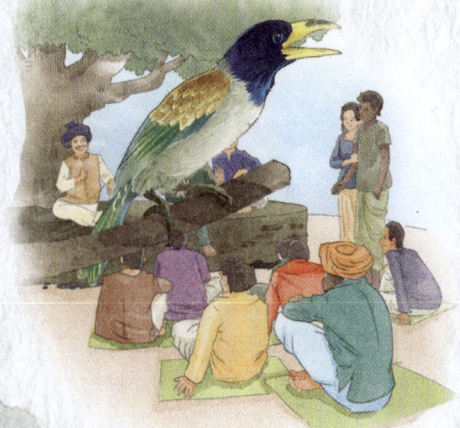

Mythology, Tales & Trivia

There is a hill-people story that the Great Barbet is the incarnation of the soul of a suitor who died of grief since he could not be with the love of his life, as his request was turned down by the panchayat. His soul now resides in the Great Barbet, and unceasingly cries out *anyaaya, anyaaya*, meaning 'injustice'!

Jayantika Davé

Wedge-tailed Green Pigeon

Scientific name: *Treron sphenurus*   Size: *33 cm*
Hindi name: *Kokila, Kokola*
Sanskrit name: *Kokathu, Kokadev*

Description

Mellow, warbling, liquid whistles coming from a fruiting tree or bush in the Himalayas? Look for the Wedge-tailed Green Pigeon! A gently elegant combination of shades of green, washed with blue-grey on the neck, and a rich, deep maroon patch on the wings, matched with bright pink-red feet!

Habits

The Kokila is a resident of forested wooded areas in our hills, with a great weakness for fruit and figs. It is largely an arboreal feeder, doing all kinds of acrobatic moves, even hanging upside down to get at the ripest fruit! It usually visits singly or in pairs, with sometimes a small flock descending onto a particularly attractive feeding tree. The sweet-fruited tushar in the gadera of our hill home is a big attraction, and during the fruiting season we get wonderful viewings, as a series of the Wedge-tailed Green Pigeons fly in to first sit on the sparse-leafed birch tree, and then fly into the tushar shrub, to disappear into its depths to feed.

Call

A series of melodious whoo-whoo-whoo whistle calls, sometimes described as 'why we wait here…what are we waiting for?'

Mythology, Tales & Trivia

L.J. Mackintosh (*Birds of Darjeeling & India,* 1914) tells of purchasing a mother and its chick from a woodcutter. The woodcutter brought them to Mackintosh from five miles away, and the male followed him the entire way, calling mournfully. At Mackintosh's home too, the male continued to call in the trees around the house, till Mackintosh finally released the mother and baby.

The Wedge-tailed Green Pigeon has been known to place its nest close to the nest of the aggressive drongo, who then takes on its role as kotwal and protects both the nests!

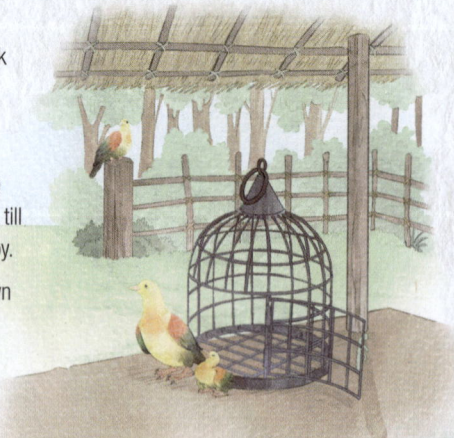

Yellow-footed Green Pigeon

Scientific name: *Treron phoenicopterus* Size: *33 cm*
Hindi name: *Harial*
Sanskrit name: *Raktakanttha Kapot, Haareet*

Description

Our morning walks in a park in Gurgaon, along a line of Ficus trees, are filled with the mellow whistles of the gentle Yellow-footed Green Pigeon. They often cluster on the top of a tree, and if the sun happens to be hitting that spot, they are a breathtaking sight, glowing a gorgeous fluorescent green-yellow, with a beautiful wash of grey-blue on the head, greenish-grey bill and prominent yellow feet!

Habits

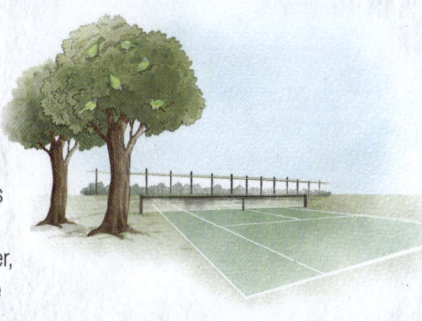

The Harial is a resident across most parts of India, staying in forests, woodlands and parks in the lowland areas. When the peepul, banyan and other Ficus are in fruit, large flocks of these birds will be seen, feeding, whistling, making short flights from one branch to another, or clambering up and around the branches like parakeets, feasting on the ripening figs!
Once, while playing tennis at the Delhi Gymkhana Club, I got chatting with a visiting Englishman, who told me that the next day he was going to a sanctuary with the single-minded aim of seeing the Yellow-footed Green Pigeon. All around us, on every peepul tree, were flocks of these birds! Of course I promptly took him for a walk, and showed them off to him… hopefully saving him a long drive!

Call

A lovely series of cooing, melodious whistles!

Mythology, Tales & Trivia

Legend has it that since Green Pigeons rarely descend to the ground, it is said that they do not like to dirty their feet, and even when they descend to drink water, they carry a twig in their feet, and perch on the twig to drink! They seek the protection of the aggressive drongo by sometimes nesting in the same tree.

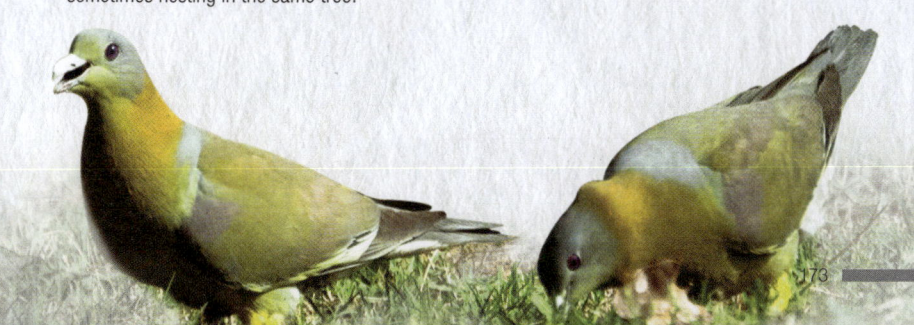

Jayantika Davé

Rose-ringed Parakeet

Scientific name: *Psittacula krameri*   Size: *42 cm*
Hindi name: *Tota*
Sanskrit name: *Kaashtthashuka*

Description

A bright green bird, with a long tail, up in a tree, or in a flock hurtling overhead, and swerving gracefully through a forest to avoid the trees will definitely be a member of the parrot family, the most common of which is the Rose-ringed Parakeet. Often seen in large flocks on old forts or buildings, they present a memorable sight of bright green daubs of paint against the warm stone.

Habits

It is most comfortable on a tree, rarely descending to the ground. But when it does, it has a charmingly awkward and sidling gait. These parakeets are peaceful and ruminative eaters, and are often seen sitting on one leg, holding up a piece of food in the other leg, delicately nibbling and peacefully enjoying the feast. The formation of their larynx and tongue helps them to imitate the human voice very well, often being able to recite whole verses. Courting parrots are a joy to watch, with much head-tickling and soothing!

Call
A loud screech-screech-screech is the most common call!

Mythology, Tales & Trivia

In villages, soothsayers keep these birds as pets. After a suitable fee has been paid, the 'far-sighted' bird will waddle out of its cage, survey the stack of pre-printed cards, and decide the recipient's fate!

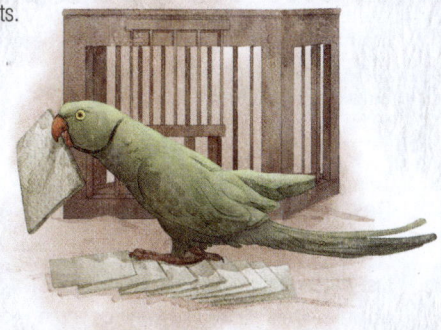

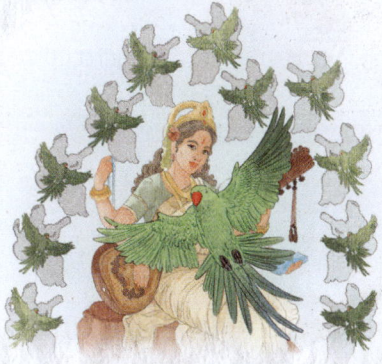

Goddess Saraswati, and her various forms of Matangi, Meenakshi or Shukapriya, all have a parrot with them, who is said to be imparting the 64 *bahyakala*s or skills to her.

The Rose-ringed Parakeet is the mount of the god of love Kamdev.

In the Puranas, Kunjal the parrot is projected as an enlightened preacher of virtues who teaches his four children devotion to Lord Vishnu, and the importance of different virtues.

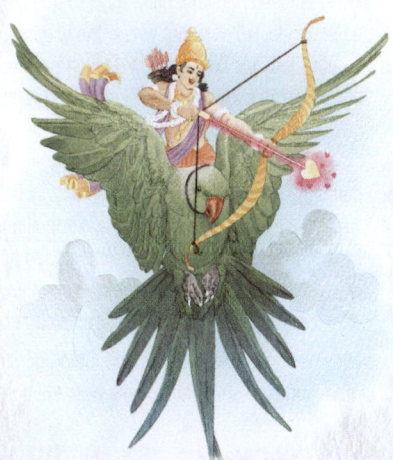

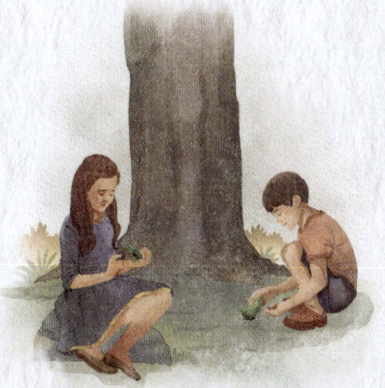

As children, our gardener taught us how to save parakeet babies that fell out of their nest, by feeding them small balls of wheat flour. If he forgot how many he had given, he would probe the stomach to count how many there were!

Jayantika Davé

Plum-headed Parakeet

Scientific name: *Psittacula cyanocephala*   Size: 36 cm
Hindi name: *Tuinya Tota, Lal-sira Tota*
Sanskrit name: *Krishnaangshuka*

Description

A soft and sweet whistling call, with the fast-wheeling flight and flash of the green of a parakeet, and we will be looking up to see where they are landing, so that we can see the beautiful plum-purple-red head of the lovely Plum-headed Parakeet in all its glory!

Habits

Moist wooded habitats, gardens with trees, and forest edges up to 1,300 m are where the widespread resident Lal-sira Tota will be found. Like all parakeets, this is a lover of fruit, berries and figs of all kinds, and will be found feasting on guavas, mangoes and figs in large community flocks. These birds have a really fast flight, and I often watch them in amazement, wondering how they can bank and wheel and still fly so fast, avoiding every tree that comes in their way, till they reach the one they want to alight on! Unlike the harsh, often screechy calls of other Parakeets, the Plum-Headed has a very sweet musical call which is an identifier even when the bird cannot immediately be seen. This is one of the parakeets that has not been kept as a cage bird in Indian homes.

They nest in a hole in a tree and, being gentle birds, are often driven away by the more aggressive Mynas, to take over the hole for their own nest.

Call

A lovely melodious huEET-huEET, with also a shriller toooi-toooi call, where one starts and then the whole flock joins the chorus!

Alexandrine Parakeet

Scientific name: *Psittacula eupatria* Size: *53 cm*
Hindi name: *Hiraman Tota, Rai Tota*
Sanskrit name: *Raj Shuka*

Description

The Alexandrine Parakeet is a striking, strident-voiced, large parakeet, with a distinctive, large, heavy red bill and a red patch on the wings. The Hiraman Tota got its name because Alexander the Great apparently sent over a large number of these birds to different countries in Europe and the Mediterranean, where they were highly valued and named in his honour.

Habits

The Hiraman Tota is a resident across large parts of India, but is now not as easily seen, as it is a lover of wooded areas, moist areas and forests. It has a preference for lowlands and is not usually found very high in the hills. A voracious eater of fruits, seeds, grains and nectar, it is not very popular with farmers, as a flock of the Alexandrine Parakeets can be very destructive in fields of maize and jowar. They are very intelligent birds, and can be trained to mimic human voices. Unfortunately, they are still caught and sold as captive birds in India, even though that is against the law. They are communal roosters, with large flocks collecting to roost in a grove of trees, with much chattering and exchanging of stories of the day.

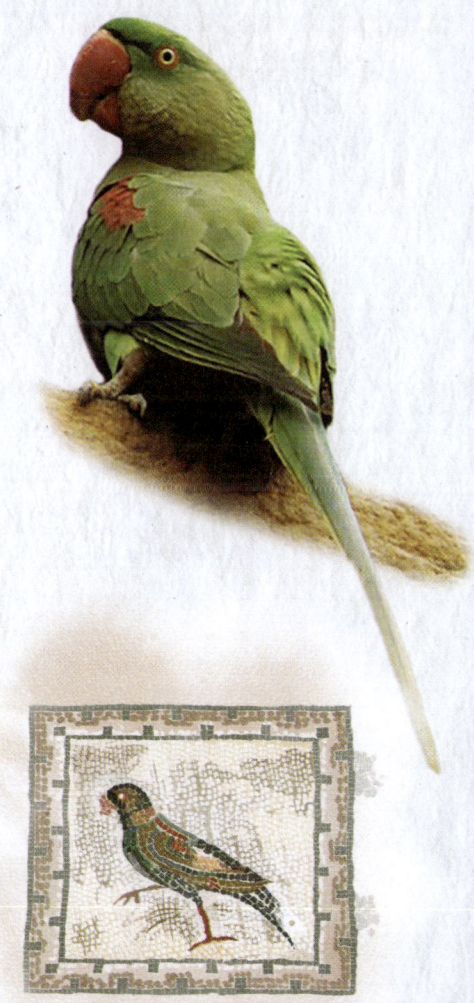

Call

A loud keeh, kyah or rolling curree call, interspersed with conversational arguing!

Mythology, Tales & Trivia

A mosaic floor inset of an Alexandrine Parakeet was made as early as 2 BC at the Acropolis of Pergamon, Turkey.

Predominantly Grey Birds

Small Pratincole

Scientific name: *Glareola lacteal*   Size: *17 cm*
Hindi name: *Abali Nudri*
Sindhi name: *Utteran*
Sanskrit name: *Haputrika (one who falls to the ground lamenting)*

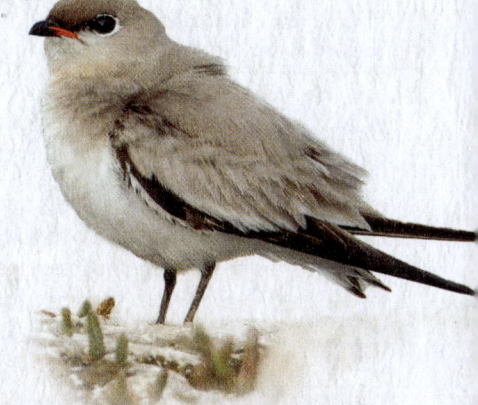

Description

The sandy banks of rivers often have a number of waders of different sizes and different heights, with many being predominantly brown...but amongst them, look out for this low-slung grey-and-white bird, with a very elongated graceful shape...the unmistakable Small Pratincole. A lovely combination of grey above, with a fawn scarf, a white shirt front, and a black bill with just a dash of dark red at the base, near the eye!

Habits

A gregarious and social bird, the Small Pratincole is a widespread resident all over India, with a particular preference for the sandbanks of streams, rivers, lakes and coastal marshes. The Abali Nudri feeds on all kinds of insects and flies, running on the ground like a plover, or hawking them by flying low over water or the ground, or even sharply banking and catching them higher up in the air. The nest is a scrape in the sand, with 2–3 greyish-brown eggs being laid.

Call

A high tirrit-tirrit call in flight!

Mythology, Tales & Trivia

During the very hot hours of the day, the little Utteran will wet its stomach feathers before returning to the nest, so that the eggs are cooled off.

Whistler beautifully describes what happens if an intruder comes near their nest – 'the birds flutter down on to the sand, gasp and flutter, lie exhausted with outstretched wings, and drag themselves along, in the apparent throes of a mortal wound' – consummate acting indeed, to divert attack!

Dewar too described the wounded-bird broken-wing tactics, saying that 'the pratincole has a singularly unbalanced mind while it is in breeding!'

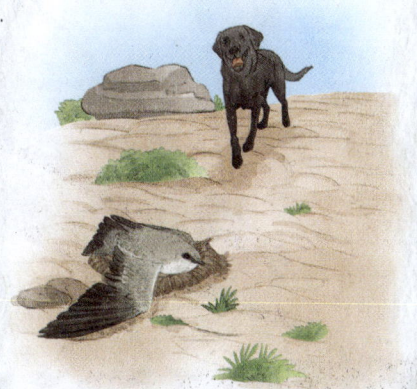

Jayantika Davé

Chestnut-tailed Starling

Scientific name: *Sturnia malabarica*   Size: 20 cm
Hindi name: *Pawei, Bhoori Myna*
Sanskrit name: *Sweta Saarika*

Description

One year, we went to Goa in winter, and stayed in a beautiful old home that had this huge semul tree in front, in full bloom, with every branch bursting with fleshy nectar-filled red flowers. And what a riot of feasting and squabbling – with the Rosy Starlings creating the most chaos, and the lovely, dignified Chestnut-tailed Starlings staying out of their way, but still making sure they got their share of nectar! A daily feast for the eyes!

Habits

The Pawei is a resident of the Northeast, a summer visitor to parts of the Himalayas, and a winter visitor to South India. It enjoys habitat that has scattered trees, preferably laden with nectar-filled flowers or fruit. It forages for insects, seeds, sometimes soft flower buds, and nectar and fruit. These birds are arboreal feeders, moving around with great dexterity amongst branches thick and thin, dropping down into lantana bushes to get their fruit, and sometimes even to the ground to pick up fruits or insects. While feeding, they keep up an incessant chatter, sharing many stories with each other, and occasionally squabbling too! They are social beings, always in pairs and often in small flocks.

Call

A series of pleasant whistles, and noisy chatters and churrs!

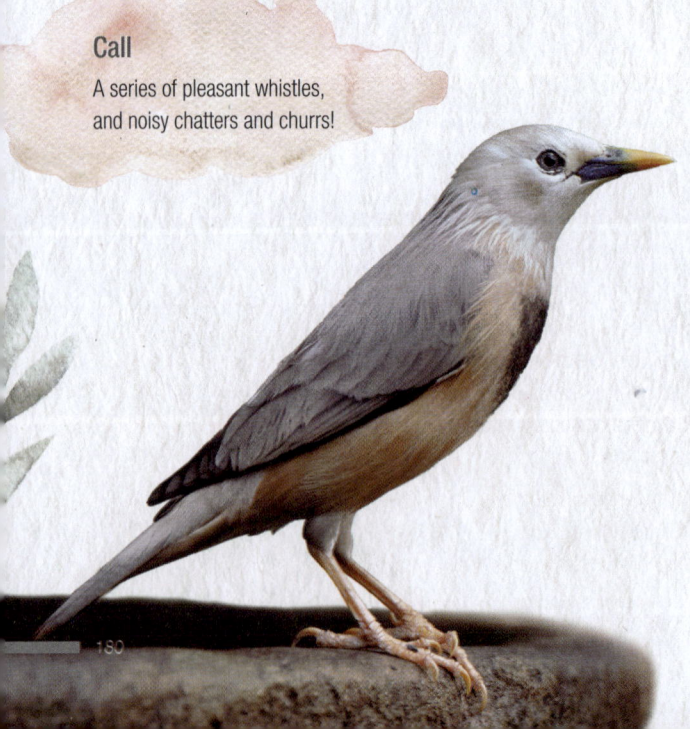

Southern Grey Shrike

Scientific name: *Lanius meridionalis*   Size: 24 cm
Hindi name: *Dudiya Latora, Safed Latora, Bada Latora*
Sanskrit name: *Bharat Sit-bhasma Latushak*

Description
The Southern Grey Shrike is a black-and-white photograph – no rufous tones anywhere, which distinguishes it from most of the other shrikes. A widespread resident across the north and western parts of India – look for it in dry shrubby countryside.

Habits
Like most shrikes, the Dudiya Latora likes open countryside, with small thorny trees and shrubs, in warm, dry lowland areas. This is the kind of cover it needs to perch on to be able to spy its prey, to use the thorns to impale the victims for later consumption, and to be able to place its nest. Large crickets and grasshoppers, beetles, reptiles, small birds and rodents are caught, often on the ground, and then carried away to be eaten safely on the perch. It sits and waits patiently, neck tucked back into its shoulders, looking as if it is just biding its time, but the quick swoop, grab and return to its perch with unsuspecting prey gives the game away! Interestingly, it lays one egg a day, till it reaches its total of 3–6 eggs!

Call
Harsh call of shrrik-shrrik, interspersed with chattering and mimicry!

Mythology, Tales & Trivia
One study in Spain found that food that is impaled in its larder is usually consumed within nine days!

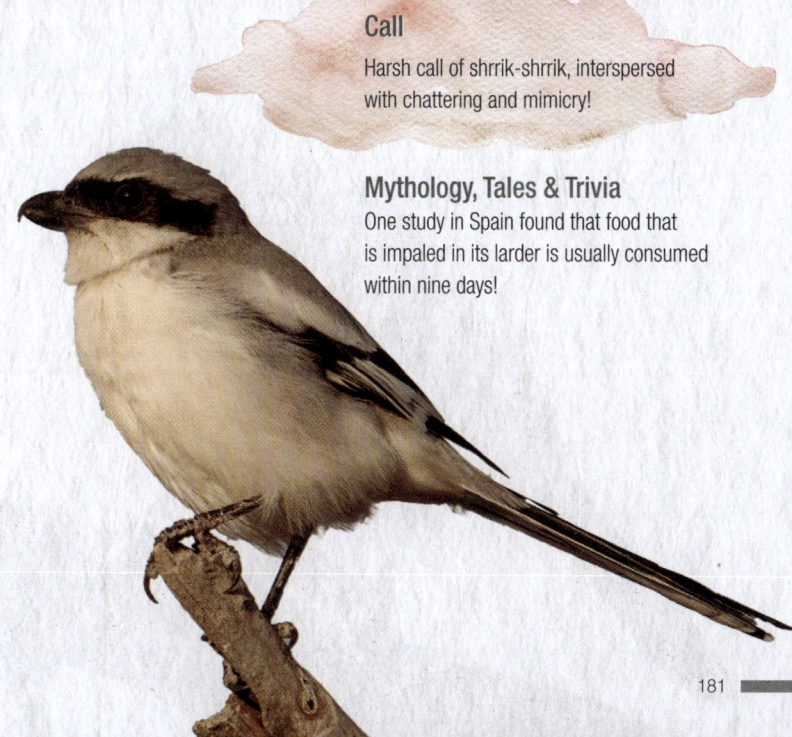

Jayantika Davé

Jungle Babbler

Scientific name: *Turdoides striata*   Size: 25 cm
Hindi name: Saat bhai, Pengya Myna, Jangli-khyr, Ghaughai
Sanskrit name: Aranya Haholika, Bhoosaarika

Description

Loud rustling amongst the dried leaves in shrubby undergrowth, and then the sight of a small flock of grey birds, turning over leaves with incessant industry, all the while moving with a clumsy hopping gait? Yes indeed, the Jungle Babbler! E.H.A. describes their behaviour beautifully – 'There is a regular flow of small talk, a good deal of mirth and laughter, and occasionally an eager dispute. In appearance – it reminds you of old Jones, who passes the day in his pyjamas!'

The very similar **Yellow-billed Babbler** is present in South India, distinguished by its light head, lovely blue iris and a very yellow beak.

Habits

Gardens, parks and open forests all across India are bound to provide sightings of the garrulous Saat Bhai or Saat Behen, as they are colloquially called. While primarily lowland birds, they can be seen up to about 1,500 m in the foothills and ghats. They are brave, and don't hesitate to attack even a small falcon that may have got hold of one of their own. The Haholika is an eminently gregarious bird, so if one of them is in trouble, it only needs to complain, and immediately there is a swarm of others to help. A wide range of all kinds of insects are looked for, with the diet being varied with seeds, berries, grains and nectar.

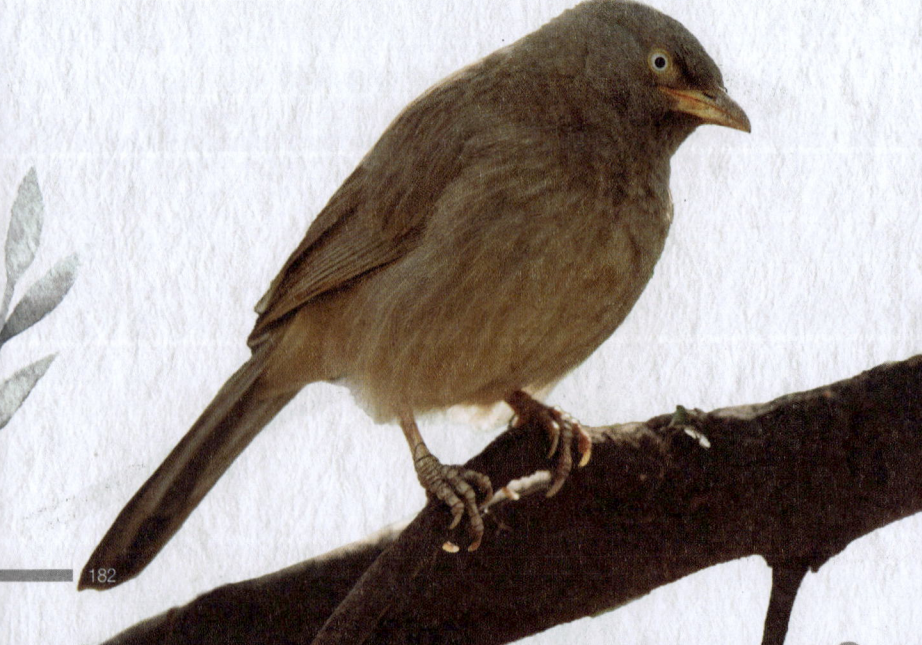

Call

A constant muttering ke-ke-ke uttered as they work the ground, interspersed with excited chattering!

Mythology, Tales & Trivia

Once upon a time, a king hired the Saat Bhai to dig a well. They completed the job, and after resting, flew to the king asking for their payment. Meanwhile, an opportune imposter had already collected the payment, and the king refused to pay them. And so the animated altercation continues to this day, as they remember the vile trick that was played on them!

One of the names used for the Jungle Babbler in ancient times used to be Gokirati, which was amalgamated from *gavi* + *bhumao* + *kir* + *iv* + *atati* = a bird that moves and works on the ground like a pig — which aptly describes their behaviour.

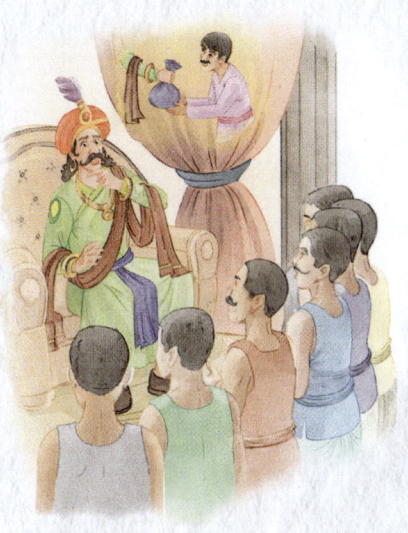

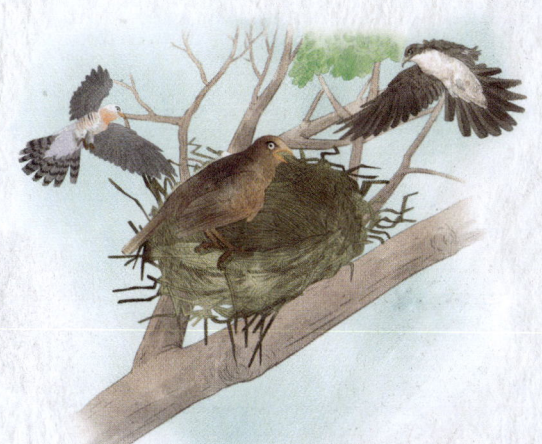

Its nest is often parasitized by the Jacobin Cuckoo and the Common Hawk Cuckoo.

Jayantika Davé

Long-tailed Shrike

Scientific name: *Lanius schach*   Size: 25 cm
Hindi name: *Mattiya Latora, Kajala Latora*
Sanskrit name: *Aarakta-prushtha Latushak, Krishna Latushak*

Description

The beautifully patterned Long-tailed Shrike, with a smart grey coat, a rufous-and-white waistcoat, and a black eye mask, is a fairly common sight in gardens and parks with some trees and shrubs, differentiated from the others by its predominantly grey-and-rufous back and sides and longer tail.

Habits

The Kajala Latora is a lowland bird that moves between 1,700 m and 3,000 m in the Himalayas in summer, living and hunting in open country, cultivated areas and shrubs and bushes with some trees. Favourite foods are grasshoppers, crickets, other insects, frogs, lizards and occasionally small birds and nestlings. Like other shrikes, it is pretty fearless, and swoops down and gets its prey from the ground or from wherever it is hiding. The Long-tailed Shrike also creates a larder by impaling insects on a large thorn in a shrubbery, so that they can be consumed at will later.

Call

The call is a harsh scolding scha-scha-scha, with the song being a fairly melodious warble, with so much mimicry in it that it is hard to distinguish the actual song and what is being copied!

Mythology, Tales & Trivia

Despite this being a bold and fearless bird, its nest is often parasitized by the Common Hawk Cuckoo and the Jacobin Cuckoo.

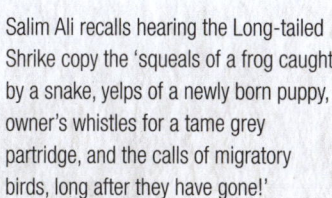

The larder habit has given this bird the name of Butcher Bird.

Salim Ali recalls hearing the Long-tailed Shrike copy the 'squeals of a frog caught by a snake, yelps of a newly born puppy, owner's whistles for a tame grey partridge, and the calls of migratory birds, long after they have gone!'

E.H.A. too describes one particularly talented individual that used to entertain him with comic dialogues between bulbuls, lapwings and other birds.

It used to be called the Rufous-backed Shrike.

Jayantika Davé

Common Pigeon

Scientific name: *Columba livia*   Size: 33 cm
Hindi name: *Kabutar*
Sanskrit name: *Neel Kapot*

Description

Ah! The ubiquitous Common Pigeon! Seen anywhere and everywhere! While not a personal favourite of mine, I do have to admit that they are good-looking birds, with their combination of blue-grey suits edged with black, and with a striking neck cravat glossed in green, blue, purple and pink!

Habits

The Kabutar is a widespread resident all over India, showing a marked preference for being near human habitation and fields during grain harvesting. They are prolific breeders, following the female around with a 'fat lady' waddle, and their heads bobbing back and forth. They have a fast, very strong flight, and easily evade raptors which try and catch them.

Call
A strutting, neck-inflating gootr-goo, gootr-goo.

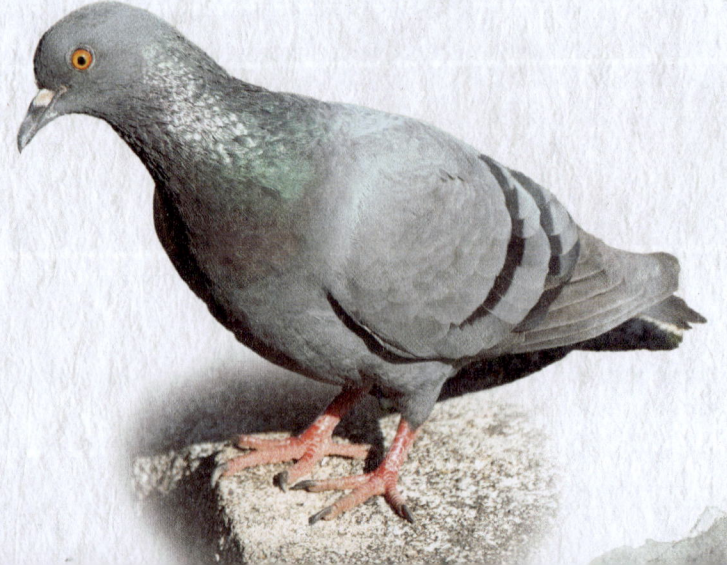

Mythology, Tales & Trivia

According to Capt. Praveen Chopra, the pigeon is deemed sacred in many religions – in Sikhism, as the follower of Guru Gobind Singh; in Islam as the saviour of Prophet Muhammed since it nested at the entrance of a cave where he was, and the persecutors therefore believed there was no one in the cave; in Buddhism as the saviour of Tarma, the son of yoga masters Marpa and Dagmema, where the pigeon acted as the carrier of the soul of Tarma to an appropriate alternate body when Tarma had a fatal accident.

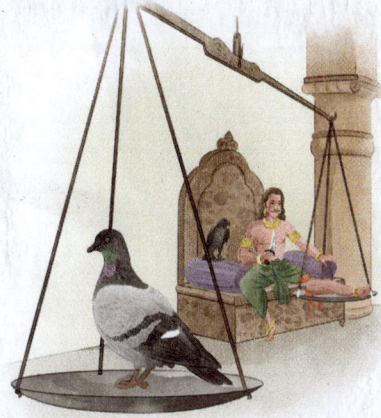

The Mahabharata, Ramayana and Jataka tales tell the story of King Shibi of the Chandravansh dynasty, who was known as a compassionate ruler and offered himself up to a hawk in place of the pigeon that had sought refuge in his lap. The gods Indra and Agni were actually testing him and had taken the form of the hawk and the pigeon, and when he passed the test, they appeared and blessed him.

Kabutarbaazi was introduced to India by the Mughals, and is still very popular. Flocks are released from different rooftops; they mingle and are then called back, and whichever flock manages to bring back rival pigeons is deemed the winner.

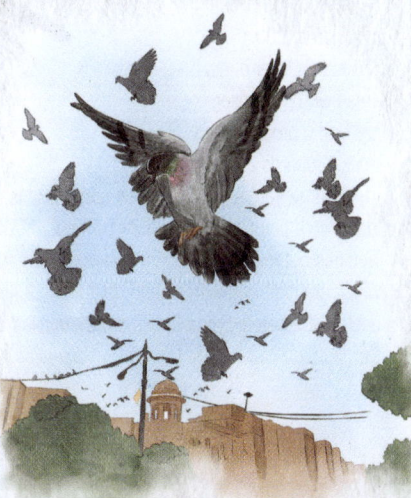

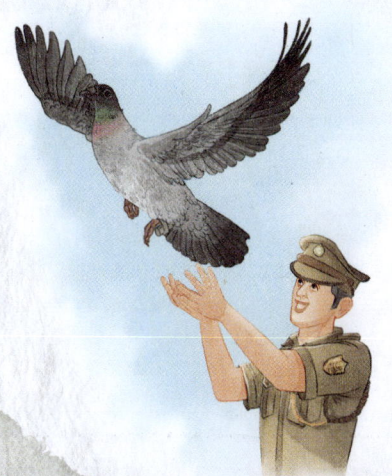

The police in Orissa used to maintain an independent P Mail service, using Belgian-bred homing pigeons to send messages during natural disasters when all other communication failed.

Jayantika Davé

Shikra

Scientific name: *Accipiter badius*   Size: 33 cm
Hindi name: *Shikra*
Sanskrit name: *Mahavir Baaz*

Description

This pretty falcon is the one most commonly seen around human habitation, so long as there are some trees around. So, do scan the skies periodically, to see the typical streamlined silhouette as it hunts from on high, or listen for the very drongo-like calls of 'titu-titu-titu', or the longer drawn-out 'iheeya-iheeya'!

Habits

A widespread resident in India, up to 200 m, the Shikra is a lover of dry areas with tree cover, preferring broad-leaved trees, orchards and the ornamental trees in our parks and gardens. It identifies a perch with good leafy cover, and from there watches out for small birds, nestlings, lizards, frogs, insects and beetles, which are captured with a short, fast flight, a flap and a glide, and carried back to the perch. In the forested park outside our apartment complex in Gurgaon, no nest is safe from this sharp-eyed predator!

Call

A loud drongo-like titu-titu-titu, with a longer drawn-out iheeya-iheeya.

Mythology, Tales & Trivia

Emperor Akbar was fond of falconry, and in spring, all his falcons were sent to the villages to finish their moulting. Once they had new feathers, and were beautiful to see, they were brought back to court.

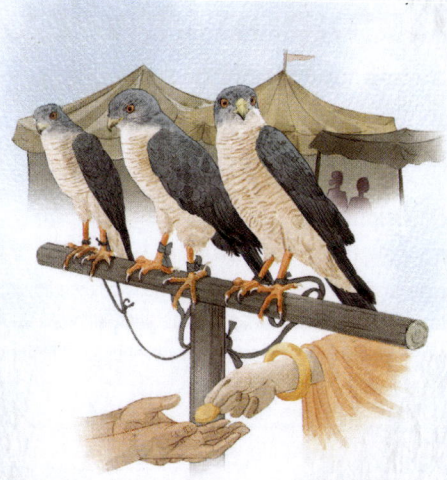

Especially good-looking males were costly – and could cost one gold *mohur* in those days.

The Shikra was a favourite of falconers, who, within 10 days, could train it to catch quail and partridge.

The Shikra is fearless, and willing to take on birds of a larger size.

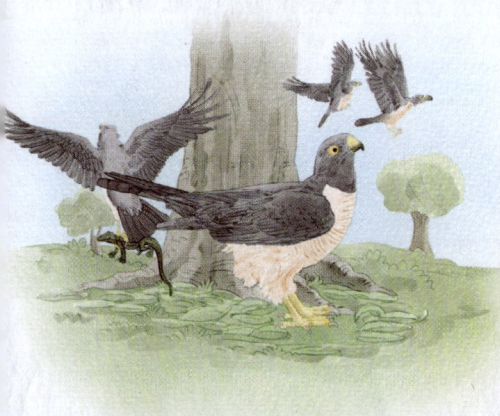

M. Krishnan tells a story of a Shikra that took on two large Jungle Crows who tried to steal a lizard it was eating. The Shikra was so angry that it dropped the lizard and, hurling invectives at the two, it seemingly grabbed one each in each talon, so that all three hurtled to the ground. When they untangled themselves, the two crows fled, and like the monkey story, the lizard got stolen by a third lucky crow!

Jayantika Davé

Common Hawk Cuckoo

Scientific name: *Hierococcyx varius*   Size: 34 cm
Hindi name: *Papiha, Kapak, Upak, Papiya*
Sanskrit name: *Babhru Chatak*

Description

A hot summer night, and the incessant call of pi-pee-ha…pi-pee-ha…pi-pee-ha…rising in scale and becoming louder and louder, and then trailing off with a series of tumbling notes… that is the Common Hawk Cuckoo…more often heard than seen! When we were young and slept outside under mosquito nets, the heat and the incessant hysterical calls were enough to drive sleep away!

Habits

The Papiha is a lowland resident across India, frequenting wooded country, forests and parks and gardens with trees. Its diet consists of all kinds of insects, grasshoppers, ants, caterpillars and lizards, together with the fruit and berries of wild and cultivated trees. It stays well hidden in tree canopy and is not easy to sight.

It is a parasitical nester, and lays its eggs in the nests of babblers, leaving them to raise its young.

Call

A rising, scaled call of pi-pee-ha…pi-pee-ha…pi-pee-ha or brain fee-ver…brain fee-ver, becoming positively shrill at the end! Another pretty interpretation of the call is *pee-kahan* or 'where's my love?' And when the Britishers first heard the call in India, they described the whole sequence as – 'Oh, lor, oh, lor, how very hot it's getting – we feel it, we feel it, WE FEEL IT!'

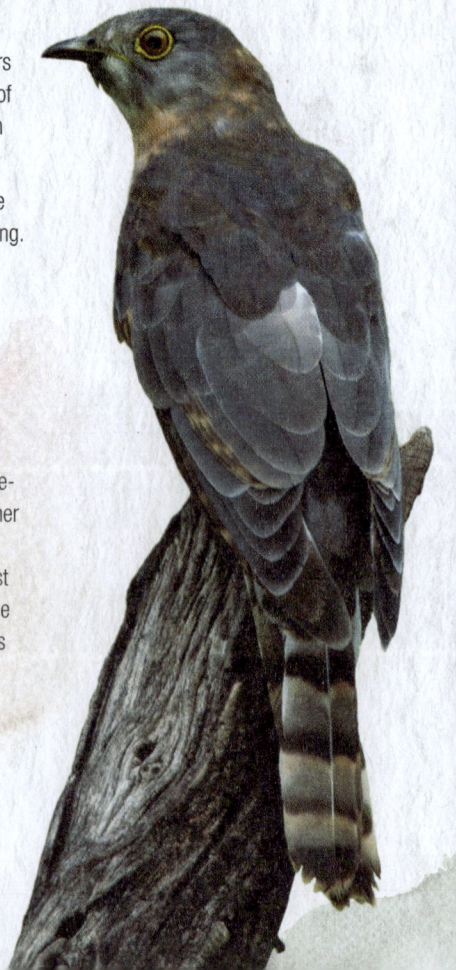

Each Little Bird That Sings

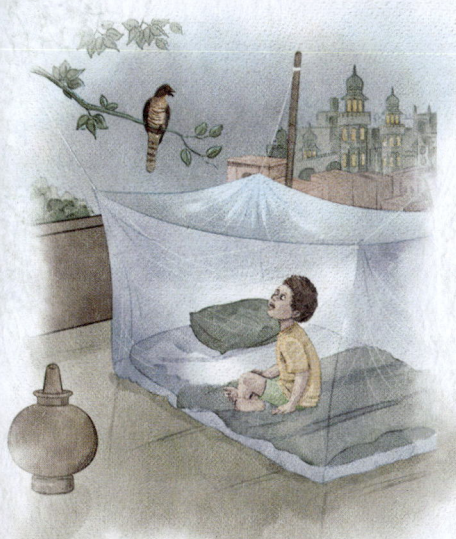

Mythology, Tales & Trivia

According to K.N. Davé, *Manusmriti* 12.7 says that the theft of drinking water would result in the thief being reborn as a Hawk Cuckoo, constantly calling and begging for a few drops of rain water.

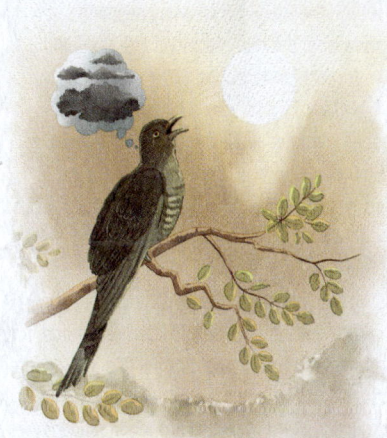

The Papiha is the subject of many a Hindi poem or song, as it signifies the yearning for a loved one who is not there.

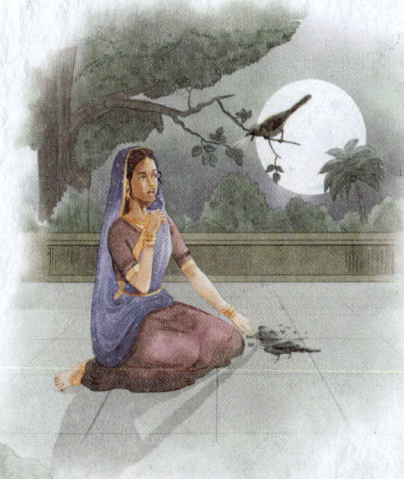

K.N. Davé also talked about another tale involving the Common Hawk Cuckoo. The poet Jamaal wrote a verse in Hindi, in which a lovelorn damsel is missing her love even more due to the moonlit night, the cool breeze, and the call of the Papiha. So, on the ground she draws a crow to silence the cuckoo; Rahu to swallow the moon; a python to swallow the breeze; and Lord Shiva to suppress the God of Love. But as soon as she hears her love returning, she quickly rubs them out.

Jayantika Davé

Black-headed Jay

Scientific name: *Garrulus lanceolatus*   Size: *33 cm*
Hindi name: *Ban Sarrah, Ban Bakra*
Sanskrit name: *Vanchaash*

Description

The Black-headed Jay is a beautiful resident of the Himalayas. An unmistakable bird, with a pinkish-fawn long coat with blue, black and white barred lapels, a black-and-white cravat, with the whole being topped off with a smart black cap! A noisy bird, this – rightfully earning its scientific name 'Garrulus'!

Habits

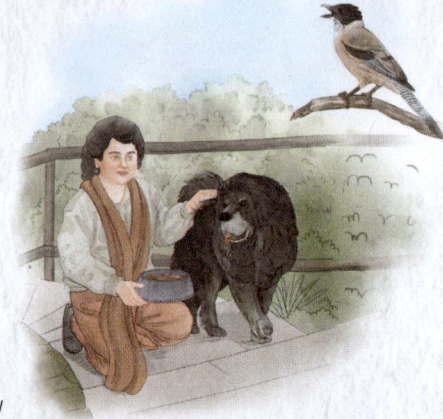

A resident of the Himalayas, from 1,500 m to 3,000 m, the Black-headed Jay descends somewhat in the harsh winters. The Ban Bakra loves forests, preferring a mix of coniferous and oak, and is also very comfortable in wooded gardens and around human beings. In Glen Haven, it waits for me to put out the grain in the feeder, or for us to mix up the food for our dogs Shogun and Buddy, and if there is a delay, it will call out raucously, raising its untidy black crest, asking us to hurry it up! Food in the wild is fruits, berries, lizards, rodents and the eggs and fledglings of small birds. When the oak trees are full of acorns, there is a lot of Black-headed Jay activity in them, as they hold the acorns with their feet, and hack them open with strong blows of their beak. A gregarious bird, it moves around in small flocks of 4–10 individuals.

Call

A harsh skaaak-skaak call, with much crest-raising when alarmed!

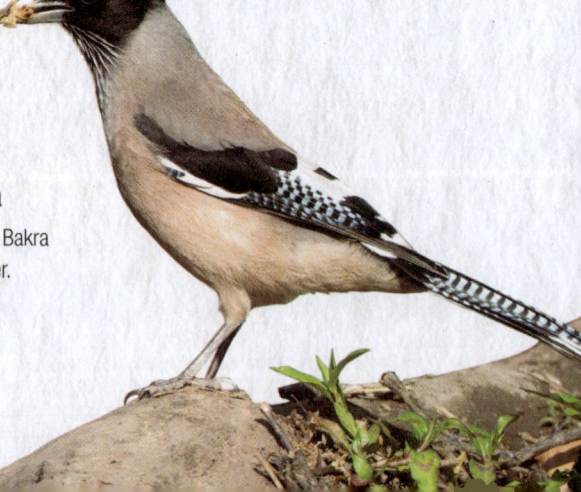

Mythology, Tales & Trivia

A great lover of acorns, the Ban Bakra stores them away for eating later.

It used to be called the Black-throated Jay!

Black-winged Kite

Scientific name: *Elanus caeruleus* Size: 33 cm
Hindi name: *Kapassi, Masunwa*
Sanskrit name: *Shablira Chilli*

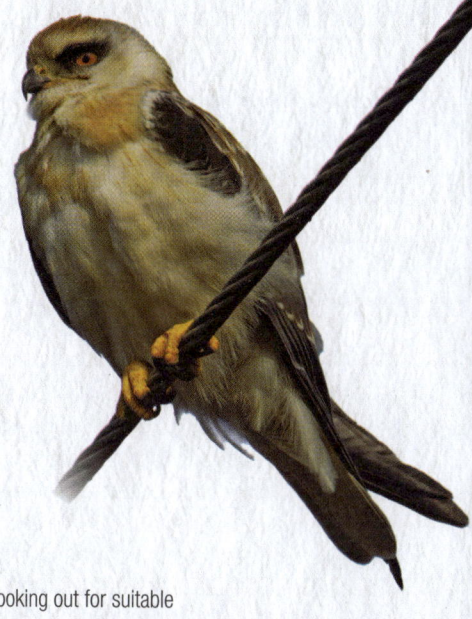

Description

A slim, elegant, dainty, grey-and-white kite, with distinctive black shoulder epaulettes, and black kajal outlining a red eye! Look out for the Black-winged Kite on electric lines in cities, with many more sightings as you drive out into the countryside, where the sit-and-tail-wag behaviour catches the eye!

Habits

The favourite haunts of the Kapassi are open grasslands dotted with small trees and bushes, or dry open areas, where prey can be sighted easily. It identifies a perch on a wire or a tree, looking out for suitable prey, periodically wagging its tail. Having seen something interesting, it will sally forth, making quartering flights as it descends lower and lower, often hovering with wings held high, somewhat like a Kestrel, till it does the final plunge-and-grab. It eats its prey on the ground or carries it back to the perch, sometimes even finishing it in flight. Favourite foods are rodents, small birds, insects and reptiles.

Call

Generally silent, with a soft, thin pee-oo call when it is courting or approaching the nest!

Jayantika Davé

Partridge, Chukar

Scientific name: *Alectoris chukar*   Size: *38 cm*
Hindi name: *Chukor*
Sanskrit name: *Chakor*

Description

One of the highlights of a trip to Ladakh or the upper reaches of the Himalayas is the sighting of the dapper Chukar Partridge. Imagine a stout matron, in a soft greyish-brown coat with smart black stripes on the sides and a black-edged scarf, making a splash with bright red shoes and red lipstick!

Habits

A resident of the Himalayas, up to 5,000 m, is the Chukor, a lover of craggy, stony bare ground, with some shrub cover. These birds are ground feeders and forage for roots, new shoots of grass, berries, insects and grains, working their way steadily up a mountain. While they progress with the usual waddling gait of the partridges, if alarmed, they can break into a fast run, and are also strong fliers, preferring to fly downhill to hide amongst the rocks. Often seen in the proximity of water, they also frequent patches of cultivated land for easy access to grain.

There is an elaborate courtship display by the male, involving head-tilting, displaying the barred flanks, circling the female, and finally begging with lowered head and wings!

Call

A chuk-chukor-chuk-chukor call is used, becoming more anxious and quicker when alarmed!

Mythology, Tales & Trivia

There are many myths about the Chukar – that it is passionately devoted to the moon and thrives on moonlight for food; that it feeds on burning charcoal and hence its beak is so red; that it eats only stones!

Kabir and Surdas have famous couplets dedicated to the Chakor, and there are many folk songs in regional languages that describe its devotion to the moon.

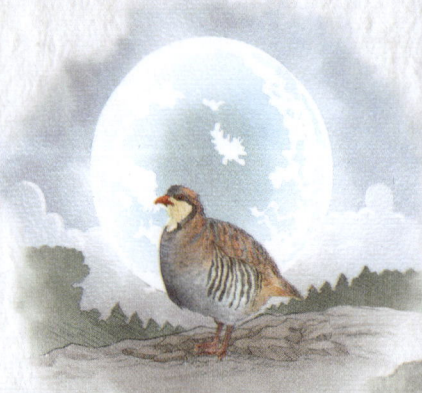

Brown-headed Gull

Scientific name: *Choicocephalus brunnicephalus*   Size: 42cm
Hindi name: *Bhuri Ganga Chilli*
Sanskrit name: *Babhru Shirsha Gangachilli* (The Sanskrit name for gulls is Veechi-kaak or Wave-bird or Wave-crow, because of the way they bob happily up and down on the waves, even on the roughest sea days.)

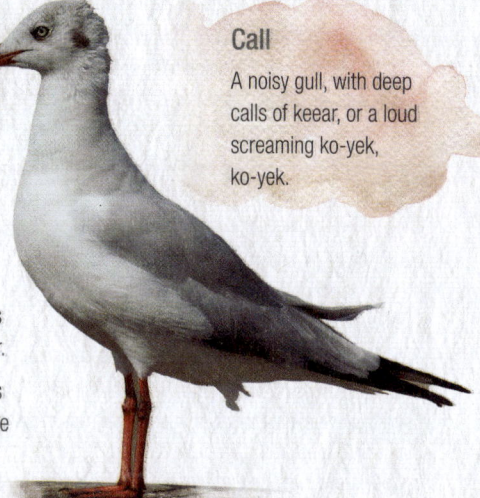

Description

In winter, along our coastline, and over large lakes and water bodies, can be seen the Brown-headed Gull, unmistakable in breeding plumage with its clear brown head atop a grey-and-white body. A little harder to identify when it is not breeding and loses the brown on its head…but then the triangular white mirrors on its black wing tips are the other identifier.

A slightly smaller, though very similar, gull is the **Black-headed Gull**, with a distinct white 'mirror flash' on its upper wing.

Call

A noisy gull, with deep calls of keear, or a loud screaming ko-yek, ko-yek.

Habits

A widespread winter visitor, gangs of often a few hundred of the Bhuri Ganga Chilli can be seen flying over large water bodies and our coastline areas, head moving left and right as it surveys the water for whatever prey it can find. Its favourite diet is fish and shrimps, with insects and worms also being occasionally taken with a quick swoop, and then the searching flight again after the prey is eaten. They swarm around fish markets and fishing boats, waiting for the offal that is thrown away.

They breed in summer in Ladakh, where upwards of 50 pairs congregate on islands on high-altitude lakes, and build large bulky nests of plant stems.

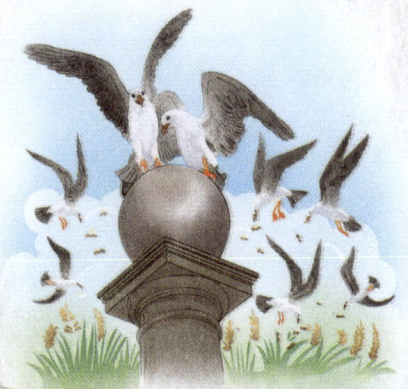

Mythology, Tales & Trivia

In Salt Lake City, there is a memorial of the bronze figures of two gulls, with the citation 'In grateful remembrance'. This was erected because from 1848 to 1850 in Utah, there was an invasion of black crickets, and the crops would have been completely decimated if it were not for the California Gulls that devoured the crickets and saved the crops.

Jayantika Davé

River Tern

Scientific name: *Sterna aurantia*   Size: 42 cm
Hindi name: *Dariai Taheri, Kurri*
Sanskrit name: *Nadi Kurri*

Description

A trip to any large water body, or wide stream or river, is incomplete without a sighting of the large, streamlined River Tern, with its bright yellow beak, and with or without a black head depending on whether it is breeding season or not. Terns are distinguishable from gulls by their relatively slimmer bodies, deeply angled wings, and deeply forked tails.

Habits

A widespread resident across India, it is found on all large inland water bodies. It feeds on fish, insects and small crustaceans, hovering, and then plunging into the waters to quickly catch its prey, often swallowing it in flight. On Chambal River, these birds make a pretty sight, as they fly along behind our boat, swooping for prey that has been disturbed and therefore surfaces. River Terns never settle on the water or perch on trees. Once they are fully fed, they sit in groups on the water edge. They nest together with Pratincoles and Skimmers on river sandbanks.

Mythology, Tales & Trivia

Sometimes called the Sea Swallow due to its habit of collecting food from the surface of the water, like a swallow!

It does not have a back toe, and hence is unable to perch.

Since they nest at a time when the sand is already very hot, they don't need to brood but instead fly around feeding.

If the nest gets flooded out due to a sudden rise in water levels, a second clutch will be laid.

Call
A short, sharp kiuk-kiuk as it flies!

Grey Hornbill

Scientific name: *Ocyceros birostris*   Size: *50 cm*
Hindi name: *Dhanesh, Chalotra, Dhanmar, Dhand, Dhanel, Lamdar, Selagilli*
Sanskrit name: *Vadhreernas, Matrinindak* (meaning 'one who puts the mother to shame', reflecting the care that the male takes of the female and the chicks)

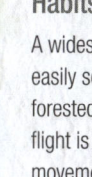

Description

When I am in the vicinity of a peepul or banyan tree in fruit, and I catch sight of the ungainly, heavy flight in of a few large grey birds, accompanied by loud pieu-pieu ringing calls, I know that the Grey Hornbills are visiting! The beak is its most significant feature – big and heavy, and with a large casque over the top of the bill.

A very similar resident of the Western Ghats is the **Malabar Grey Hornbill,** which lacks the casque and has an orange or yellow bill.

Habits

A widespread resident across India, it is easily seen in parks, woodlands and lightly forested areas with fruiting trees, as their flight is noisy and flapping, and all their movements are pretty clumsy and ungainly! Their flight is typical – a series of rapid strokes, followed by sailing.

The tennis courts at the Delhi Gymkhana Club are ringed with ancient peepul, banyan and other fig trees…so in the fruiting season, they are host to large numbers of the Dhanmar…usually flying overhead in a follow-the-leader fashion, at the very time that one of us is throwing up a ball to serve! Joyful distraction!

The nest is made in the natural cavity of a tree. The female seals herself off in the nest, closing off the entrance with a mix of droppings and mud, and emerges only after the fledglings have grown. Once she seals herself in, only a narrow slit is left through which her beak emerges, so that the dutiful male can regurgitate food and feed her.

Mythology, Tales & Trivia

The eyelids have lovely long eyelashes.
The casque or protuberance on top of the bill develops with age.
In ancient times, the flesh was used medicinally to alleviate the pangs of childbirth.

Call

A penetrating ka-kak-kak or gentler ringing pi-pi-pipipieu-pipipieu.

Jayantika Davé

Western Reef Egret

Scientific name: *Egretta gularis*   Size: 60 cm
Hindi name: *Kala Bagla*
Sanskrit name: *Krishna Bak*

Description

When you are visiting the coastal areas of India, mainly the west and southeast coasts, look out for this very dark egret (or heron as it was earlier called), waiting patiently on the sea shore at high tide for the tide to ebb, or actively foraging at the seashore and in low waters. The distinct leggy look, and uniformly dark-grey colouring with a bright white chin, make it easy to identify. It does have a white morph too, when it can be confused with the **Little Egret**. I enjoy looking at these birds, particularly at dawn or dusk when, with their dark colouring and still stance, they look like statues set amongst the dark seaside rocks.

Habits

An inhabitant of sea coastlines, it forages in shallow waters, looking for fish, worms and crustaceans. When it is high tide, it waits patiently in a hunched-up posture, and as the tide ebbs, it strides forth, picking at what has been left on the shore, moving quicker than other herons do. The Kala Bagla is active during the day, and often uses foot-stirring to unearth buried food, which it captures with a quick dash.

Call
A grunt or a harsh squawk!

Each Little Bird That Sings

Grey Junglefowl

Scientific name: _Gallus sonneratii_   Size: 75 cm
Hindi name: _Jungli Murgha, Ban Murgha, Bhoori Ban Murgi_
Sanskrit name: _Yavgreev Tamrachood_

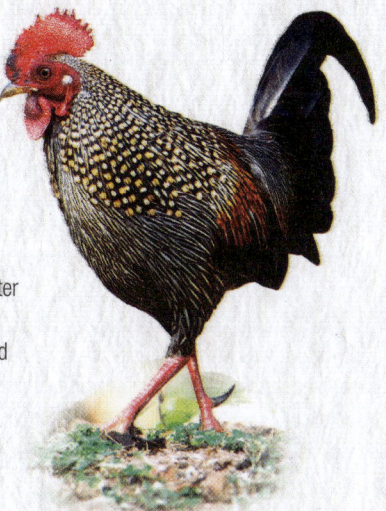

Description

While I had earlier got quick sightings of the Grey Junglefowl, my first leisurely sighting of this gorgeous bird was in Thattekad, where we kept hearing the call but couldn't see the bird. After a patient wait, out strutted this large male in full breeding plumage – the white-and-black-speckled neck shining against a grey-and-gold body, finished with a long, arched, purple-black, iridescent tail – what a sight!

Habits

The favourite habitat of the Jungli Murgha is scrubby undergrowth in evergreen and mixed forests in the Ghats and peninsular India, where it is found up to a height of 2,400 m. The berries of lantana are a particular favourite, and these plants are a good place to wait for a sighting. Young grass, berries, figs, insects and reptiles are the other food it enjoys, sometimes seeking out cattle and elephant dung and picking through that. Grey Junglefowls move around in pairs, or small groups of 5–6 birds, though sometimes an even larger number can be seen in the vicinity of a particularly prolific berry bush. The Grey Junglefowl is a shy and wary bird, scuttling off into undergrowth with a typical neck-stretched-out and drooping-tail action!

Call

A loud kuk-ka-kurruk-ka, sometimes accompanied by wing-flapping, like that of the domesticated cock!

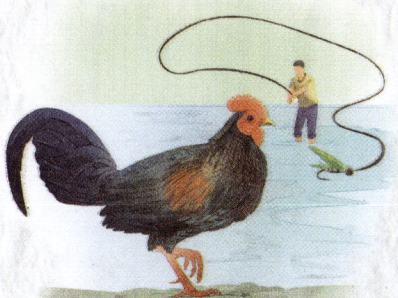

Mythology, Tales & Trivia

The hackle feathers of the male cock, at the back of the neck and upper back, are a shiny black, marked with metallic yellow spots and streaks, and are much in demand by anglers for making the flies in fly fishing.

Jayantika Davé

Demoiselle Crane

Scientific name: *Anthropoides virgo*   Size: *95 cm*
Hindi name: *Karkara, Koonj, Karkatiya*
Sanskrit name: *Khar Kronch, Kurkretu*

Description

Every time I see the elegant Demoiselle Crane, I can just see it beautifully represented as a painting by a Japanese artist! A particular favourite of my father, these beautiful cranes are a study in grey and white…the white plumes sweeping out beyond the eye, and the black neck plumes cascading out well beyond the curve of the breast…unforgettable!

Habits

The Karkara is a winter visitor, primarily to the Western part of India. Its favourite habitat is open semi-arid grasslands, with some proximity to water. It feeds on seeds of grasses, grains, other vegetation, insects, worms and lizards. A highly gregarious bird, it moves in large flocks, flying in typical V formation, and rests up during the heat of the day on sandbanks alongside jheels.

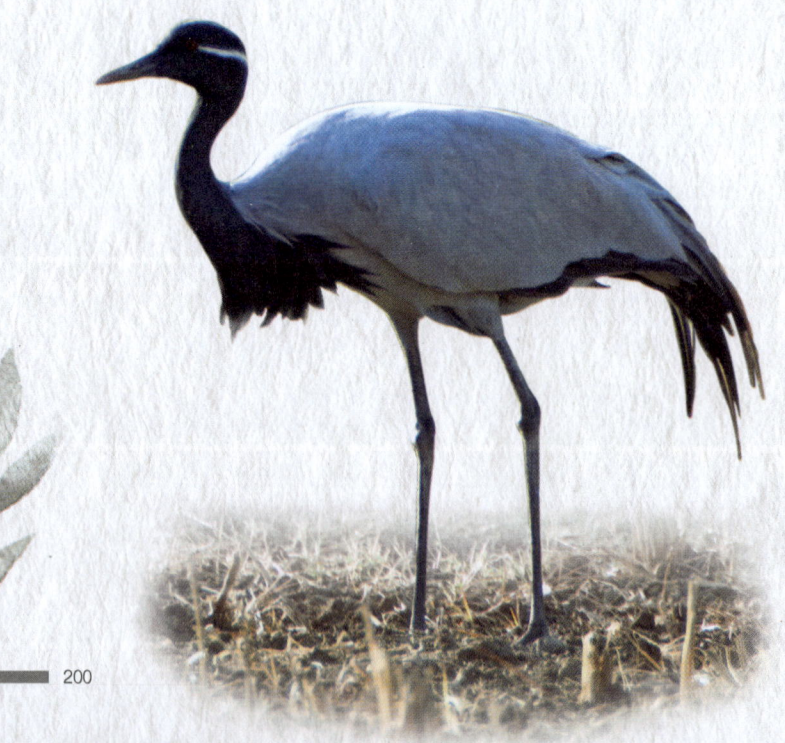

Call

A husky, loud, trumpeting garrooo-garroo in flight. Salim Ali describes this beautifully – 'the din of a great concourse of koonj taking off from the ground, with their kurr-kurr calls uttered in varying keys, has been aptly likened to the distant roaring of the sea!'

Mythology, Tales & Trivia

Khichan, a village in Rajasthan, is famous for the number of Demoiselle Cranes it attracts. In the 1970s, a local couple had started putting out grain for pigeons, and found that they were attracting Demoiselle Cranes too. Soon other villagers joined in, and now, from late August to March, more than 30,000 cranes are fed daily!

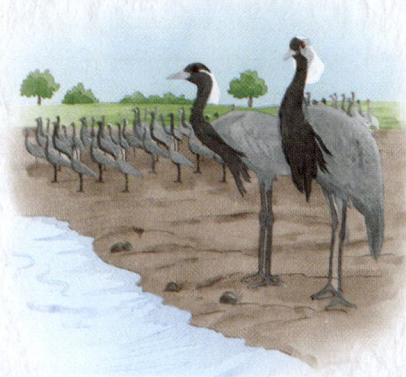

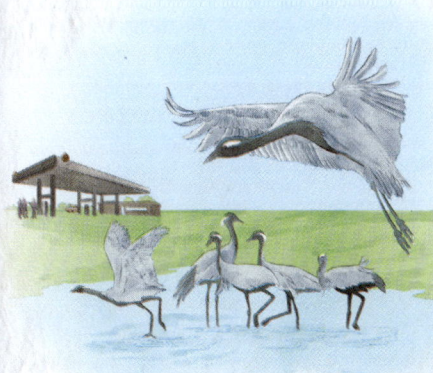

Once, we were birding in the Great Rann of Kutch, and soon it was time to leave. And while the beauty of the Karkara still filled my heart, I was sad that we wouldn't see them for a long while. We stopped to fill petrol at a petrol pump…and suddenly, with loud 'garrooo-garroo' calls, a whole flight of Demoiselle Cranes landed at a small water body just behind the pump, and we could watch them again! I felt like a wish had been granted!

Jayantika Davé

Grey Heron

Scientific name: *Ardea cinerea*   Size: 94 cm
Hindi name: *Anjan, Nari, Sain, Kabud*
Sanskrit name: *Parssik Anjan Bak*

Description

Tall, long-legged, plumed elegance in grey, black and white, with a dash of black buttons down the breast? The Grey Heron has it all! A widespread resident and winter visitor across all of India, the Anjan frequents water bodies, lakes and rivers, standing still and statuesque, till it does a sudden jab to spear a tasty morsel of fish. During breeding season, it is an even lovelier sight, with the neck and head plumes becoming thicker and more elongated, and the legs turning a deep orange-red.

The **Purple Heron** is similar in silhouette to the Grey Heron, but perhaps more striking, with a deeper blue-grey colouration, and a distinctive chestnut neck.

Habits

The Grey Heron is very easy in its choice of habitat, so long as there is enough shallow water present. It prefers areas with borders of trees, shrubs, islands and low vegetation, but is equally at home in large open bodies of water, canals, rivers and irrigated fields. While primarily a lowlands bird, it has been recorded in Ladakh at 3,500 m. Its diet is mainly fish, crabs, eels, crustaceans, snakes, small mammals and sometimes small birds and chicks. It is a day heron, and is usually a solitary bird, standing quiet, hunched up, seemingly asleep, but always watchful, as the quick successful jab of the powerful neck and beak at unsuspecting prey shows!

It nests colonially, in mixed colonies with storks, cormorants, spoonbills and ibis.

Call
A loud guttural frarnk or gwark.

Common Crane

Scientific name: *Grus grus* Size: *115 cm*
Hindi name: *Kraunch, Kronch, Kulang*
Sanskrit name: *Kraunch, Lakshman Sarus*

Description

During winter, in the Little and Great Ranns of Kutch, look overhead to see these tangled skeins of birds, flying high in a V formation. One bird calls, and all the others answer, drawing the eye upwards to see where these resounding krrroah-krrroah calls are coming from! And what an elegant sight the Common Crane is…grey suit, with a black polo-neck, a lovely plumed tail and a red beret!

Habits

A lover of open grasslands with sufficient shallow water around, the Common Crane has a particular preference for the rhizomes of grasses. This combination makes the Little and Great Ranns of Kutch a very attractive habitat for them. I will never forget two sights…one was when on our first trip to the Little Rann of Kutch, the air suddenly filled with these deep calls, and then flight after flight of the Kraunch took off and kept wheeling overhead, till the sky was dark with hundreds of them!

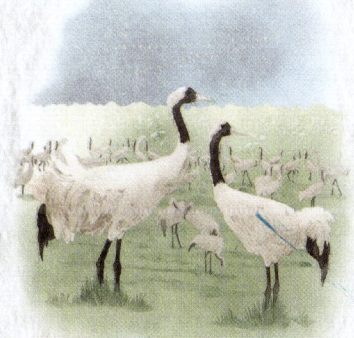

Another time, we were in the Great Rann of Kutch, and in one huge open grassland, there were thousands and thousands of these cranes, probing, picking and feeding busily on the grass rhizomes…so many that there wasn't an empty patch on the horizon! And to top it all, as we left, endless flights went overhead, heading out to the fields to feed at dusk, filling the evening with their calls! A day completely filled with wonder!

Call

A deep, throaty, far-carrying krroah-krooah call!

Mythology, Tales & Trivia

The Common Crane arrives in winter from West Siberia, travelling a long route through Afghanistan and Pakistan, to finally winter in North, West and Central India.

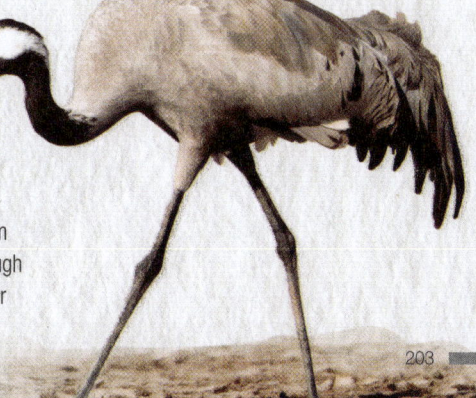

Jayantika Davé

Sarus Crane

Scientific name: *Antigone antigone* Size: *156 cm*
Hindi name: *Sarus*
Sanskrit name: *Lakshman Sarus*

Description

A really large, unforgettable crane, the Sarus Crane is a study in grey and white, with a striking red head and orange-red legs. When we were children, my father took us to visit a friend of his who lived on a farm, and as we entered, this Sarus came striding up, looked us straight in the eye, approved, and let us in! It was a pet Sarus – aptly named Colonel – and we were completely enthralled!

Habits

The devotion of a Sarus pair is legendary, and because of that, villagers protect them and their young. They are quite comfortable with human presence, feeding and nesting in fields, shallow wetlands and ponds. Their primary diet is grasses, grains, snails, crustaceans, frogs, fish and snakes. Even though the Sarus is globally endangered, at certain times of the year, and in the right environs, it is possible to see up to 100 birds in one morning!

The mating display is absolutely spectacular, with the pair facing each other, bowing, and then leaping, prancing and dancing – a beautiful sight!

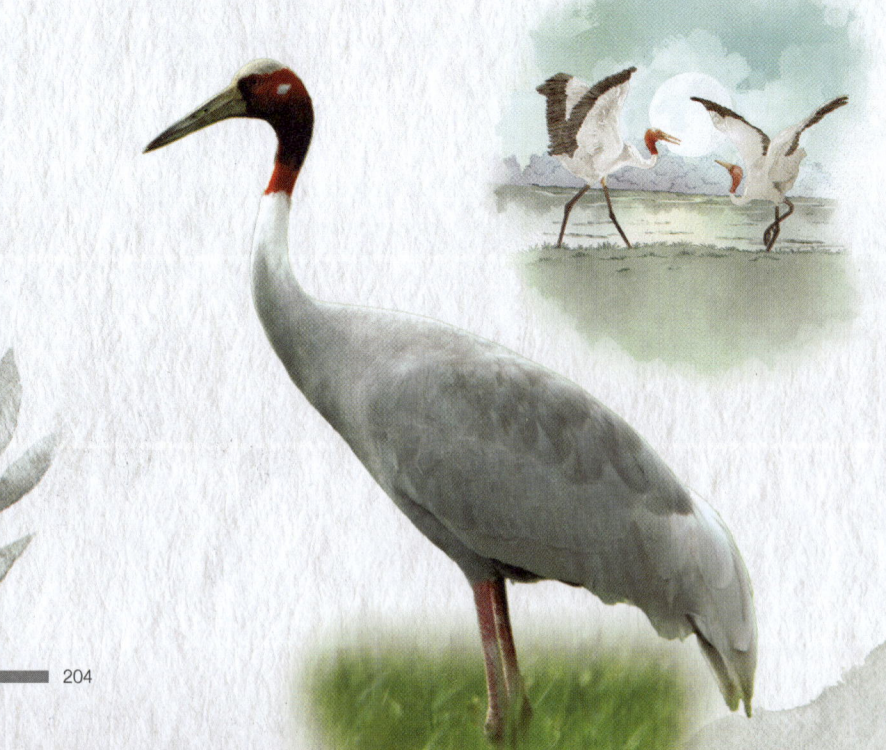

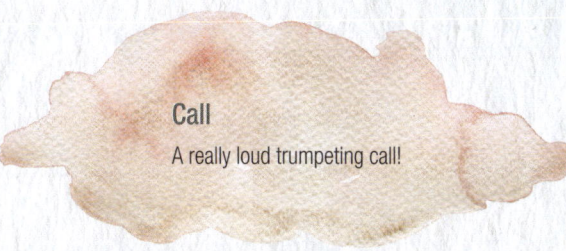

Call
A really loud trumpeting call!

Mythology, Tales & Trivia

A legend about the creation of the Ramayana attributes it to the devotion of a Sarus pair. The sage Valmiki once saw a female sarus, loudly wailing at the loss of her mate who had just been killed by a hunter. Valmiki was so outraged that from his mouth poured a curse on the fowler, set in a four-part metre. He marvelled at what he had said, and pronounced that these should be called shlokas (Ramayana 1.2.9-12). When he returned to his hermitage, Lord Brahma appeared, and told him that the shlokas had emanated from him at Brahma's will, and that he should now create the story of Rama, calling it the Ramayana, which would endure till times immemorial. And that is how the Valmiki Ramayana came into being!

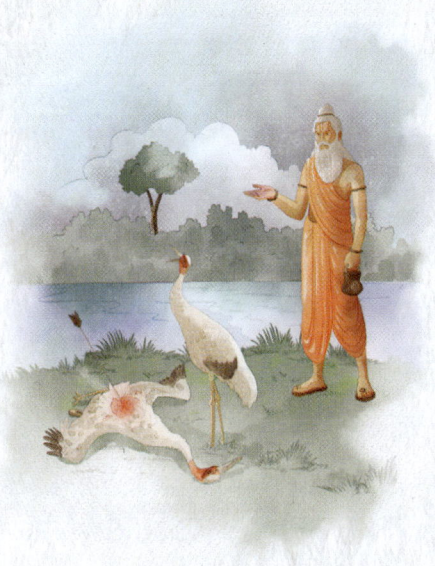

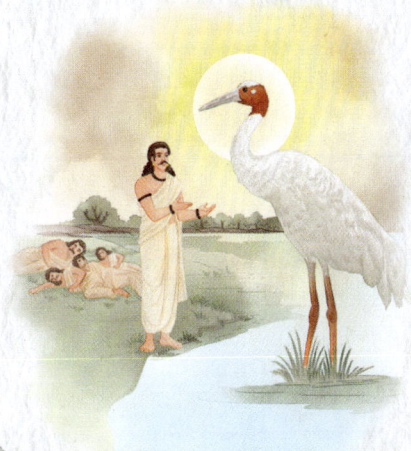

During the Pandavas' 12-year exile in the forest, Yudhishtir sends his brothers, one by one, to fetch water from a nearby lake. They all fail to return, and when he goes himself, he sees them all dead. He then hears the voice of a crane, which asks him to answer 18 questions on dharma, which his brothers had refused to answer. He answers correctly, and his brothers come back to life.

These 18 questions are appended in the Mahabharata as Dharma Baka Upakhyan – The Legend of the Virtuous Crane.

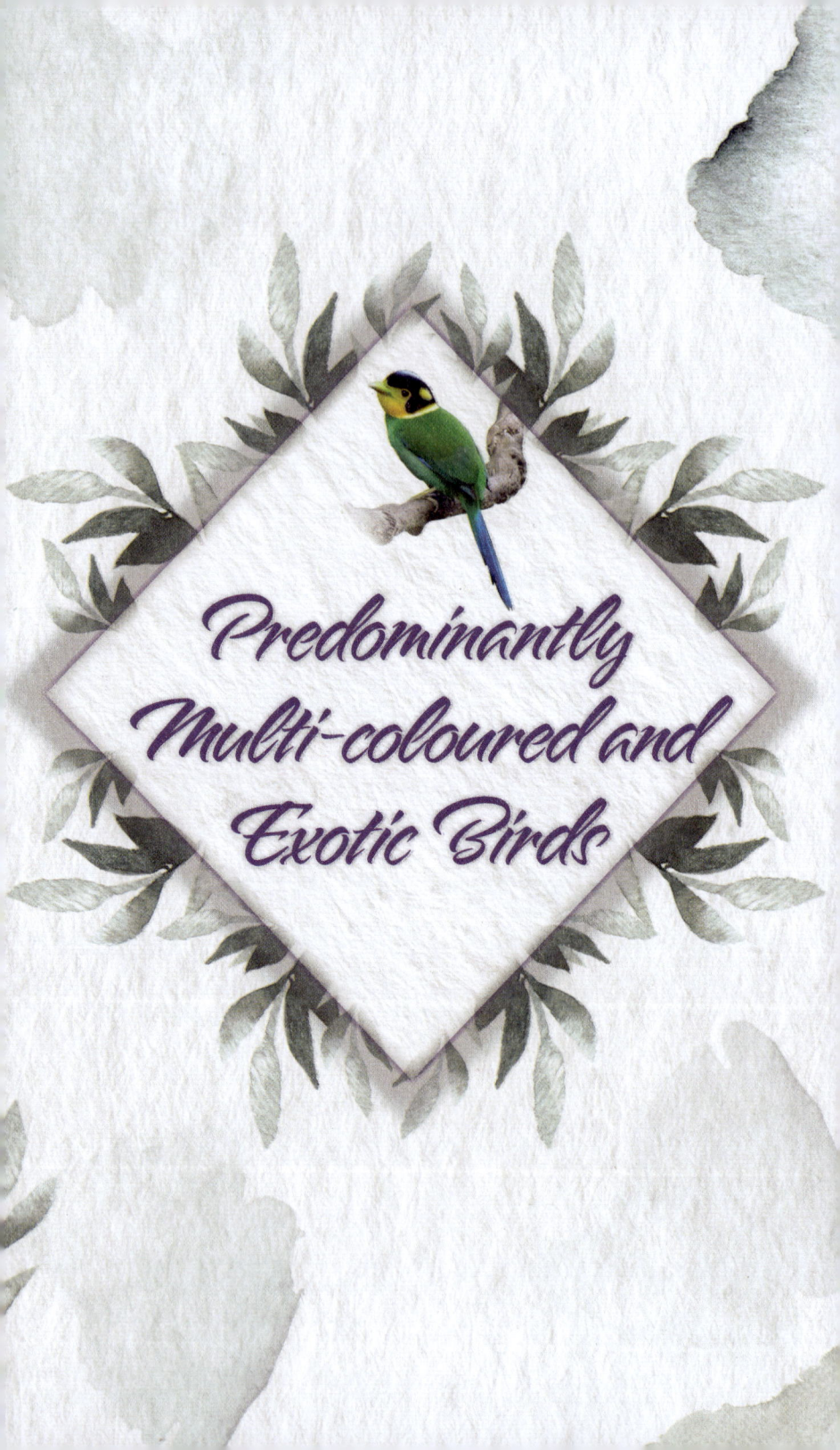

Each Little Bird That Sings

Red-billed Leiothrix

Scientific name: *Leiothrix lutea*   Size: *13 cm*
Hindi name: *Jharjhari, Nandan-chiri, Nandani*
Sanskrit name: *Rochishnu*

Description

The Red-billed Leiothrix is a pretty little beauty – a study in grey, highlighted with flaming shades of gold and orange, and topped with a bright red beak! In the Himalayan hills, up to 4,000 m, this secretive bird looks dull as it moves amongst the foliage of trees, but as it emerges into the light, the breast flames gold and orange, the wing bars in black, gold and orange are in full display, and the bright red beak completes the picture!

Habits

The Jharjhari is a gregarious bird, found always in flocks of at least five birds, often going up to 10–15 or more. It forages for fruit, berries and insects amongst thick vegetation, conifers and the lower branches of evergreens. It is a busy little beaver – always on the move – hopping, seeking in the cracks of bark, and always singing! At 'The Hide' in Sat-tal, a place affectionately named by all birders who know Sat-tal, it is possible to get very clear sightings of the Red-billed Leiothrix, as it bathes in a small stream there, and preens on a strategically placed branch just above!

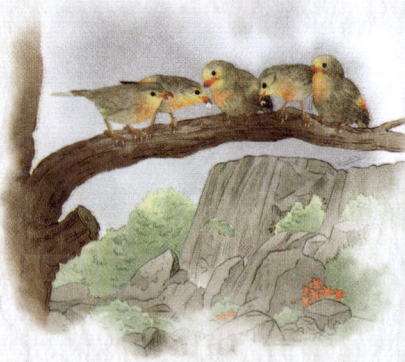

Call

A clear series of pepe-pe-pa and a faster pu-pu-pu-pu.

Mythology, Tales & Trivia

The males show off their singing prowess, particularly in the breeding season, and have been known to use up to 99 different sounding syllables in their song!

A native of the Himalayas, Southeast Asia and Southern China, the Leiothrix was imported into the Hawaiian Islands in 1911, and then deliberately released into the wild from 1918 onwards.

In the cage bird trade, it used to be known as the Peking Nightingale.

Jayantika Davé

Indian Pitta

Scientific name: *Pitta brachyura*   Size: *19 cm*
Hindi name: *Naorang*
Sanskrit name: *Padmapushpa*

Description

The Hindi name of Naorang is the perfect description for this almost tail-less, small, upright carriage bird! So, colour a bird a soft, glowing pinkish-beige, add dark blue-green to the back, blue to the rump, a splash of a glossy turquoise green-blue on the wings, a bright scarlet red belly and undertail and a black eye-mask – and you have the exotic Indian Pitta! Much like one of the favourite Indian jewellery designs – the Navratna.

Habits

Breeding in the Himalayas, and descending to Central and West India in the summer, and further to the coastal South Indian areas in winter, the Indian Pitta is found amongst the undergrowth of forested areas. It forages for earthworms, insects, snails and worms, behaving very much like a thrush, tossing dried leaves aside as it digs underneath them, with much rustling, and wagging its stumpy tail up and down! We had some lovely uninterrupted sightings of the Indian Pitta in the Thattekad Bird Sanctuary, where it was easy to see in the undergrowth of the areas surrounding the home of Eldhose, who is an amazing bird guide and host!

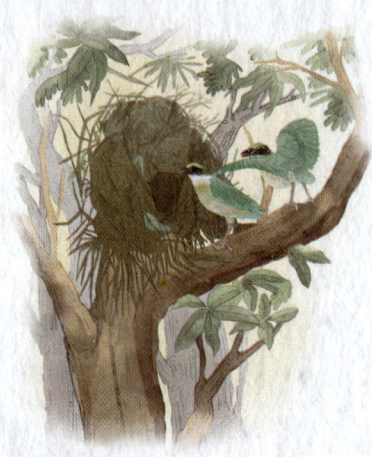

Breeding season coincides with the rains, with a large football-shaped nest being made of twigs, leaves and grass, placed in a small tree, and with a side entrance being created.

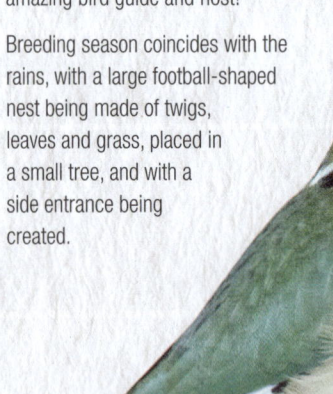

Call

A clear whistling pree-teee, pree-teee, sometimes sounding like 'quite clear, quite clear!'

Each Little Bird That Sings

Long-tailed Broadbill

Scientific name: *Psarisomus dalhousiae*   Size: 28 cm
Local name: *Dang Mo-mith*
Sanskrit name: *Rajishuk*

Description

The Long-tailed Broadbill is a bird dressed up for a fancy-dress party! It chose a bright green coat with blue edging, added a sunshine-yellow scarf, and for some reason, topped off its costume with a black skull cap with a blue spot on the crown! It is a resident of the Himalayan foothills, and not very common – so a sighting is always wondrous!

Habits

The Long-tailed Broadbill is typically found in forested areas in the Himalayan foothills, with a weakness for forested ravines, usually with some running water around. I have seen it only singly, or in pairs, but up to six individuals can inhabit one area.

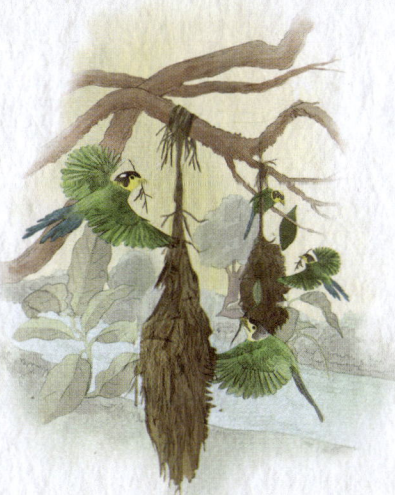

They feed in the trees, and down to thick undergrowth, often climbing up creepers, constantly gleaning for insects, bugs, butterflies, caterpillars and spiders. For me, my 'flash upon the inward eye' moment has been when we watched two pairs building their nests. The nests were big round balls, hung from a really long woven rope, looped and secured to a branch of a tall tree at the edge of a ravine, and so the balls swung free! We sat on a neighbouring slope, and watched for over an hour, while two pairs of these beautiful birds kept flying back and forth – building…building…building! An unforgettable sight!

Call

A loud whistling pseew-weeiuw-weeiuw repeated at quick intervals!

Jayantika Davé

Amur Falcon

Scientific name: *Falco amurensis*   Size: 29 cm

Description

In October, the little Amur Falcon begins to arrive in Nagaland and Manipur, and moves patchily to other parts of India later, having flown a distance of around 20,000 km! A sturdy, courageous warrior, this is one bird that every bird lover should make a special trip to see!

Habits

On arrival in India, they congregate in open areas bordered by some wooded areas, foraging for insects and grasshoppers, sometimes small birds and frogs. The Indian Ocean crossing can take up to three days, all without food, so eating and building body fat is important for these little falcons. They roost colonially in the trees, and are noisy and vocal, filling the air with their shrill kew-kew-kew calls! During early morning and late evening, the air fills with huge numbers of them either taking off to hunt or return, and the sight of so many of them is absolutely exhilarating!

Call

A shrill kew-kew-kew, particularly while in the communal roost!

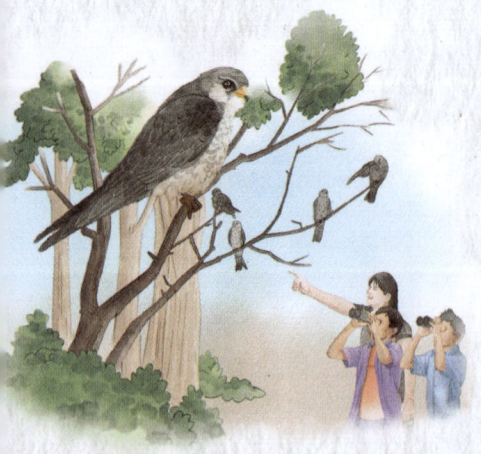

Mythology, Tales & Trivia

In Nagaland, these birds used to be captured in huge numbers for food, by placing large nets in their flight path. This came to the attention of Bano Haralu, a journalist and conservationist, who got a group of eminent conservationists together, and launched a TV campaign to draw the attention of the world to this annual massacre. The government then stepped in to stop this, and many people got together to educate the local people on the need to protect the Amur Falcons as a source of tourism income. This has proved to be a very successful conservation programme.

Their name has originated from Amur River.

Malabar Trogon

Scientific name: *Harpactes fasciatus* Size: 31 cm
Hindi name: *Kufni Chiri*
Sanskrit name: *Lohpakshi, Lohprishttha*

Description
In the forests and hills of the Western and Eastern Ghats is found this beautiful bird with a dignified demeanour, and a smart dress combination of a grey-black head and neck, a brown coat and a lovely red waistcoat!

Habits
The Malabar Trogon is a resident, and inhabits broad-leaf and semi-evergreen and moist forests up to 2,000 m. It picks up insects, beetles, moths and caterpillars and also enjoys some berries, continuing to hunt even after dusk.

As a hunting strategy, it sometimes follows mixed flocks of birds. We have seen this in the Thattekad forest, and it is such a still, silent bird that, despite its fairly brilliant colouring, it took us some time to locate it! But once we did, we were able to enjoy great viewings, since it continued to sit peacefully, its blue beak and blue eye ring gleaming in the dappled light.

Call
A throaty, pretty 'cue-cue-cue...'

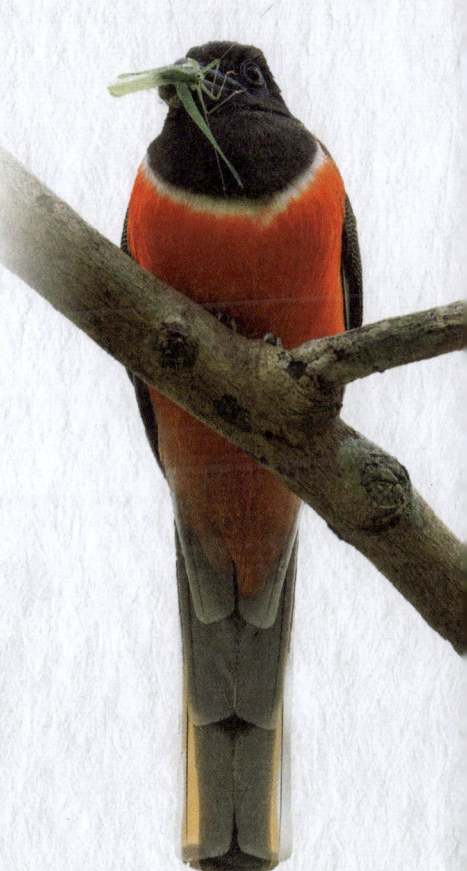

Jayantika Davé

Blood Pheasant

Scientific name: *Ithaginis cruentus*   Size: 38 cm
Local name: *Chiku, Same, Siri*
Sanskrit name: *Seerpaad*

Description

The Blood Pheasant is aptly named! A medium-sized plump pheasant, with a ragged crest, red bare skin around the eyes, blood-red throat, grey-white plumage splashed with blood, and fluorescent pale green undersides! Once, we were birding in Bhutan in end-February. It was freezing, there was snow all around, and there were beautiful icicles hanging off the conifers. We were at a fairly open snowy plain which was dotted with rocks, and suddenly a flock of the beautiful Blood Pheasants appeared, feeding unconcerned as we watched without moving! The sight of their fluorescent green-white plumage, splashed with blood red, will always stay as one of my 'flash upon the inward eye' moments!

Habits

A high-altitude resident of the Northeast Himalayas, the Blood Pheasant inhabits coniferous forests, rhododendron and other sub-alpine scrub, and can be seen up to 4,500 m. It feeds on grass shoots, insects, small fruits, seeds, bamboo shoots, berries and young leaves. It is a gregarious bird, and moves in small flocks of 5–20 birds, feeding in a very hen-like fashion, scratching, pecking and constantly moving.

The nest is a primitive small depression in the ground, lined with soft grass.

Call

When guarding its territory, a strident piercing kzeeuk-cheeu-cheeu-chee, otherwise a series of short clucks and long, trilling sree calls!

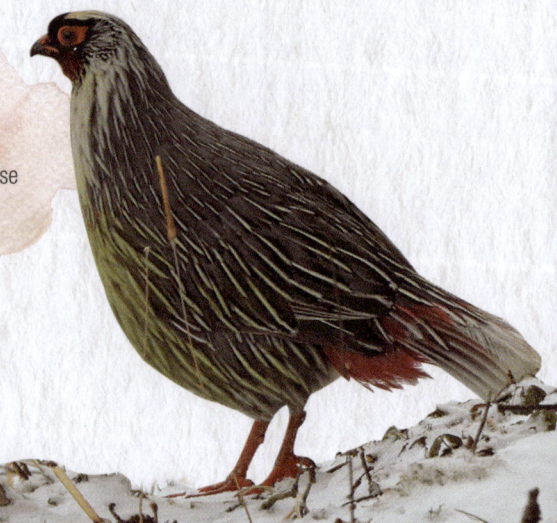

Satyr Tragopan

Scientific name: *Tragopan satyra*   Size: 70 cm
Hindi name: *Lungi*
Sanskrit name: *Jignu Juhuraan*

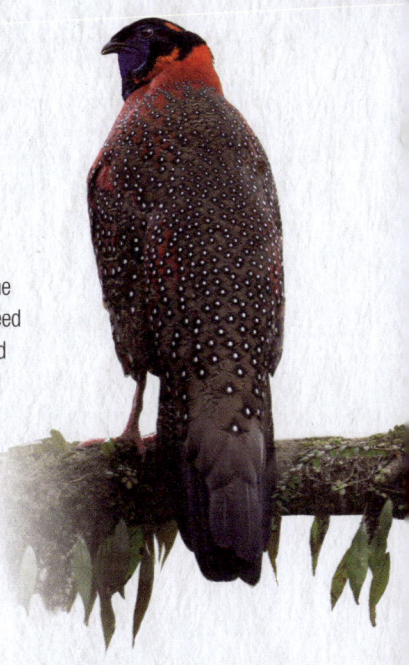

Description

A call that's the bellow of a bull, plumage that is as red as the depiction of the satyr (devil), and what you are seeing is indeed the stately Satyr Tragopan! The Tragopan has been described as the Ruby of the Himalayas in a newspaper article written in 1936, which I found tucked into my grandfather's book. A Bhutan trip, a 4.30 a.m. start, and there it was…sitting on a stump on the side of the road, deciding what to do with its day! And what it did that day was to saunter across the road, climb up the hill, and saunter back again, settling down always in clear sight, intermittently letting out the loud, bellowing 'moo-aaah, mooo-aaah' call! We were spell-bound… another of my 'inward eye' moments!

Habits

The Lungi is a resident of Central and East Himalayas, through to Nepal, Sikkim, Bhutan and Arunachal. A lover of broad-leaved forests up to 4,000 m, with an especial love for oak and rhododendron, with dense undergrowth and bamboo thickets. It forages for insects, grasses, roots and fruit, and is most active from the early morning till the afternoon. Its favourite haunts are wet spots near streams, where it overturns leaf litter looking for tasty morsels.

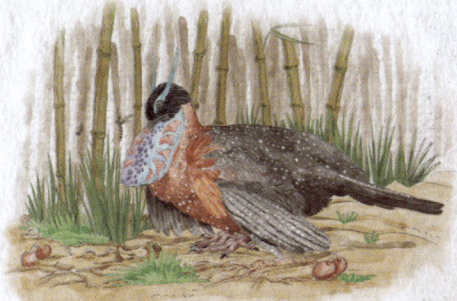

Call

Calls most often early in the morning, with a loud, echoing, deep 'moo-aaah, moo-aaah' repeated a number of times!

Mythology, Tales & Trivia

One of its Hindi names, Jiguraan, comes from a fusion of Persian and Sanskrit descriptions: *jaiga* = Persian for head ornament, *jignu* = fire in Sanskrit, *rana* = beautiful, *juhuran* = goat. So the complete description is—beautiful fiery bird, with a head ornament, horns and a bleat like a goat.

Jayantika Davé

Himalayan Monal

Scientific name: *Lophophorus impejanus*   Size: 70 cm
Hindi name: Monal, Neel Mor
Sanskrit name: *Suvarna-mayoor*; has a pretty analogue in Persian – 'Murgh-i-Zarreen' or the Golden Cock

Description

Take the colours of a peacock – iridescent blue, green, purple and copper – paint on a rufous-brown neck and tail, and complete the picture with a prominent rounded crest – and you are looking at the magnificent Himalayan Monal! And when we saw this beautiful Monal against a backdrop of pure white snow, it just took our breath away!

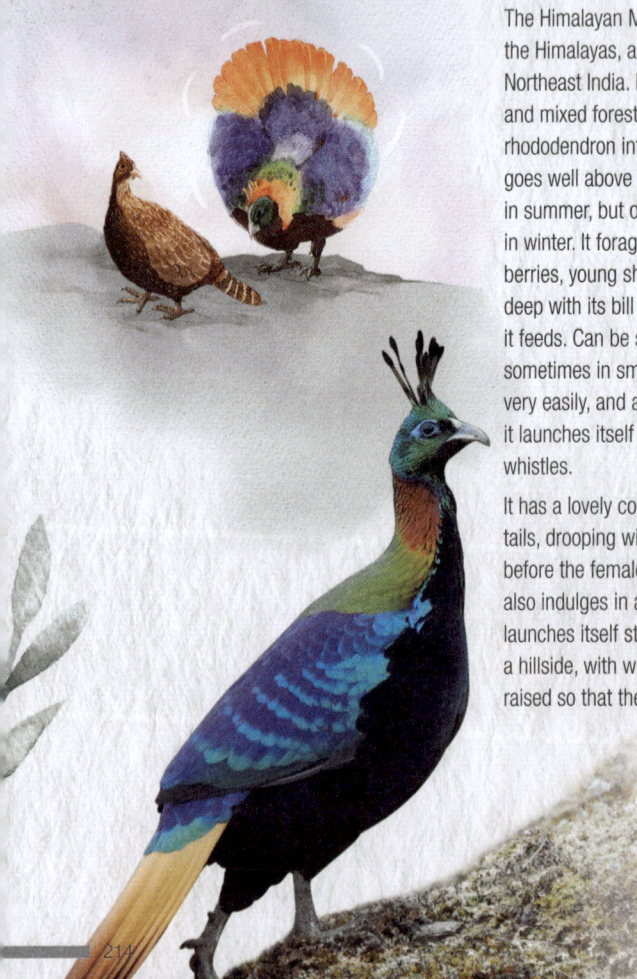

Habits

The Himalayan Monal is a resident of the Himalayas, all the way to Bhutan and Northeast India. It favours coniferous and mixed forests, particularly enjoying rhododendron interspersed with bamboo. It goes well above the tree line up to 4,000 m in summer, but descends to about 2,500 m in winter. It forages for seeds, tuberous roots, berries, young shoots and insects, digging deep with its bill and constantly moving as it feeds. Can be seen singly, or in pairs, and sometimes in small groups too. It alarms very easily, and at the slight hint of danger, it launches itself down the hillside with loud whistles.

It has a lovely courtship display of fanning tails, drooping wings, and much parading before the female. To impress a female, it also indulges in an aerial display, when it launches itself straight up into the air from a hillside, with wings held high, and the tail raised so that the white rump is very visible.

Call

A strangely curlew-like call – cur-lewww, cur-lewww, with the alarm call being described by Mackintosh as 'quick-quick-quick'!

Mythology, Tales & Trivia

In our scriptures, the name Indrabh has been used for the Monal, which was considered a fit gift for Kartikeya.

Its whistling calls, morning and evening, were noticed by the ancients, and interpreted as praying to the sun.

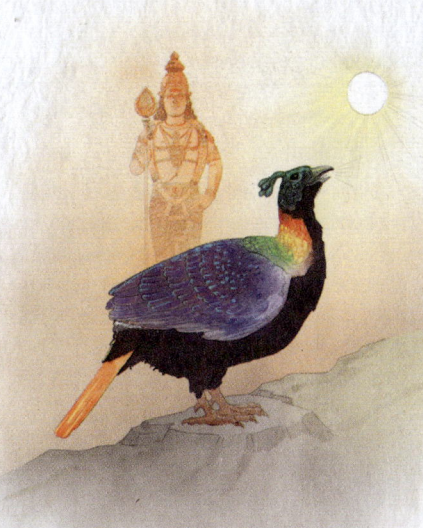

In Tibet, the Himalayan Monal has become comfortable enough with unthreatening human presence, and visits monasteries to take grain put out by the monks.

The name 'Monal' comes from the Prakrit *mrinal* = eating roots and tubers.

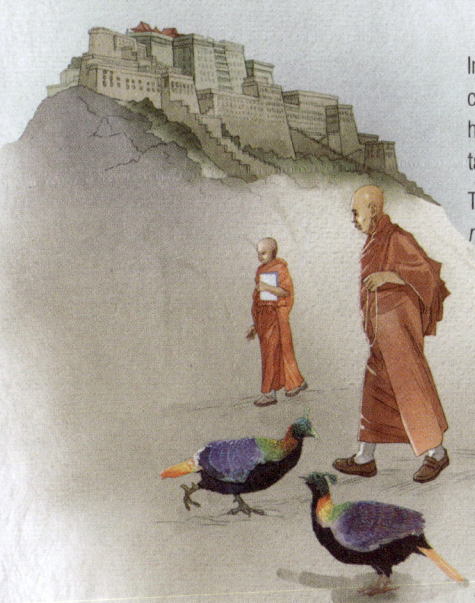

Jayantika Davé

Indian Peafowl

Scientific name: *Pavo cristatus*   Size: 200 cm
Hindi name: *Mor, Mayura*
Sanskrit name: *Mayura*

Description

The large, resplendent Indian Peafowl is a study in how all the colours of the rainbow can be put together in one gorgeous bird! Protected both by religious sentiment and the fact that it is our national bird, the Mor is a reasonably familiar sight around our villages and larger parks. The beauty of the Peafowl attracted many admirers, and from India, they were introduced to many parts of the world – to the Middle East during the tenth century BCE, and to Rome and Britain by the fourth century BCE. This spread is depicted in varied illustrations in manuscripts, paintings and inclusion in architecture elements.

Habits

A fairly gregarious bird, it moves around in groups of 4–5. Its loud screaming call and dance is a predictor of the monsoons, and the dance is a lovely sight, with a single male showing off all its colours, tail raised, slow pirouette, with a paroxysm of quivering, and all this effort directed at a bevy of completely uninterested drab females! The dance is so spectacular that it has been incorporated in various forms, in our classical as well as folk dances.

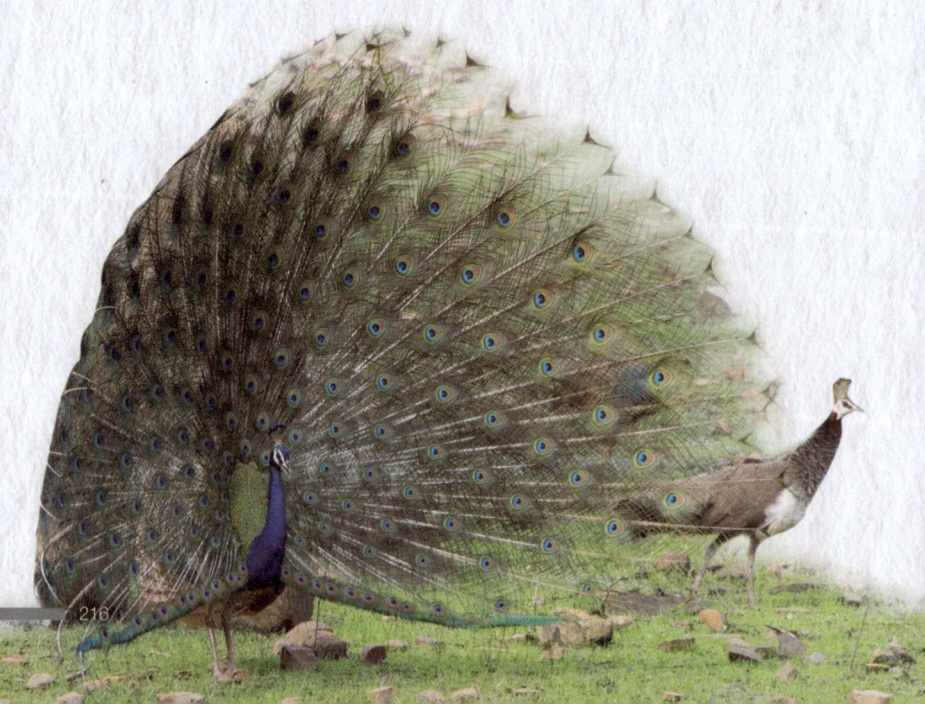

Call

A loud, braying call, may-awnh or '*minh* = rain + *aao* = come'.

Mythology, Tales & Trivia

Long years ago, the peacock had dull brown tail feathers. During a battle that Indra waged against the asuras, the peacock raised its long tail feathers as a screen from behind which Indra could fight and defeat the asuras. Indra, in gratitude, blessed the peacock with the beauty of many colours!

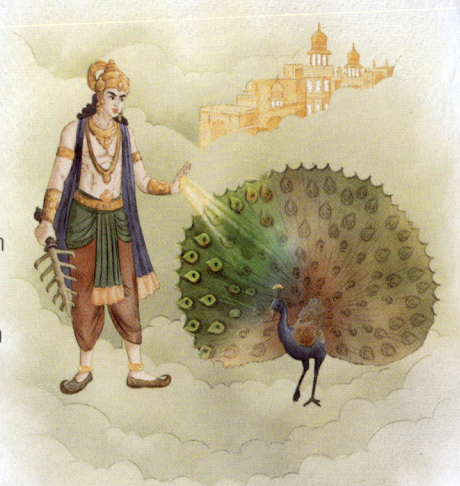

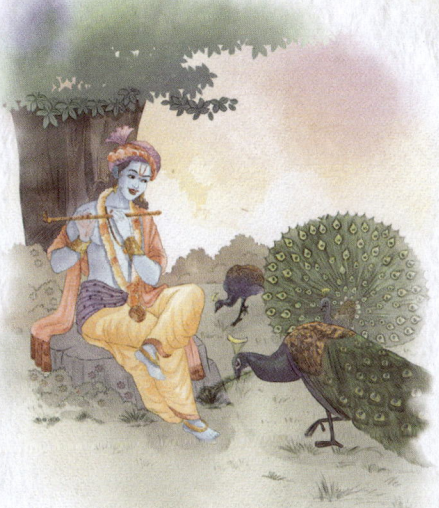

In another story, Krishna was playing the flute in the forest, and all the peacocks of the forest, mesmerized by the sound, danced with him for days. When he stopped, the king of the peacocks laid his feathers at Krishna's feet, as homage. Ever since, Krishna has worn peacock feathers in his hair.

Mackintosh describes how, at a temple in Kuntinagar, up to 100 peacocks and chicks would gather to eat grain when the elderly priest called them from the forest with calls of 'aa aa aa'!

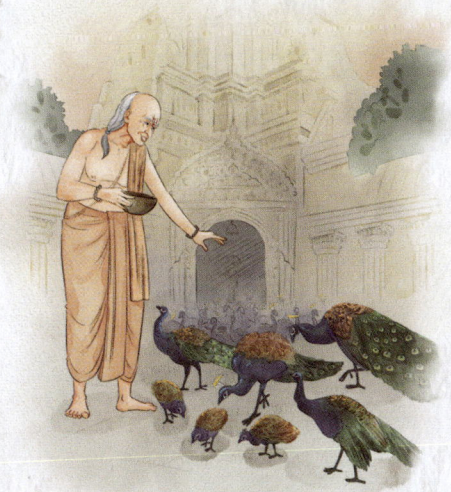

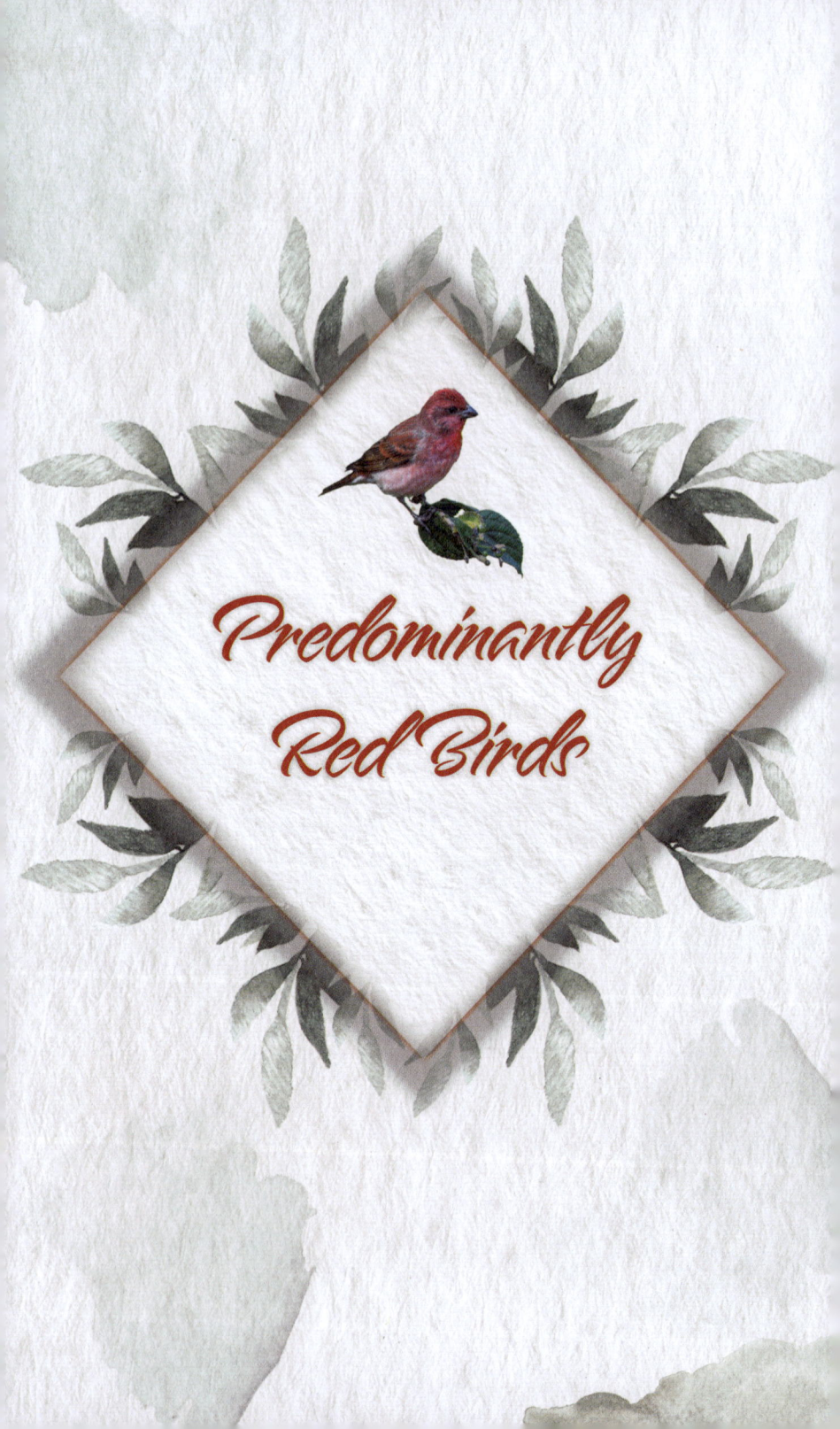

Each Little Bird That Sings

Red Avadavat

Scientific name: *Amandava amandava*   Size: *10 cm*
Hindi name: *Laal Munia*
Sanskrit name: *Sevya Kalvinka*

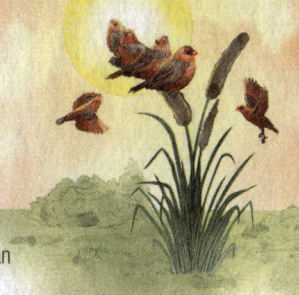

Description

The lovely little red jewel that is the Red Avadavat can be seen in its full red glory from around June to December, which is its breeding season. Good places to see it are areas with tall grasses and reeds and scrubby areas across India. The bright red colouration with white spots is an unmistakable sight!

Habits

The Laal Munia is a gregarious mover in flocks, and loves small grass seeds, often climbing up tall stems of flowering grass to pick the seeds right from the top. Sometimes, at just the right moment, the sun lights them up, and it looks as if the blonde grasses have ruby tips – which then take flight in a glittering red cloud – a breathtaking sight!

The courtship display is an elaborate affair, with the male holding a feather or a grassy stem as an offering, fluffing up its feathers, fanning its tail, singing, bowing to different sides, and performing a little circle of hops.

Call

A thin piping tsi-teei, as also a descending series of whistles!

Mythology, Tales & Trivia

Dewar suggests that the English named this bird Amadavat due to the fact that it was from Ahmedabad that the first set of birds was exported to England. Its colouring, and its cheerful confiding manner made it a favourite cage bird, and large numbers used to be exported to Europe.

The trapping method in olden times was to place captive birds in a cage, with a net flap in front of the cage on which seed was sprinkled. When wild birds came, attracted by the singing of the captive birds and the birdseed, the net flap was jerked up, trapping the birds.

Jayantika Davé

Crimson Sunbird

Scientific name: *Aethopyga siparaja*   Size: *11 cm*
Hindi name: *Phulchuiya, Shakarkhora*
Sanskrit name: *Suvarnapushp*

Description
The lovely little Crimson Sunbird is a resident of our Himalayas, and some parts of lowland India. It appears on the bottle brush in our home in the hills, and is such a striking sight, with the top half of the body shining red, and the iridescent green head and long green tail, making a beautiful picture against the feathery red flowers of the bottle brush!

Habits
The Phulchuiya appears wherever there is nectar in flowers – in forests, large gardens or scrubby areas. It goes up to 2,000 m in the Himalayas, and descends to lower elevations during winter. While nectar is its primary diet, it also takes spiders and insects. A family-minded bird, we always see them in pairs, though the two may forage separately. The pretty psip-psip-psip call is a clear announcement that the nectar-stealing has started!

A long-tailed oval nest is made with fine grass and other leaves, woven together and bound with cobwebs, and tied onto a thin branch of a small tree. A side entrance with a small porch is made, through which the bird makes a quick entrance and exit.

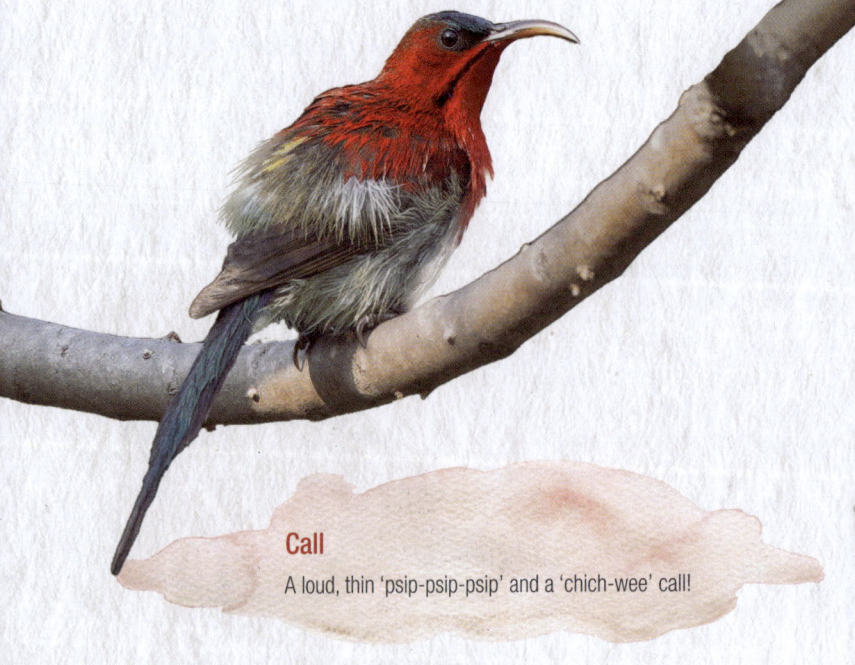

Call
A loud, thin 'psip-psip-psip' and a 'chich-wee' call!

Common Rosefinch

Scientific name: *Carpodacus erythrinus*   Size: 14 cm
Hindi name: *Tuti, Lal Tuti, Surkhab Tuti*
Sanskrit name: *Raktsheersh Kalvink, Var Chatak*

Description

Winter heralds the arrival of this lovely red-headed visitor! It breeds in the Himalayas, and as winter arrives, it spreads across most of India. It looks a lot like a very streaked sparrow that decided to dress itself up by tipping some dull pink-red paint over its head and chest!

Habits

The Lal Tuti can most often be seen in shrubbery at the edges of forests, orchards, cultivated fields and also amongst bushes and reed beds near small running streams. During breeding it is seen up to 4,000 m, but in winter it will stay below 2,000 m. It forages on the ground and amongst trees, looking for seeds, berries, fruits, nectar, young shoots and insects. It is very adept at stripping the outer core of harder fruit or seeds, and quickly getting to the soft and tasty core. They are loners and unobtrusive birds, most often seen alone or in pairs, and very rarely in a small group.

The male courts the female by raising its head-feathers and tail, drooping its wings, and doing quivering circles of the female, which may then also join in the dance. Sometimes he is so carried away that he will also burst into song!

Call

A pretty 'oo-eeet? oo-eet?' call!

Mythology, Tales & Trivia

The Common Rosefinch seems to need salt minerals, finding them in mortar from walls, or from animal urine.

The full-plumage males are usually in a minority, since they attain their full colouring only after Year Two.

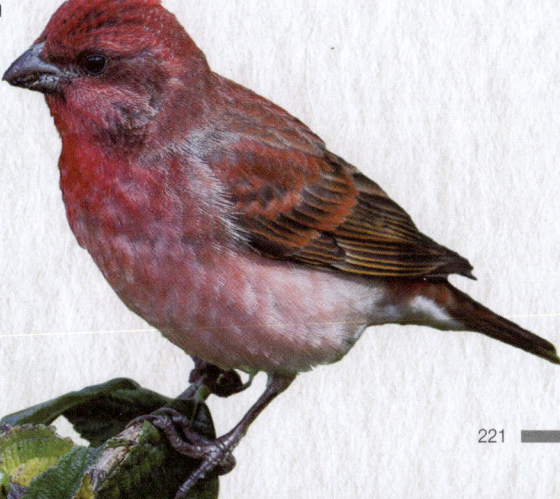

Jayantika Davé

Scarlet Minivet

Scientific name: *Pericrocotus (flammeus) speciosus*   Size: 22 cm
Hindi name: *Lal Saheli, Pahari Bulalchashm*
Sanskrit name: *Shoon Vishfuling*

Description

A visit to the Himalayas, or the hills of Central and East India, is incomplete without a sighting of a small flock of the bright red Scarlet Minivet – red silhouettes against a clear blue sky, or scarlet splashes of paint on the top of a tree. In Glen Haven, I can set my watch with them – 8.00 a.m. on a winter morning, the sun begins to hit the pines behind the house, and a small flock of Scarlet Minivets will definitely arrive!

Habits

The Lal Saheli enjoys the forest cover of tall trees – conifers, evergreens and deciduous – and can be seen up to 2,000 m. While it is a resident, it moves to slightly lower altitudes in winter. Its diet is insects, spiders and grasshoppers, and in the pursuit of active flying insects, it takes on an acrobatic flycatcher-like pursuit. The Scarlet Minivet also has an interesting habit of hovering close to foliage to frighten lurking insects into taking flight, and then quickly catching them. Usually seen in small flocks of 5–15 birds, they do a follow-the-leader act as they go from tree to tree. Fruiting trees are an attraction, seemingly to get at the insects that are attracted by the ripe fruit.

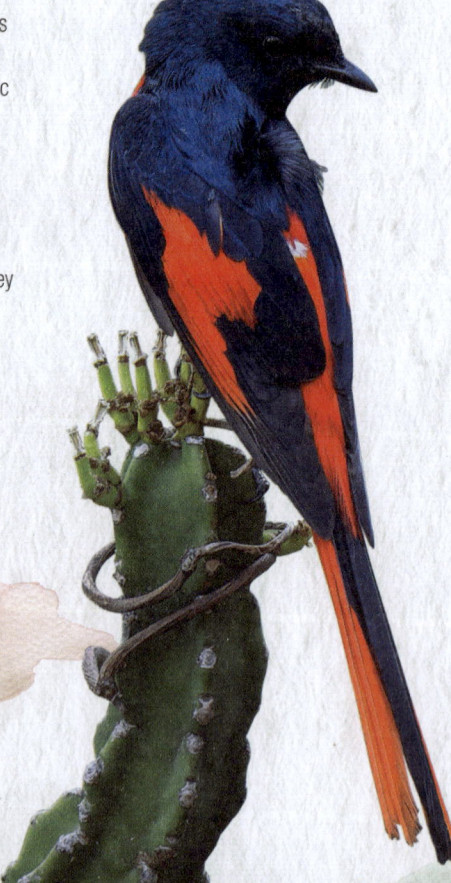

Call

A loud tweetwee-tweetywee-tweety-tweety-wee.

Each Little Bird That Sings

Rufous Sibia

Scientific name: _Malacias capistratus_   **Size:** 21 cm
Local name: _Sambriak Pho_
Sanskrit name: _Shreevad_

Description

Our arrival at our hill home is marked by the sight of the lovely Rufous Sibia – a lively presence in the bushes and bamboos around the veranda – sitting fearlessly on the railings, waiting to steal Buddy's food, showing off its beautiful rufous colouring, glossy, striking black head, and subtle blue-grey wings.

Habits

An inhabitant of mixed forests, cultivated areas and gardens in the Himalayas – broad-leaved, conifers, chestnuts, rhododendrons and the Padam (the local cherry) – the Rufous Sibia is found between 1,200 m and 3,000 m. Its diet is berries, nectar and insects, which it gets by seeking these in tree canopies, in shrubs and in bamboo groves. These birds get very comfortable around human beings, and in Glen Haven, as soon as I put out Buddy's food, a few of them will gather in the surrounding bamboos, calling out impatiently, and waiting for him to leave at least some of his food for them!

Call

A clear and repeated tee-dee-dee-dee-dee-o-lu, descending at the last two notes, and with the flock doing a softer, chattering ti-te-te amongst themselves as they forage!

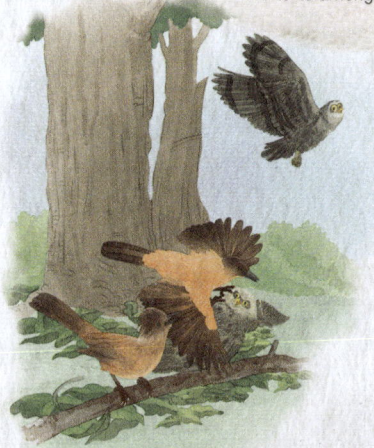

Mythology, Tales & Trivia

The Rufous Sibia is a fearless defender of its brood. Mackintosh describes an incident where a Collared Owlet was eyeing young Sibias that were attempting their first flight. The parent attacked the Owlet, tumbling with it to the ground, pinning it down with one leg, while 'boxing' it with the other leg, till the Owlet gave up and flew off.

Jayantika Davé

Orange-headed Thrush

Scientific name: *Zoothera citrina*   Size: 21 cm
Hindi name: *Safed Gala Kasturi, Dama*
Sanskrit name: *Shwet-kanth Bhu Kasturika*

Description
The Orange-headed Thrush is a summer visitor, a resident, and a winter visitor to different parts of India. This gorgeous orange-and-grey thrush is always a joyful sight. The best chances of sightings are early morning and late evening, as it tends to be most active during those hours.

Habits
The Orange-headed Thrush (earlier aptly called the Ground Thrush) is a big skulker! It is almost always found amongst the undergrowth of moist forests, bamboo thickets and cultivated groves, usually near running water and overgrown ravines. It is seen up to 2,300 m in the Himalayas, and my favourite sighting places are the forests around Panna Tal in Uttarakhand, or the greatly overgrown shrubby parts of the Keoladeo Sanctuary (in what used to be called the Nursery). Favourite foods are earthworms, slugs, snails, fruit, berries, figs and grass seeds. It does the thrush thing of rummaging around dried leaves, tossing them over to uncover what lies beneath, and is so often rummaging in the damp earth that its beak will always be muddy!

Call
A long, complicated, melodious song with many trills and some imitations!

Mythology, Tales & Trivia
The Hindi (Safed-gala) and Sanskrit (Shwet kanth) names strangely refer to the white throat of the bird, which is the least striking part of such a bright-coloured bird!

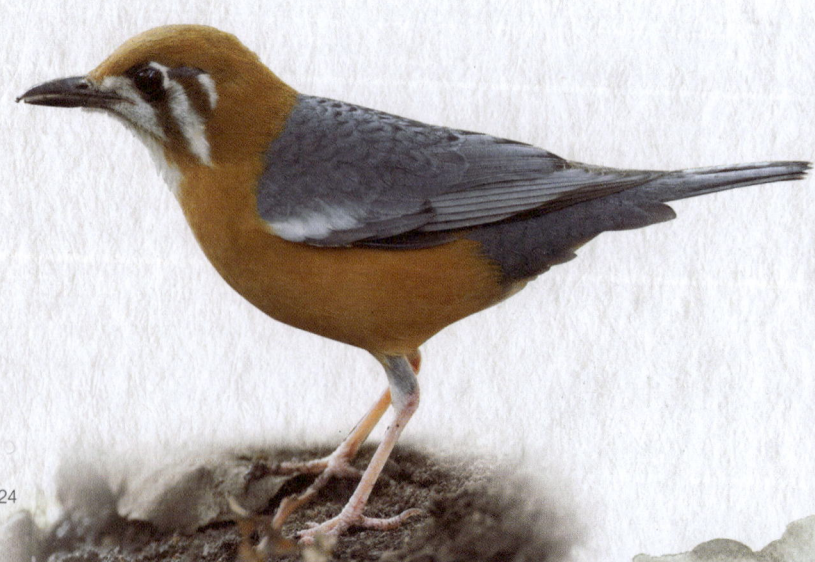

Each Little Bird That Sings

Common Kestrel

Scientific name: *Falco tinnunculus*   Size: *33 cm*
Hindi name: *Karontia, Koruttia, Khermutia*
Punjabi name: *Lal Shikra*
Sanskrit name: *Aakash-yogini, Lohandi-Shakuni*

Description

As our plane landed in Vadodara recently, and we were taxiing in, on one of the large signboards right next to the runway was this slim, elegant falcon, bright chestnut back contrasting with the grey head…sitting still, and watching the aeroplane go by! It was in an open grass field, a favourite prey site, and it had decided to wait out the aeroplane's arrival, and get right back to hunting! Lovely!

Habits

Favourite habitats are open grasslands with some shrub vegetation, semi-desert with scrubby growths, wetlands and the outskirts of villages and habitation. A widespread winter visitor, and a resident in some areas, the Lal Shikra can be seen up to 5,500 m. The hunting flight of the Common Kestrel is one of the identifiers. A strong flier, it hovers on quivering wings above a good hunting ground, staying almost stationary in the air, descends halfway and hovers again for a second look, and then swoops down quickly and noiselessly to capture terrestrial rodents or small birds.

It uses craggy ledges, and holes in trees or rock faces to make a sketchy nest.

Call

A shrill, piercing kee-kee-kee-kee.

Mythology, Tales & Trivia

The Common Kestrel uses its beak to disable the nervous system of a rodent it has caught, and then the tight grip of its claws to suffocate the victim.

It used to be called the Windhover, due to its habit of hovering and hunting.

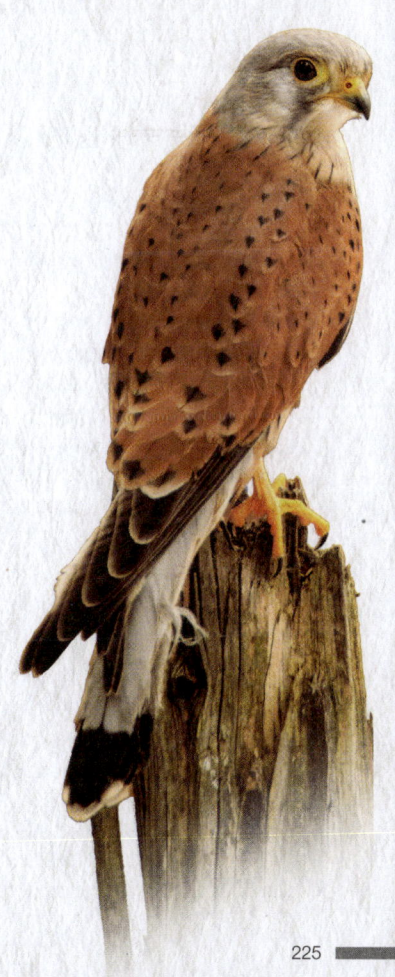

225

Jayantika Davé

Common Hoopoe

Scientific name: *Upupa epops*   Size: *31 cm*
Hindi name: *Hudhud*
Baluchi name: *Murgh-i-Suleiman*
Sanskrit name: *Putrapriya (referring to the parents' love for their offspring. The female does not leave the nest till the fledglings are ready to fly, and the male feeds them till then.)*

Description

I love the very descriptive Baluchi name of Murgh-i-Suleiman for this unmistakable russet black-and-white-striped beauty, with the long, downward-curved, slim, swordlike beak! When it is startled, when it alights, and when it spies something especially interesting, the crest feathers expand into a lovely corona of cinnamon red, bordered with black! A widespread resident, and a visitor to our gardens, parks, and other open country areas, the Common Hoopoe is always a delight to see.

Habits

It is a frequenter of open areas with short grass or broken ground, which provide it easy access to its main diet of insects, crickets, grasshoppers, ground-dwelling grubs and worms, with an occasional lizard, frog or snake. Common Hoopoes forage alone or in pairs, waddling along energetically on the ground, and probing and digging deep into the earth for prey. When I was young, our house had a huge peepul tree behind the kitchen, and wedged between the peepul and the wall, someone had left a large iron pipe upright. A pair of Common Hoopoes used this as their nesting site for years, and I spent many a happy hour watching the bringing up of this family! While the Murgh-i-Suleiman is a widespread resident across India, it also moves up to 4,000 m in the summer.

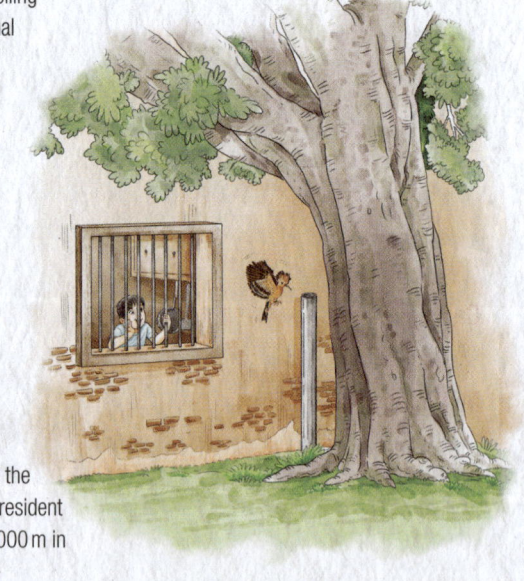

During the breeding season, I have seen the male being exceptionally caring to the female… digging out worms from the ground, and feeding her with the really plump ones.

Call

A mellow hoo-poo, hoo-po-po series of notes, repeated often.

Mythology, Tales & Trivia

Portraits of the Hoopoe have been found in mural paintings in ancient Egypt.

Some Eastern countries regard the Hoopoe as the favourite and confidant of Solomon, who bestowed it with its crown!

Ancient medical prescriptions, from the Egyptian days to the *Pharmacopoeia* of Dr R. James (1752), have recommended the use of different parts of the Hoopoe for improving the memory or stopping hallucinations.

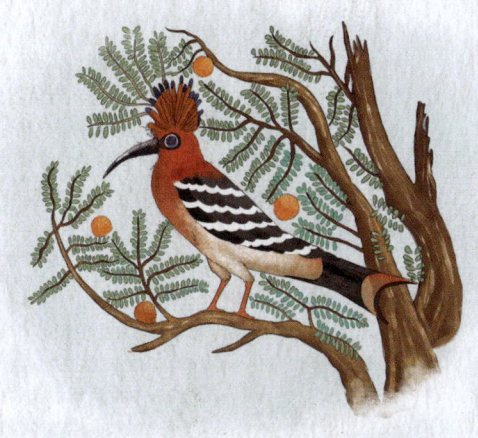

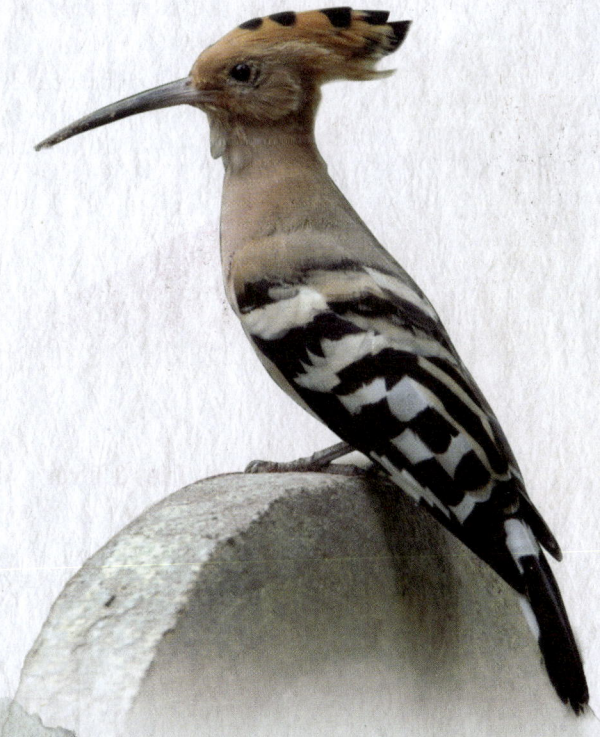

Every Little Bird that Sings

Southern Coucal

Scientific name: *Centropus (sinensis) parroti* Size: 48 cm
Hindi name: *Mahoka, Kuka*
Sanskrit name: *Kukkubh, Kumbharar Kukkut*

Description

When we are out walking in a wooded park or in open scrubby areas, and we hear a deep, resounding 'hoop-hoop-hoop' call, a quick scan of vegetation low on the ground will usually show us the Southern Coucal—a medium-large bird with its head, back and stomach glossed in a deep blue-purple black, and the wings a gorgeous rich chestnut! The tail is long and broad, and its earlier name of Crow Pheasant was an apt descriptor for this very striking bird—always a treat to see!

The very similar **Greater Coucal** is much larger in size, and is a resident of the Himalayan foothills and northern India.

Habits

A widespread resident across a lot of India, the Mahoka loves grasslands, open forests, cultivated areas and scrub, preferably near a stream or swampy area. It is a lowland bird, and is seen up to 1,200 m in the hills. A great skulker, and fairly clumsy in its movements, it avoids flying wherever possible, preferring to do a stately walk. When forced to fly, it is a laboured flap-and-glide process! Its favourite diet is insects, snails, slugs, rodents, frogs, snakes, bird eggs and nestlings.

It builds a large circular nest of twigs, leaves and grass, and hides it inside a bush, or places it in a small tree.

Call

Deep hoop-hoop-hoop resounding calls!

Mythology, Tales & Trivia

Was sometimes called Hedge Crow due to its habit of skulking in hedges.
Another apt name was Crow Pheasant, due to its long and spread-out tail.

Brahminy Kite

Scientific name: *Haliastur indus*   Size: 48 cm
Hindi name: *Brahmini Cheel, Safed Cheel, Shankar Cheel, Dhobia Cheel, Roo Mubarak, Khemkarni*
Sanskrit name: *Kunkumarakt, Dharmchil, Arishtkank*

Description

A water body or stream, a tall tree next to it, and somewhere in the upper branches, you should see the medium-sized, glorious Brahminy Kite – a blaze of rufous-chestnut, with a striking white head! If not on their perches, these birds can be seen wheeling overhead, and are easily recognizable due to their distinctive colour combination.

Habits

The favourite habitat of the Dhobia Cheel is near water – lakes, rivers, coastal areas and water bodies. They hunt for fish, and small rodents, animals and birds. In ports, they are largely scavengers, perching on ships and lifting refuse from the water. They sometimes eat carrion, and around villages, they have been known to steal domestic fowl. They are lowland birds, and can be seen up to 1,800 m in the Himalayas.

Call

While normally fairly silent, the call is a drawn-out kite-like kyerrrh.

Mythology, Tales & Trivia

The Brahminy Cheel is said to be sacred to Vishnu and is also considered a descendant of Garuda as it has the same colouring of white head and red wings, and is therefore deemed sacred to Hindus.

Even in France, it is called Milan Sacre, meaning 'sacred kite'.

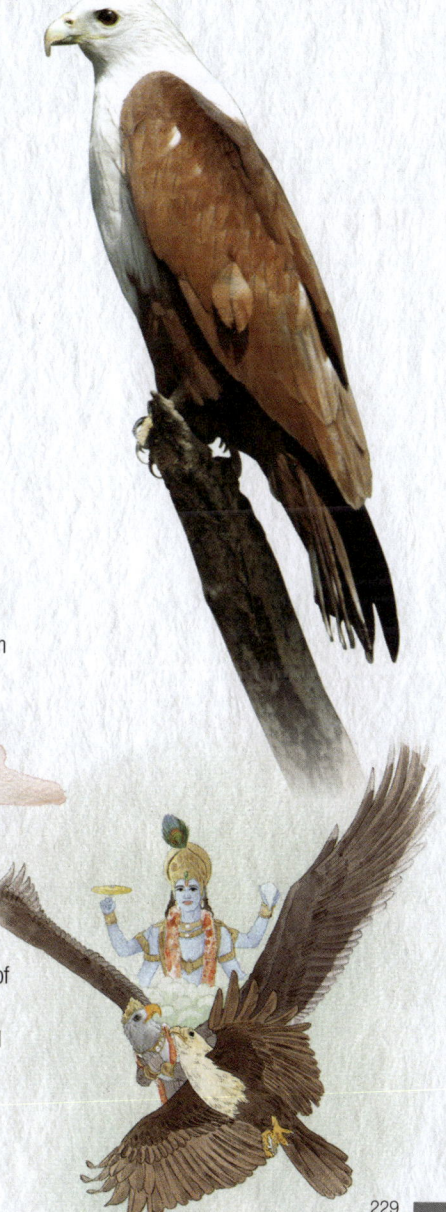

Jayantika Davé

Red Junglefowl

Scientific name: *Gallus gallus*   Size: 70 cm
Hindi name: *Jungli Murgha, Ban Murgha, Laal Murgha*
Sanskrit name: *Tamra Chood Kukkut*

Description

A loud but gentle melodious cock-a-doodle-doo in the Himalayas, and there is a Red Junglefowl around! A very dressed-up version of the domestic cock, the Jungli Murgha is resplendent in flaming bronze-gold, reds, glossy green-blue-purple, with a long and curved greenish-black tail. They are very shy birds, and not easy to see, but if you hear the call and sit very still, you may be in for a treat!

Habits

A resident of the Himalayas and the Northeast, the Red Junglefowl can be seen in forested areas, often near cultivation, sometimes entering fields to feed. Their favourite diet is seeds, grains, fruit and insects, and they forage like domestic fowl, by scratching the ground with their feet, and then picking out items. They are a lot more visible during early morning and evening, and can be seen in small groups, usually with one male accompanied by a few females. During our recent visit to Kaziranga, every morning a glowing male Red Junglefowl, accompanied by a bevy of females, would make a dramatic appearance from the forest edge to forage out in the open, retreating strategically at any disturbance – truly lovely!

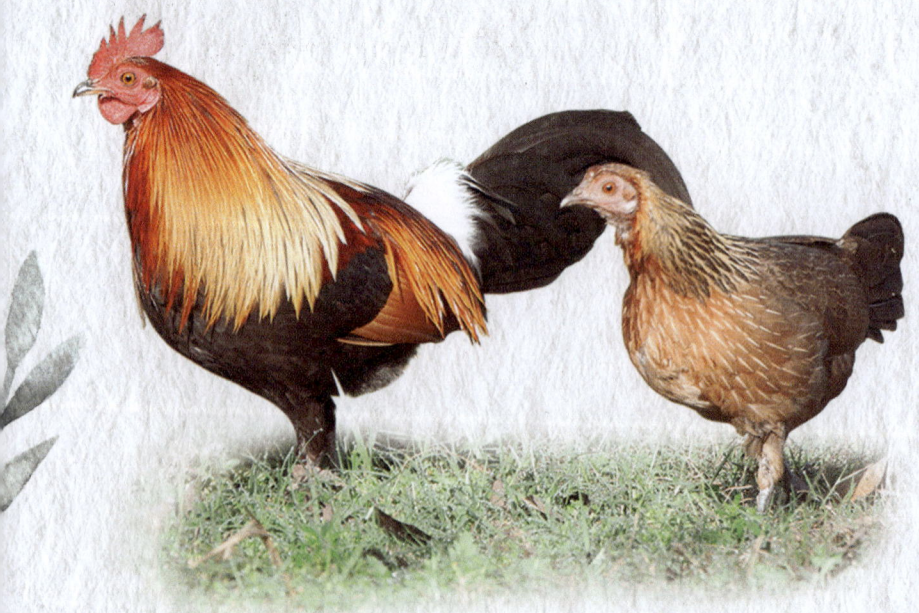

Call
A clear, loud, melodious cock-a-doodle-doo call!

Mythology, Tales & Trivia

The Red Junglefowl is believed to be the ancestor for all domestic poultry in India. This fowl is depicted on seals, going back to 2700–2500 BCE, found in the Indus Valley Civilization excavations. .

Tutankhamun's tomb also contains a drawing of the head of a cock.

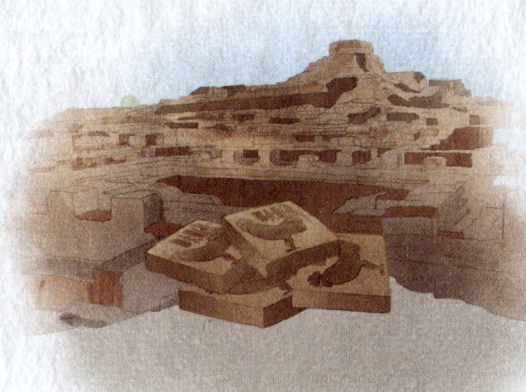

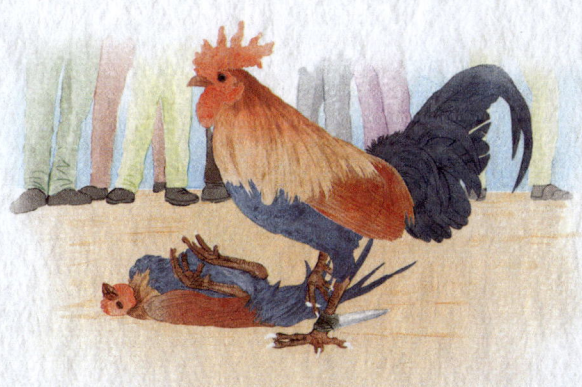

During cockfights, the majestic male was equipped with iron spurs, with the vanquished quickly being put to death by the stronger cock. Blake's description is apt – 'A gamecock clipped and armed for fight, doth the rising sun affright.'

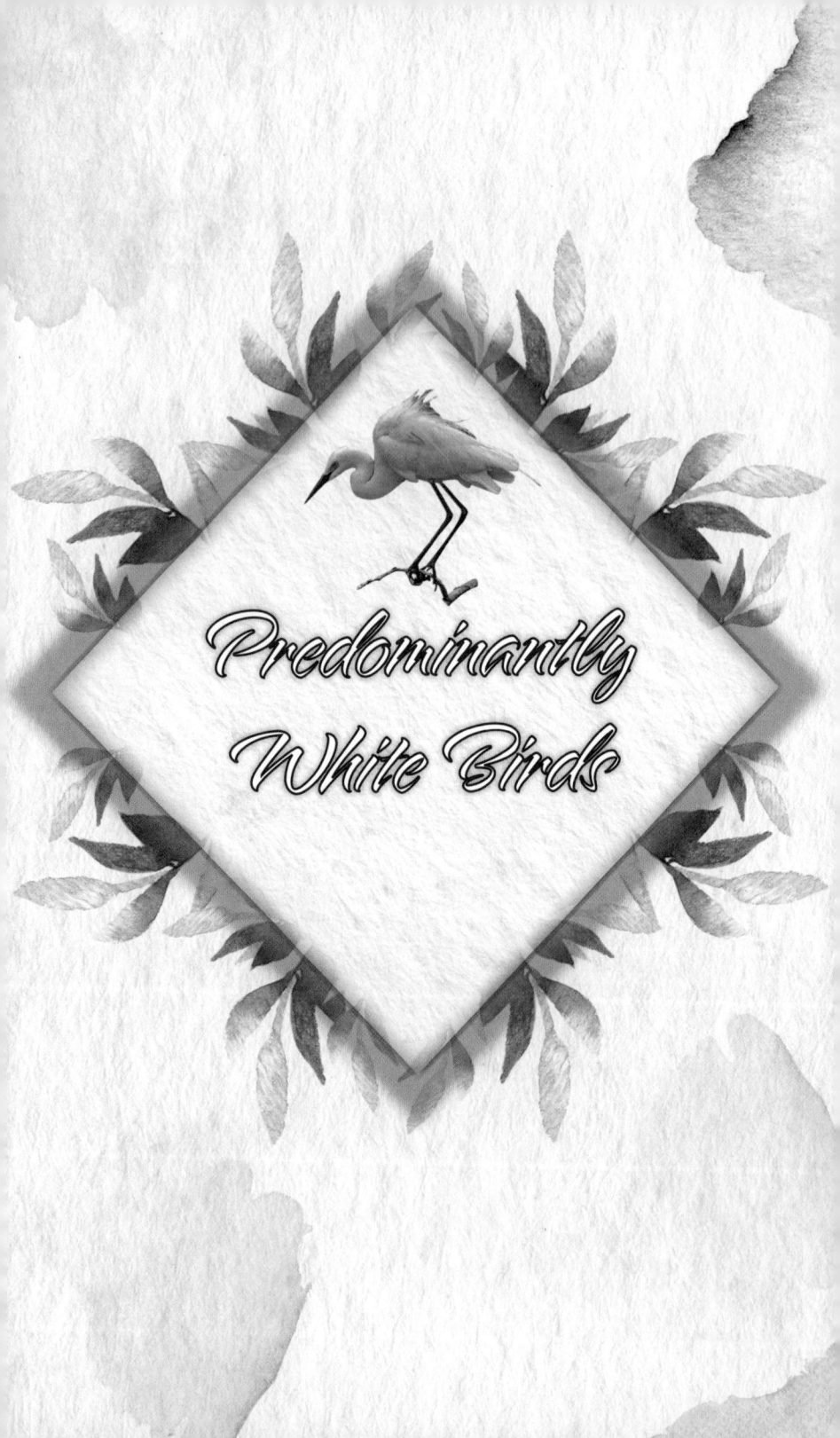

Asian Paradise Flycatcher

Scientific name: *Terpsiphone paradisi*   Size: 20 cm
Hindi name: *(Rufous Plumage) Shah Bulbul, Husaini Bulbul; (White Plumage) Sultan, Doodh Raj*
Punjabi name: *Pari Tik Tiki*
Sanskrit name: *Shwetvanvasin, Rajjuvaal*

Description

Shady forested glades in summer, with some water nearby, and a white fairy floats past, trailing long white robes?! No, you are not imagining things – it is the lovely Asian Paradise Flycatcher in its breeding plumage! In this phase, the Punjabi name of Pari Tik Tiki is so apt! Its other avatar is a smart rufous, with a smart black crest in both phases!

Habits

The Asian Paradise Flycatcher is a widespread summer visitor and resident in some coastal areas. Its primary diet is small winged insects, spiders, grasshoppers, butterflies and moths. It forages either alone or in pairs, but never in large numbers. It identifies an appropriate perch on a shady tree or in a glade, and then sallies forth after insects, often looping back to land on the same perch. In the dappled sunshine of these glades, this vision in white is particularly ephemeral – flashing white in a patch of sunlight, and then gracefully disappearing into shadow, with the undulating white streamers still catching some light as they too then disappear into stillness!

The beautifully constructed nest is a deep cone of grasses and thin fibres, bound together with cobwebs, so that it glows silvery white!

Call

A pretty peety-to-whit or a harsher weep-poor-willie.

Mythology, Tales & Trivia

The Paradise Flycatcher was once an even more glorious bird, clad from top to toe in dazzling white, and with a magnificent tail of snowy plumes – so much so that it began to compare itself with the Birds of Paradise! For this pride, it was shorn of its tail and utterly disgraced. It repented, however, and God was kind, and allowed it to retain two of the feathers of its tail, but He blackened its face, so that it may never forget its shame.

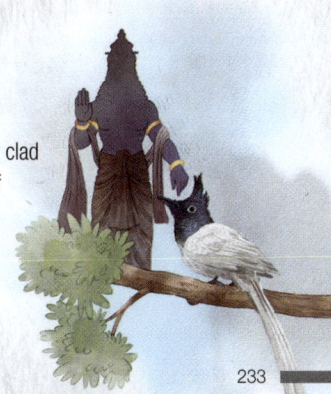

Jayantika Davé

Cattle Egret

Scientific name: *Bubulcus ibis*   **Size:** 50 cm
Hindi name: *Surkhia, Badami, Dorai, Gai Bagla*
Sanskrit name: *Gau Balaka*

Description

A drive-out into the countryside, and as soon as you see grazing cows or buffaloes, you will definitely see an army of the white, or gold and white (if in breeding plumage), Cattle Egrets, strutting along behind the cattle, and taking advantage of all the insects that are being flushed out!

Habits

The primary diet of the Gai Bagla is insects, frogs and sometimes fish. Its favourite habitats are cultivated fields, because it is very comfortable with human presence and thrives on the disturbance of insects by man or tractor. Gregarious by nature, these birds feed in flocks, and will always be seen in groups of 10 to maybe 100 birds. A lovely sight is to see the Badami Bagla perched on the back of cattle as they move through grazing areas – using the cattle themselves as 'beaters' to flush out prey, and the cattle's back as a vantage point to quickly sight and grab prey.

The Cattle Egrets have an elaborate courtship ritual, in which the males will bring twigs, erect their plumes, move from foot to foot, and simultaneously spread and flap their wings. They nest communally in heronries, with a messy twig nest being made.

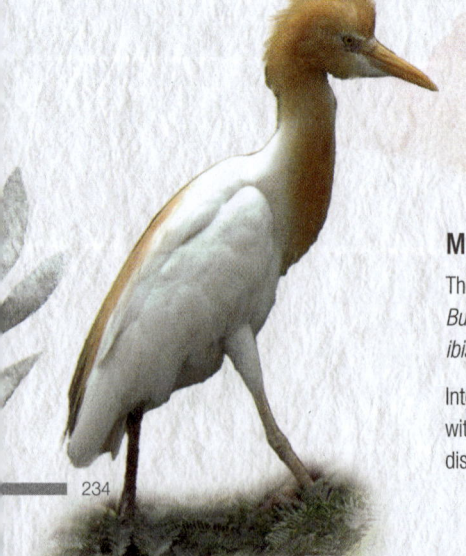

Call

A relatively silent bird, with sometimes a quiet, hoarse rick-rack murmuring call!

Mythology, Tales & Trivia

The scientific name is descriptive of the bird – *Bubulcus* from the Latin 'belonging to cattle', and *ibis* from the slightly downward-curved bill.

Interestingly, they often feed in a leapfrog manner, with each wave flying over the others in front to dislodge insects for the whole flock.

Little Egret

Scientific name: *Egretta garzetta*   Size: 60 cm
Hindi name: *Kilchia, Karchia Bagla*
Sanskrit name: *Balakika, Shikhini-balaka*

Description
The countryside, anywhere in India, near water of any kind – and the large flocks of slim, delicately built, long-legged white birds that you see are the Little Egret. In breeding, it adds feathery white plumes to the lowest curve of its neck, to its crown, and to its tail. Truly reminiscent of a pretty princess, dressed all in white! A very similar – though slightly larger – version is the **Intermediate Egret**, with black, not yellow, feet.

Habits
The Karchia Bagla frequents wetlands of any kind – freshwater or salt, river or lake, marshy wetland or salt pans, sandy beaches or cultivated flooded fields. It is a widespread lowland resident, but can be seen up to 2,200 m in Bhutan. The Little Egrets' primary diet is insects, aquatic life, small fish, worms, reptiles, rodents and small birds, which they get by walking around and picking, or foot-stirring in flooded areas, and sometimes getting spurred to quick runs or semi-flights to catch faster-moving prey. They are a particularly lovely sight when the early morning sun bathes bright green fields of paddy in a golden glow, and they are dotted with white egrets, as if someone had spattered a green canvas with white paint.

They are colonial nesters, often nesting with other egrets, cormorants, spoonbills and ibises. A large messy nest of twigs is made and placed in a tree.

Call
A loud kark-kark-kark.

Mythology, Tales & Trivia
The breeding plumes were used as decorative additions to a head-dress in the East, or for fancy ladies hats in the West. This resulted in many Little Egrets being killed during breeding. This practice has now been stopped.

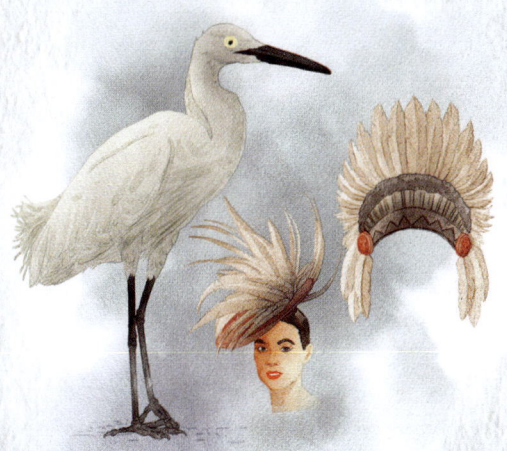

235

Jayantika Davé

Egyptian Vulture

Scientific name: *Neophron percnopterus*   Size: *70 cm*
Hindi name: *Safed Gidh, Kol Murghab, Kal Murgh*
Sanskrit name: *Alikachav, Bhasak*

Description

The Egyptian Vulture is an unmistakable, predominantly white vulture, with a yellow face, beak and neck feathers, looking a lot like an old, ruffled, disreputable hen! It is on the Globally Threatened list.

Habits

It frequents dry, arid, open areas, as well as the outskirts of habitation, where garbage heaps and slaughterhouses are a favourite haunt. It tends to appear alone or in pairs, and waits to be the last feeder. The Safed Gidh occurs in the lowlands, and goes up to 2,600 m in the Himalayas. Cliffs and crags are the preference for nesting sites.

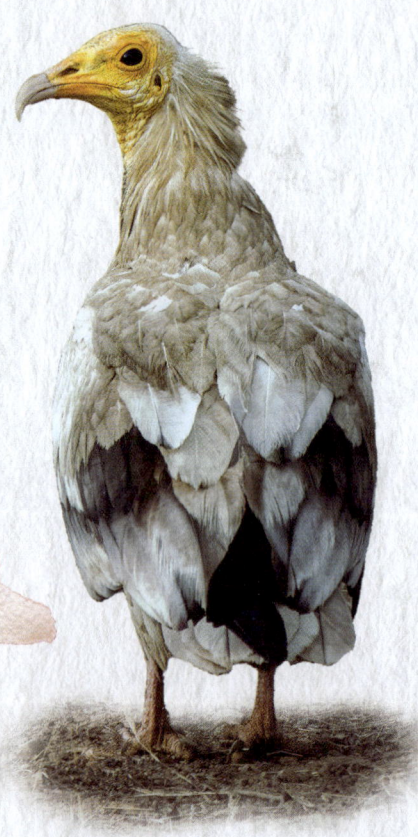

Call

Normally a very silent bird, with a few hisses and groans!

Mythology, Tales & Trivia

L.J. Mackintosh in his *Birds of Darjeeling and India* tells an amusing story about these vultures, where they had taken to using a municipal ropeway to a garbage dump for both a joyride and a feast! So 20–30 of these vultures would ride down the ropeway, and whenever the pulley approached, the leading bird would utter a warning 'kok kok kok', and hop nimbly over the pulley and settle down again. Alerted by the warning, the whole line would do their nimble hop-and-settle-down routine...a quaint sight!

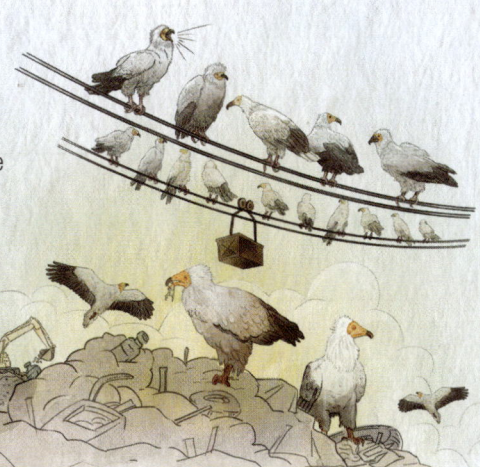

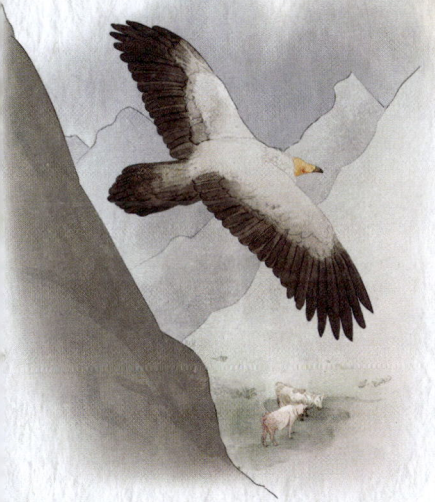

In the *Jaiminiya Brahmana* II.438, there is a legend that the Asura-Panis, who were the keepers of the cows of Indra, once stole them and hid them in a deep valley. The gods asked the vulture to find them. The vulture tracked them down, but accepted a bribe of *aamiksha* from the Asuras, and lied to the gods. Indra suspected what had happened, and squeezed his neck, and out came the aamiksha! Indra then let him go with the curse 'May thy sustenance be of bad origin', and that is why the Egyptian vulture feeds on dung!

M. Krishnan tells of a shrine at Tirukkalukunram, where a pair of Egyptian vultures appear exactly at noon to partake of the *prasad* placed on a shelf of rock by the resident priest. They are believed to be two immortal saints (white clothes), who first bathe and then come to take prasad.

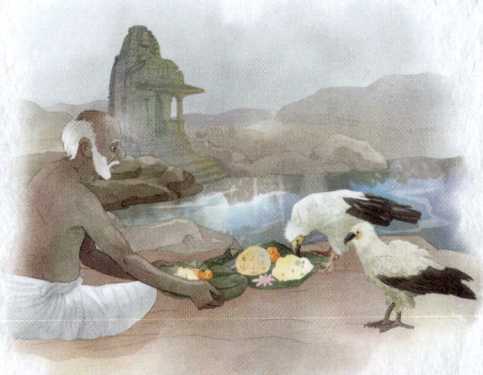

Jayantika Davé

Black-headed Ibis

Scientific name: *Threskiornis melanocephalus*   Size: 75 cm
Hindi name: *Safed Baza, Didhar, Munda*
Sanskrit name: *Shwet-kaak, Shwet-bak, Shartika*

Description

Looking like it has stepped straight out of Egyptian mythology onto our wetlands is the distinctive Black-headed Ibis – a leggy, medium-sized white Ibis, with a black bald head, and a heavy downcurved black bill! It is a resident across large parts of India, and can be seen in open areas, near water, wetlands or flooded fields.

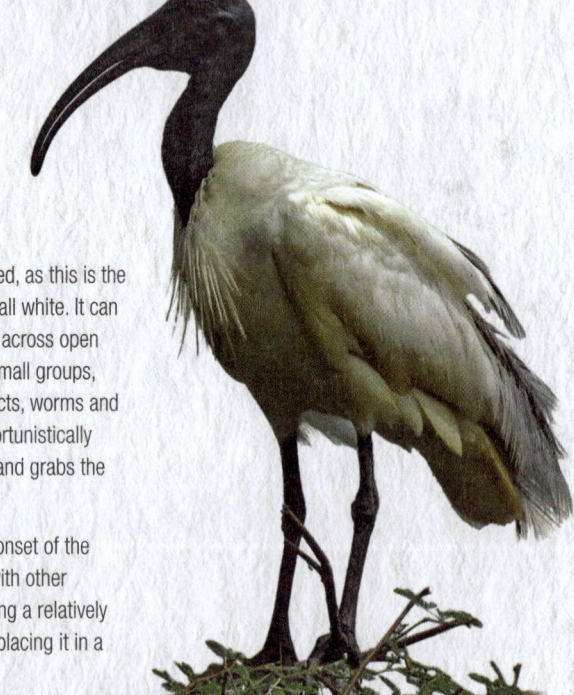

Habits

The Safed Baza is aptly named, as this is the only one of our ibises that is all white. It can be seen walking majestically across open countryside or wetlands, in small groups, feeding on frogs, snails, insects, worms and small fish. It sometimes opportunistically follows cattle as they graze, and grabs the insects they flush out.

Breeding coincides with the onset of the monsoon. It nests together with other storks and cormorants, making a relatively small platform of twigs, and placing it in a medium-sized tree.

Call
A silent bird, occasionally grunting and croaking!

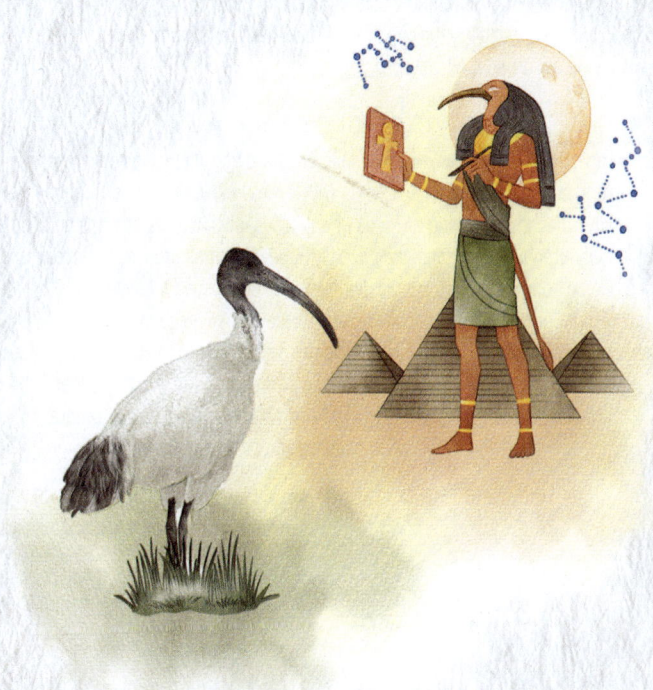

Mythology, Tales & Trivia
The Ibis was venerated by the ancient Egyptians, and their god Thoth, the god of knowledge, writing and wisdom, was depicted as an Ibis-headed god.

Jayantika Davé

Eurasian Spoonbill

Scientific name: *Platalea leucorodia*   Size: 85 cm
Hindi name: *Chamach Baza*
Sanskrit name: *Darvida, Darvi-mukh (Darvi = spoon)*

Description

Water bodies in the entire northwest and western parts of India are incomplete without the sighting of the Eurasian Spoonbill…looking like a tall, leggy, though large, egret, till it turns, and you see the long spoon-shaped yellow-tipped bill!

Habits

The Chamach Baza, as it is aptly named, enjoys larger, shallow wetlands, including marshy areas next to rivers, and coastal lagoons. It feeds with a remarkable open-beak, continuous sweeping-sideways motion, ensnaring all kinds of aquatic insects, worms, frogs, small fish and plant matter. A fairly gregarious species, they usually appear in small groups. The spoon shape of the bill has been a source of much speculation, with the suggestion that perhaps it creates suction to pull prey in, or that it reduces water disturbance and so helps to catch more prey – but there has been no conclusive diagnosis. During the day, they tend to stand around sleepily on the banks, taking flight to feeding grounds in the evening. When a flock of the Eurasian Spoonbill is in flight overhead, in their typical V or straight line formation, the clear spoon shape of the bill is very visible!

The breeding season is tied to the presence of good water conditions, and a platform twigs nest is placed either in a reed bed or on small trees.

Call

Usually silent, with grunts and bill-clattering sometimes!

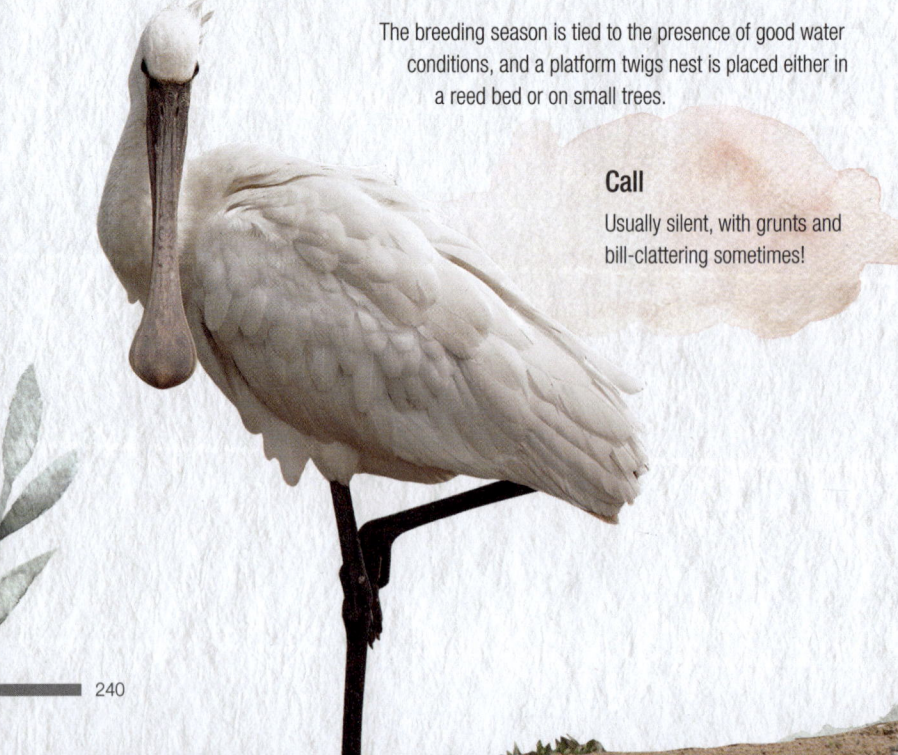

Lesser Flamingo

Scientific name: *Phoenicopterus minor*   Size: 85 cm
Hindi name: *Chhota Raajhans*
Sanskrit name: *Balaka*

Description

The salt pans and wetlands of the Greater and Lesser Ranns of Kutch in Gujarat are a 'must visit' in India, because it is here that you see the Lesser and Greater Flamingos. Against the stark landscape of the Rann, a tightly clustered big ball of white and pink, shifting, turning, moving…and then suddenly, the ball takes flight, and the white turns to a deep pink cloud, with trailing bright pink legs – a 'take your breath away' sight! The **Greater Flamingo** is significantly larger, and is distinguished by its size, overall paler colouring, and black-tipped larger bill.

Habits

The main habitat for the Chhota Raajhans is saline lakes and lagoons, which are host to their diet of tiny algae and invertebrates. They feed with the head tipped upside down, and the bill sweeping from side to side, sifting out edible portions from the saline water. The Flamingo feeds by inverting its head completely, submerging its beak and sometimes part of its head in the water, using the upper scoop-shaped beak to fill with mud which is then filtered out, leaving tiny food particles.

Call

A very low murmuring murr-err, which is almost a continuous sound when a large flock is feeding together, and a loud goose-like honk!

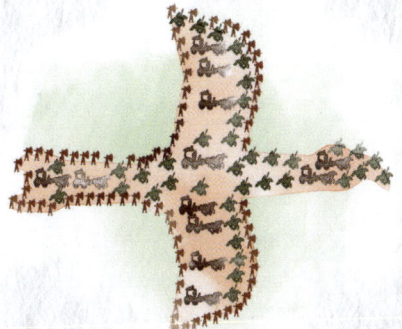

Mythology, Tales & Trivia

In the Mahabharata 6.50.40, the flamingo is referred to as Aruna-Kronch due to its red colour. The sage Brihaspati designed an effective army formation called Arunkronchvyooh, using the outline of a flamingo in flight.

Jayantika Davé

Great Egret

Scientific name: *Casmerodius albus*   Size: *95 cm*
Hindi name: *Tar Bagala, Bada Bagala, Malang Bala, Turra Bagla*
Sanskrit name: *Prasch Jesht Bagla*

Description

The Great Egret is an unmistakably large egret – tall, stately, dignified… usually standing in solitary splendour! Its size and a slim neck with a distinctive S-shaped kink are distinguishing features. During the breeding season, it becomes a showy beauty with a large number of long white plumes drooping from its tail. While it is a widespread resident across India, it is not present in large numbers, and so a sighting is always a joy!

Habits

Favourite habitats are wetlands, both inland and along the coast, the shores of lakes and salt pans, and flooded fields. It has been recorded up to 3,750 m in Tibet. It forages for fish, aquatic invertebrates, rodents, reptiles and opportunistically even small birds. It proceeds slowly with a majestic walk, and catches its prey with a quick extension of the long neck, periodically stopping and standing still, till a tasty morsel is sighted.

A large untidy nest of twigs is made, placed at the top of a tree near water.

Call
Dry croaking sounds!

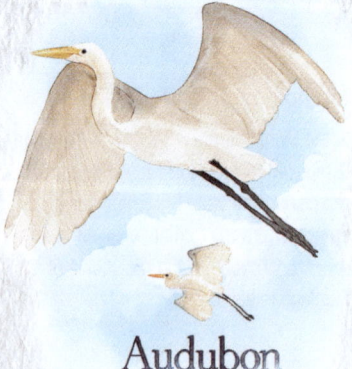
Audubon

Mythology, Tales & Trivia
The statuesque Bada Bagla is the symbol of the famous National Audubon Society.

Great White Pelican

Scientific name: *Pelecanus onocrotalus*   Size: 160 cm
Hindi name: *Hawasil*
Sanskrit name: *Jal-sinh (water tiger), Maha-plav, Mahapakshi (due to its large size)*

Description

The Great White Pelican is a large, stocky pure-white bird, with a huge, heavy wedge-shaped yellow bill, and a pouch extending below the bill – unmistakable! It is a winter visitor to the lakes of North India, and to the salt pans of Gujarat…so our winter visits to Gujarat have three amazing target sightings – the Lesser and Greater Flamingos, and the fat, squat White Pelicans! A very similar bird is the **Dalmatian Pelican**, distinguished by a dirtier appearance, a tufted crest, and grey (instead of yellow) legs and feet.

Habits

The Great White Pelicans prefer lakes that are deeper, as their diet consists mainly of fish. They appear alone, in pairs or in small flocks, and then proceed to hunt, sometimes communally creating an arc, and driving fish to shallow areas, where they can be quickly gulped. A flight of the Hawasil is lovely to see – with these birds unmistakable for their outline of the neck tucked tightly in, the huge beak in full silhouette, and a strong deliberate flight!

Call

A silent bird that growls and grunts and croaks aggressively only during the breeding season!

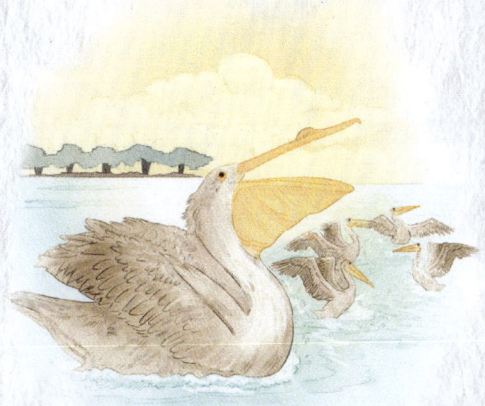

Mythology, Tales & Trivia

Research has shown that a single bird eats between 900 and 1,200 gm of fish a day!

Flocks of Pelican have been seen to capture their prey by forming a line across the water, and herding the fish into the shallow water by beating the water with their wings. The fish are then scooped up – a scoop of the great lower mandible, with its elastic, naked membrane hanging below the neck.

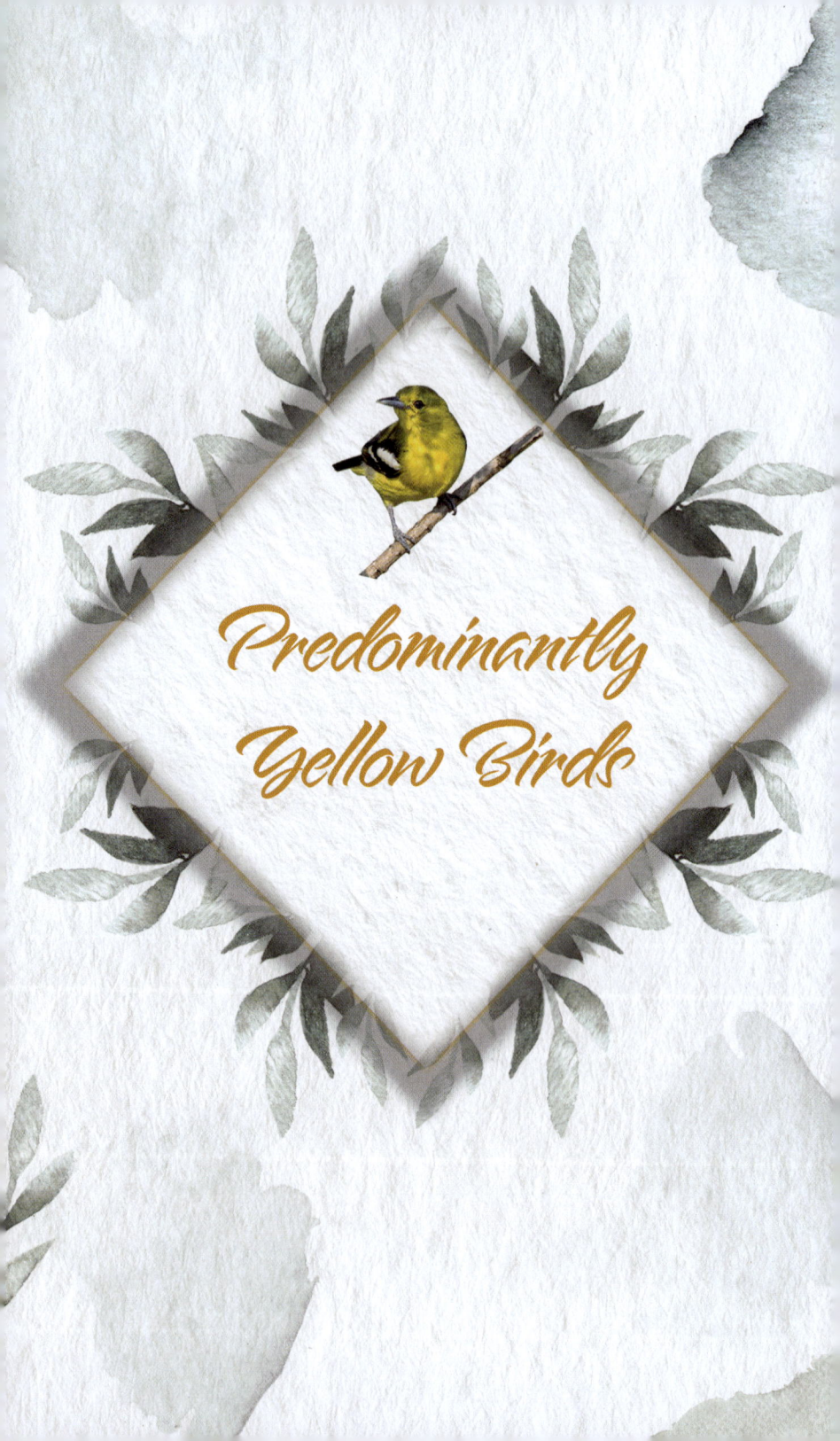

Purple-rumped Sunbird

Scientific name: *Leptocoma zeylonica*   Size: *10 cm*
Hindi name: *Shakar Khora, Man-changi*
Gujarati name: *Pachrangi Phul Chakli, Pacharangi Shakkarakhoro*
Sanskrit name: *Shinjirika*

Description

Central and southern India are home to the lovely resident Pacharangi Shakar Khora, so aptly described in the colloquial name – five colours, and a lover of nectar! A typical sunbird with its gleaming colours and long, sharply curved beak, and its face always inside a flower!

Habits

Its favourite habitats are lightly wooded areas at the edge of a forest, or in parks and gardens, preferably with an abundance of flowering trees. The Purple-rumped Sunbird is a bird of the lowlands, occasionally heading up to about 2,000 m. Its preferred diet is mainly nectar, insects of all kinds, caterpillars and sometimes small fruit. It appears singly or in pairs, and is very active, flitting from flower to flower, hanging upside down to look into crevices in the bark for insects, continuously twittering and fluttering. With its nectar-feeding habits it is a great cross-pollinator, which is very useful, but it also spreads the difficult-to-get-rid-of tree parasite Loranthus.

The male and the female work together to create the pear-shaped nest, made of grass, fibres and other strips, and decorated on the outside with leafy, cobwebby material. The male is an active parent, guarding the female when she is in the nest, and later helping to feed the chicks and carrying away the faecal sacs.

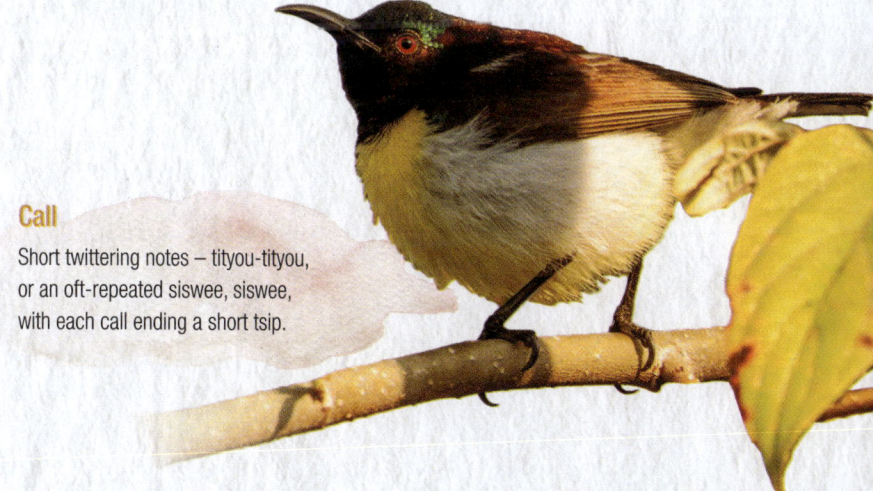

Call

Short twittering notes – tityou-tityou, or an oft-repeated siswee, siswee, with each call ending a short tsip.

Jayantika Davé

Oriental White-eye

Scientific name: *Zosterops palpebrosus* Size: 10 cm
Hindi name: *Baabuna*
Sanskrit name: *Chatkika, Putrika*

Description

A pretty and gregarious bird is the Oriental White-eye…seen in groups in the trees, actively moving around, seeking…seeking, and singing its happy 'cheer-u, cheer-u' call! The main colours you see are the olive-yellow above and bright yellow throat, and as soon as you get it in your binoculars, the clear white eye-ring jumps out at you!

Habits

The Baabuna loves broad-leaved and open mixed forests, or parks and gardens with lots of trees, preferably trees with small berries, fruits and flowers. It frequents the lowlands, and hills up to 2,800 m. In our garden in Glen Haven, it is a cheerful common visitor, with flocks visiting our Padam (wild cherry) tree all through the year, but definitely when it is in bloom, and again when it is full of the red wild cherries. The diet of the Oriental White-eyes is supplemented with insects too. They move in small flocks, hunting energetically, hanging upside down, peering into likely nooks and crannies, and all the while cheerfully singing away!

A small, delightfully woven nest of grasses, cobwebs and fibres is made, and hung between two thin twigs in a small bush or low tree, or in a bamboo grove.

Call

It is a cheerful chatterer – and the flock constantly communicates with a series of cheuw or cheer or prreee-u calls!

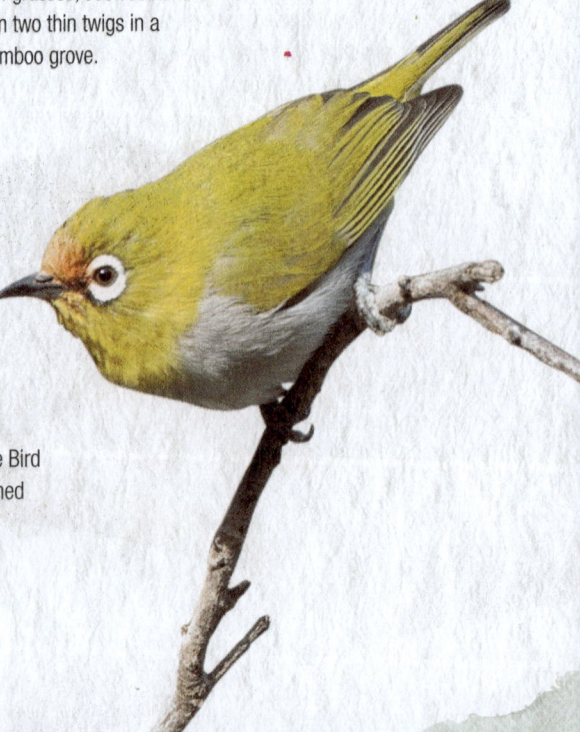

Mythology, Tales & Trivia

It used to be called the Spectacle Bird because of the round white-rimmed glasses it seems to be wearing!

Each Little Bird That Sings

Indian Yellow Tit

Scientific name: *Machlolophus xanthogenys*   Size: *13 cm*
Hindi name: *Peela Ramgangara, Sabz-roshan*
Sanskrit name: *Valguli*

Description

A cheeky, cheerful sight across Peninsular India is the Indian Yellow Tit, an olive-green, yellow-and-black bird, with a perky and uptilted black crest. A very similar, brighter-coloured tit that shows up in the Himalayas is the **Black-lored Tit**. Cheerfully singing as it diligently searches through the trees for insects, both these tits are lovely splashes of sunlight in a tree!

Habits

Open forested areas of oak, pine, bamboo or other evergreens are the favourite haunts. In the Himalayas, the Black-lored Tit is seen up to 2,400 m, and in Peninsular India, the Indian Yellow Tit is seen up to 1,800 m.

Their favourite foods are small insects, spiders and fruits – with mulberries and raspberries being favourites, together with nectar, soft flowers and buds. It feeds by constantly moving in the top half of a tree, hanging upside down, peering behind leaves, and sometimes doing a short quick flight to catch an insect that is getting away. The Peela Ramgangara is a sociable little bird and forages in small flocks, together with other similar hunters. It has a particularly loud and cheerful call, which draws the eye to see what is lighting up the foliage – a true Sabz-roshan bird!

Call

A loud cheerful tsee-tsee-wheep-wheep-wheep or tsi-tsi-pit-tui.

Mythology, Tales & Trivia

The vernacular names for the tits are very apt:
1. Sabz-roshan or 'the light of green trees'
2. Ramgangara = the sweet-voiced bird

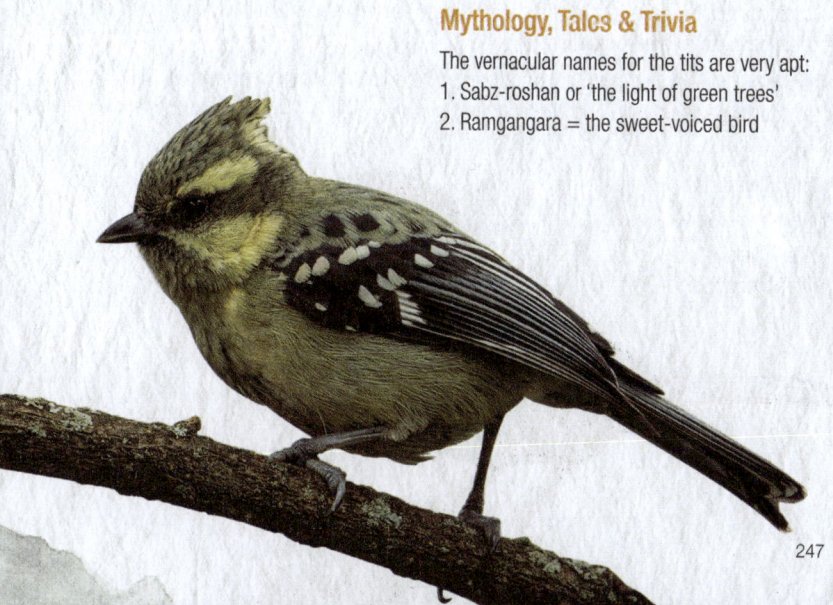

Jayantika Davé

Green-backed Tit

Scientific name: *Parus monticolus*   Size: *13 cm*
Hindi name: *Hara Roshan, Ras Ramgangara*
Sanskrit name: *Kshudra Valguli*

Description

Breakfast on the deck in Glen Haven in the Himalayas always came with the ringing 'whitee-whitee' call of the Green-backed Tit! And a look into the wild cherry next to the deck will always be rewarded with the sighting of this lovely olive-green and bright yellow tit, with a neat black cap and black shirt front.

Habits

The Hara Roshan is the most commonly seen tit of the Himalayan hill stations. Its favourite haunts are open forests of oak, rhododendron and conifers, and bamboo thickets and scrub, up to 2,800 m in the Himalayas. It easily comes into wooded gardens and is not shy of human presence. Favourite foods are insects, berries, seeds, soft flowers and fruits. It moves around in pairs, and often a few pairs can be seen together. Food is sought in the middle and top half of trees, with much fluttering, peeking, upside-down peering, and clinging to the bark and looking into crevices. While the Green-backed Tit is mainly arboreal, it often flutters down into undergrowth, as well as picks food off the ground. With a cleanliness fetish, a small group of them will always be seen at our bird baths or little pond, doing a quick *snaan*!

The nest is made of soft grass, hair and fibres and placed in the hole of a tree trunk. They are happy to use the nest-box of our home, placed high in a corner of the house under the eaves.

Call

A happy, high series of white-whitee or fit-schew calls!

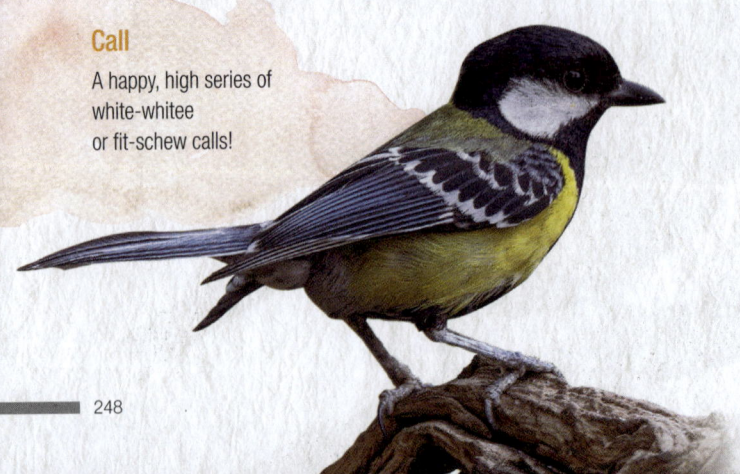

Common Iora

Scientific name: *Aegithina tiphia*   Size: *14 cm*
Hindi name: *Shaubeegi, Shaubeega*
Sanskrit name: *Bharat Shukkika, Shreevad, Shukika, Sookarika, Madhuk*

Description
A striking yellow-and-black bird, resident across India, is the Common Iora. The combinations of black and yellow are varied across regions in India, but the bird itself is unmistakable, and is usually seen in the mid-canopies of open mixed forests, woodlands and orchards.

Habits
This lovely golden-and-black beauty is found alone and in pairs, at forest edges, open woodlands, parks, gardens, orchards, and amongst trees in cultivated areas, usually amongst the lowlands, but is easily seen up to 2,000 m if the habitat is right. The Shaubeega preys on insects, spiders, beetles and caterpillars by seeking restlessly under leaves and amongst the branches in the top canopy of trees. It is a loner and moves around alone or in pairs. At my brother's re-wilding project in Corbett, we have our lunch under the canopy of a few large trees, and with an 'Oh here we are!' call, the Common Iora joins us and feeds amongst the broad leaves above our head!

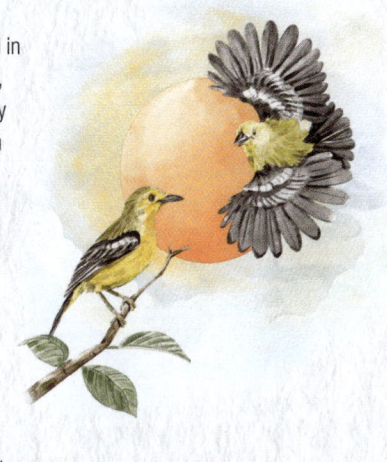

Whistler beautifully describes their striking breeding display, where the male flies up into the air, and spirals down to its perch, descending with all its feathers, especially the rump feathers, fluffed up, so that it looks like a little ball! On landing, it struts about like a little peacock, with drooped wings, uttering a sibilant note.

Call
A loud whistling 'oh here we are', or a softer 'if you please'!

Mythology, Tales & Trivia
It is one of the main nests parasitized by the Banded Bay Cuckoo in its range.

Call sounds like Shou-biga or So-be-ye…giving rise to the Hindi name of Shoubiga.

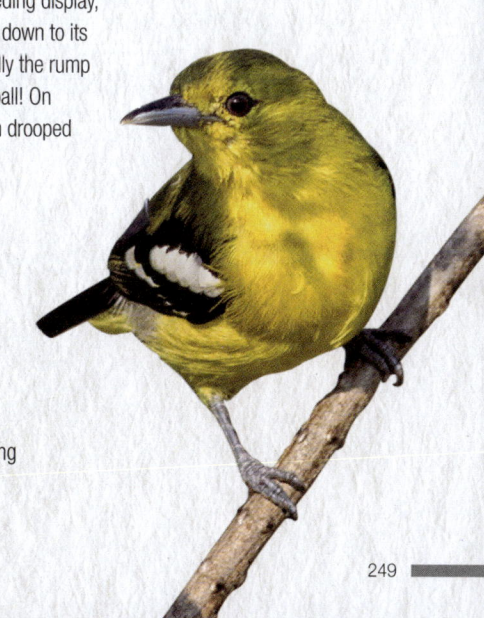

Jayantika Davé

Yellow Wagtail

Scientific name: *Motacilla flava*   Size: 18 cm
Hindi name: *Pilkya, Pani-ka-Pilkya*
Sanskrit name: *Pitta Khanjjan, Ashvakhya, Khanjkhayt*

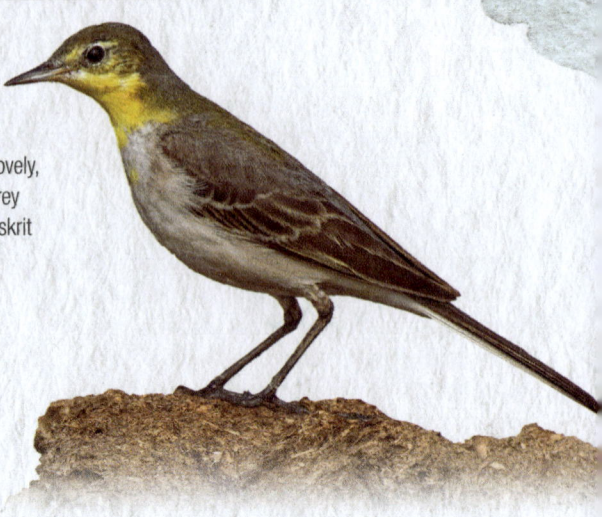

Description

Wetlands and the borders of marshy areas in winter all over India are dotted with the lovely, eye-shaped yellow and olive-grey Yellow Wagtail, giving it its Sanskrit name of Khanjjan.

Habits

Winter birding always leads to great sightings of the Yellow Wagtail, which is a highly gregarious bird in the right habitat, and can often be seen in groups of 20–30 birds. So, when we are out looking at the migratory water fowl that arrive to our wetlands in winter, a quick scan of the surrounding damp, marshy and grassy areas, bordered with reed beds or vegetation, throws up amazing sightings. It is mainly a lowland bird, but breeds up to 4,500 m in Ladakh. It forages for land and water invertebrates, seeds and soft plants by walking quickly, picking up food items from the ground or water, making quick dashes, and sometimes a little jump and flight to catch an insect in the air. The Pani-ka-Pilkya is often seen in the company of grazing animals, taking advantage of the fact that insects are attracted to these animals and their dung.

Call

A loud pseeu or tsreep srriii-srriiit.

Mythology, Tales & Trivia

Once in Basai in Haryana, we were wonderstruck at the sight of close to a hundred Yellow Wagtails busily working the ground, long and elegant yellow silhouettes with wagging tails!

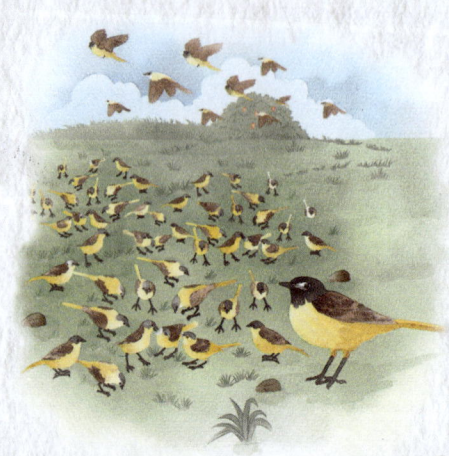

Golden Oriole

Scientific name: *Oriolus kundoo*   Size: 25 cm
Hindi name: *Peelak, Pirola, Piyarola*
Marathi name: *Haldya*
Kannada name: *Suvarna Pakshi*
Sanskrit name: *Sugreev Kanchan, Ambakmaddari, Ambaakpipeelak*

Description

Suvarna Pakshi, or the Golden One, is the best descriptor for this brilliant medium-sized yellow-gold bird with black wings, and a lovely, fluting 'weela-whee-oh' call! A similar-looking but even more striking bird is the **Black Hooded Oriole**, which is of the same colouration but has a shining black head, and is a resident across all of India.

Habits

The Golden Oriole is best seen in fruit trees in open forests, parks and gardens, and in village orchards. The bright flash of yellow as it flies past is unmistakable, as is its distinctive call. Very partial to fruits, and particularly to mangoes, as its Sanskrit names highlight, it is a fruit and berry eater, enjoying figs, mulberries, mangoes and other sweet fruits, as well as insects of various kinds and caterpillars. It usually forages alone or in pairs, seeks its food within the canopy of trees, and draws attention to itself mainly with its sweet call, or the flash of gold as it flies from one tree to another. It is a resident in the central part of India, sensitive to temperature, moving south to winter there, and in summer moving to the hills to cool off!

The nest is a fairly deep cup woven from grass stems and thin roots with cobwebs and other raggedy material draped on the outside to camouflage it. It is often built in close proximity to the nest of the aggressive drongo for protection.

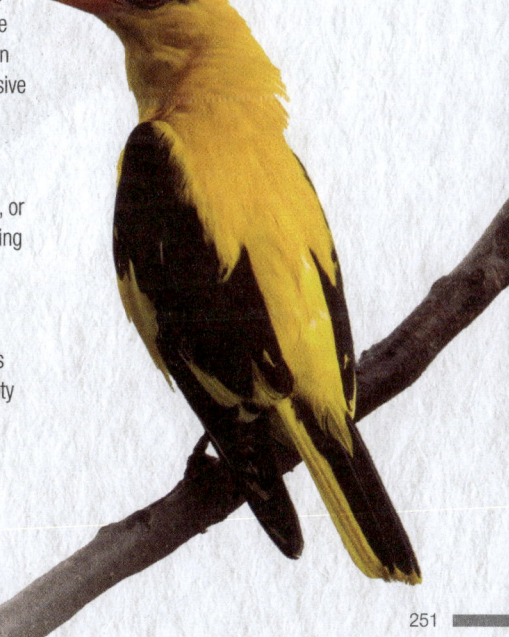

Call

A beautifully melodious pee-lo, pee-lo-lo, or weela-whee-oh with some harsh chattering too!

Mythology, Tales & Trivia

It used to be called Mango Bird due to its colouring like a ripe mango, and its affinity for mango trees!

Jayantika Davé

Lesser Goldenback

Scientific name: *Dinopium benghalense*   Size: 27 cm
Hindi name: *Sunehra Katphora*
Sanskrit name: *Kashtth-Kutat, Aaghaat, Darvaghat*

Description
A loud knocking against a tree trunk, a manic, laughing kyi-kyi-kyi, and you will see the glorious widespread resident Sunehra Katphora, with its flaming gold back and equally bright red-crested head. There are three other Goldenback Woodpeckers, which vary in size by location, but are quite similar in appearance (**Common Goldenback** – Hills of Southwest India, **Himalayan Goldenback** – Himalayas, and **Greater Goldenback** – Himalayas and hills in the South).

Habits
The Lesser Goldenback is most often seen in all kinds of open woodlands, wooded gardens, parks and village groves, particularly amongst the older trees. It forages vigorously for ants, spiders, caterpillars and beetles, sometimes also digging into fruit and taking the nectar of honey-filled flowers. Very adept at moving around tree trunks, on the undersides, peering behind the bark, moving backwards if necessary, and foraging at all levels of the tree, sometimes dropping down to the ground if an ant nest has been found.

Call
A loud shrieking klerk or a whinnying kyi-kyi-kyi-kyi

Each Little Bird That Sings

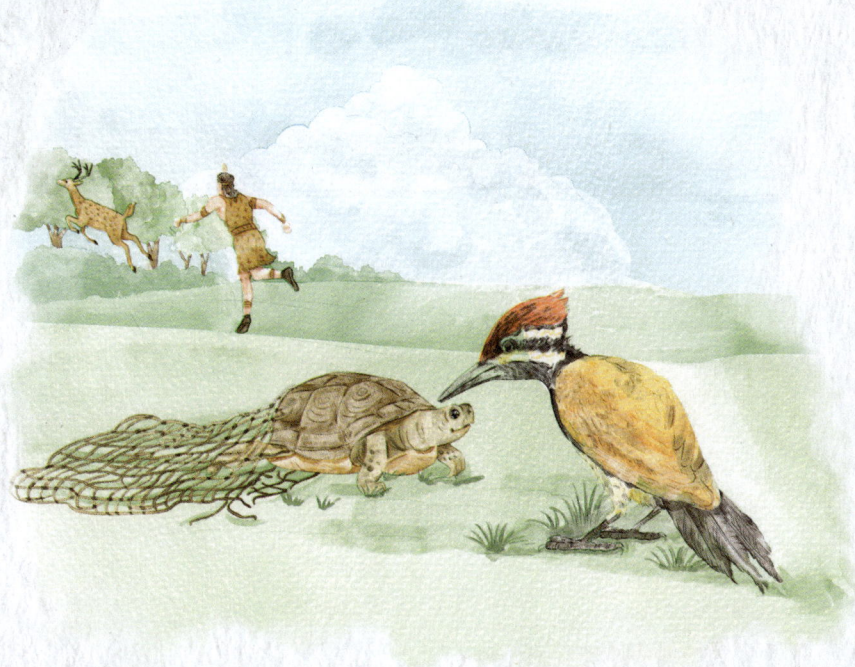

Mythology, Tales & Trivia

The Jataka tales have a lovely story about three friends – a woodpecker, a deer and a turtle. One day, the deer got caught in a net set by a hunter and called for help. The turtle immediately set to gnawing through the leather net, while the woodpecker flew to the hunter's hut, and attacked him each time he tried to emerge. The hunter finally got to the lake just as the deer got free. But the turtle was still there, and the hunter put the turtle into his sack. The clever deer then led the hunter deeper into the forest, while the woodpecker pecked the turtle free from the hunter's bag!

Bibliography

Book Title	Author	Year of Publication
A Manual of the Game Birds of India, Vol. 1–2	Eugene W. Oates (1845–1911)	1898
Birds at the Nest	Douglas Dewar (1875–1957)	1928
Birds in Sanskrit Literature	K.N. Davé (1884–1983)	1985
Birds' Nesting in India	Capt. G.F.L. Marshall (1843–1934)	1877
Birds of an Indian Village	Douglas Dewar (1875–1957)	1921
Birds of Burma	B.E. Smythies (1912–99)	1940
Birds of Darjeeling and India	L.J. Mackintosh	1914
Birds of the Indian Subcontinent	Richard Grimmett, Carol Inskipp, Tim Inskipp	2011
Breeding Birds of Kashmir	R.S.P. Bates and E.H.N. Lowther	1952
Fauna of British India, Vol. 1–8	E.C. Stuart Baker (1864–1944)	1922
Game, Shore and Water Birds of India	Col. A. Le Messurier	1904
Himalayan and Kashmiri Birds	Douglas Dewar (1875–1957)	1923
Indian Birds	Douglas Dewar (1875–1957)	1919
The Indian Ducks and Their Allies, Part 1–10	E.C. Stuart Baker (1864–1944)	1897
Indian Hill Birds	Salim Ali (1896–1987)	1949
Indian Scientific Nomenclature of Birds of India, Burma and Ceylon	Dr Raghu Vira and K.N. Davé	1949
Of Birds and Birdsong	M. Krishnan (1912–96)	2012
Pet Birds of Bengal	Satya Churn Law (1923–83)	1923
Popular Handbook of Indian Birds	Hugh Whistler (1889–1943)	1935
The Birds of India, Vol. I, II & III	T.C. Jerdon (1811–72)	1863
The Book of Indian Birds	Salim Ali (1896–1987)	1941
The Common Birds of Bombay	Edward Hamilton Aitkin (E.H.A.) (1851–1909)	1999
Common Birds of India, Vol. I & II	Douglas Dewar (1875–1957)	1925
The Fall of a Sparrow	Salim Ali (1896–1987)	1985
The Game-Birds of India, Burma and Ceylon, Vol. 1–3	E.C. Stuart Baker (1864–1944)	1930
The Waterfowl of India and Asia	F. Finn (1868–1932)	1920

Acknowledgements

Writing this book started as a dream and turned into a journey of continuous learning, lit by the wonder of our avian world, the supportive hands of friendship, and the pure joy of creation!

This book would not be what it is without the support of so many people. Beautiful photographs bring the birds to life, and I will forever be indebted to my friend and fellow birder Nikhil Devasar, who has provided 132 of the 198 photos in this book, and to my other very talented birding photographer friends Kavi Nanda and R.G. Srikanth who provided 38 and 25 photographs, respectively.

The illustrations are the other key feature of this book and bring the stories to life. They would not have been possible without Rahul and Yamini Arora who, when I spoke to them about the concept, said that they and their wonderful team at MPS would absolutely make this happen – thank you, dear friends! To the team at MPS -- Project Manager Priyanka Raheja who held this complex project together beautifully, with great competence, patience and understanding; Art/Design Team head Dalbir Singh, and his team of very talented designers and illustrators; and Sandhya Joshi, AVP Content, who ensured the team had support – I could not have done this without you!

My sincere thanks to M.K. Ranjitsinh-ji, who wrote an incisive foreword, with the weight of his wisdom behind it.

I am very grateful to Rupa Publications, and especially to Kapish Mehra for believing in me and the story this book has to tell, and to Rudra Sharma for spearheading the task of bringing this book to the reader.

The information provided is accurate to the best of my knowledge; a detailed bibliography has been provided for the antecedents of some of the stories. Photographer credits are as below:

Nikhil Devasar: Adjutant Stork, Greater, Asian Openbill Stork, Asian Pied Starling, Bar-headed Goose, Barn Owl, Bay-backed Shrike, Black Bulbul, Black Drongo, Black Francolin, Black Redstart, Black-crowned Night Heron, Black-headed Ibis, Black-headed Jay, Black-naped Monarch, Black-necked Stork, Black-winged stilt, Blood Pheasant, Blue Whistling Thrush, Brahminy Kite, Brown-headed Barbet, Brown-headed Gull, Cattle Egret, Chestnut-bellied Sandgrouse, Chestnut-tailed Starling, Cinnamon Bittern, Common Crane, Common Hawk Cuckoo, Common Hoopoe, Common Kestrel, Common Kingfisher, Common Myna, Common Pigeon, Common Redshank, Common Tailorbird, Cotton Pygmy Goose, Crested Serpent Eagle, Demoiselle Crane, Dusky Crag Martin, Eurasian Collared Dove, Eurasian Curlew, Eurasian Spoonbill, Frogmouth, Sri Lanka, Garganey Duck, Glossy Ibis, Great Barbet, Great Cormorant, Great Egret, Great Hornbill, Great Indian Bustard, Great White Pelican, Greater Racket-tailed Drongo, Green Bee-eater, Grey Francolin, Grey Heron, Grey Junglefowl, Grey-winged Blackbird, Himalayan Monal, House Crow, House Sparrow, Indian Peafowl, Indian Pitta, Indian Pond Heron, Indian Robin, Indian Roller, Indian Silverbill, Indian Skimmer, Indian Spot-billed Duck, Indian Thick-knee, Jacobin Cuckoo, Jungle Babbler, Jungle Crow, Jungle Myna, Kalij Pheasant, Knob-billed Duck, Large-tailed Nightjar, Laughing Dove, Lesser Flamingo, Lesser Goldenback, Lesser Whistling Duck, Lesser Yellownape, Little Cormorant, Little Grebe, Little Ringed Plover, Long-tailed Broadbill, Long-tailed Shrike, Orange-headed Thrush, Oriental Honey Buzzard, Oriental Magpie-robin, Oriental Skylark, Oriental Turtle Dove, Oriental White-eye, Osprey, Paddyfield Pipit, Painted Stork, Pallas' Fish Eagle, Peregrine Falcon, Pied Avocet, Pied Bushchat, Pied Kingfisher, Plum-headed Parakeet, Purple Sunbird, Purple Swamp Hen, Purple-rumped Sunbird, Red Junglefowl, Red-billed Blue Magpie, Red-billed Leiothrix, Red-naped Ibis, Red-vented Bulbul, Red-whiskered Bulbul, River Tern, Rosy Starling, Ruddy Shelduck, Rufous Treepie, Sarus Crane, Satyr Tragopan, Scaly-breasted Munia, Shikra, Small Pratincole, Southern Grey Shrike, Spotted Dove, Spotted Forktail, Spotted Owlet, Striated Laughing Thrush, Verditer Flycatcher, Western Reef Egret, White-breasted Waterhen, White-crested Laughing Thrush, White-rumped Vulture, White-throated Kingfisher, White-throated Laughing Thrush, Woolly-necked Stork, Yellow-footed Green Pigeon

Kavi Nanda: Alexandrine Parakeet, Ashy Prinia, Asian Koel, Barn Swallow, Black Kite, Black-winged Kite, Blue-throat, Bronze-winged Jacana, Brown Rock Chat, Common Babbler, Common Greenshank, Common Iora, Common Moorhen, Common Pochard, Common Quail, Common Sandpiper, Common Snipe, Common Starling, Crimson Sunbird, Darter, Egyptian Vulture, Eurasian Coot, Eurasian Marsh Harrier, Gadwall, Indian Spotted Eagle, Little Stint, Northern Pintail, Oriental Pied Hornbill, Partridge, Chukar, Pheasant-tailed Jacana, Red Avadavat, Rose-ringed Parakeet, Sirkeer Malkoha, White-browed Fantail Flycatcher, White-browed Wagtail, White-eared Bulbul, Yellow Wagtail, Yellow-crowned Woodpecker

Srikanth RG: Amur Falcon, Asian Paradise Flycatcher, Baya Weaver, Brahminy Starling, Common Rosefinch, Common Teal, Coppersmith Barbet, Dusky Eagle Owl, Golden-fronted Leafbird, Green-backed Tit, Grey Hornbill, Greylag Goose, Indian Yellow Tit, Little Egret, Malabar Trogon, Mallard, Northern Shoveller, Red-crested Pochard, Red-wattled Lapwing, Rufous Sibia, Scarlet Minivet, Southern Coucal, Streaked Laughing Thrush, Wedge-tailed Green Pigeon, Wigeon

Alamy: Golden Oriole, Lesser Florican; **Shutterstock:** Indian Nuthatch

Index

A

Adjutant Stork	78–79
Alexandrine Parakeet	177
Amur Falcon	210
Ashy Prinia	93
Asian Koel	41–42
Asian Openbill Stork	71
Asian Paradise Flycatcher	233
Asian Pied Starling	57

B

Bar-headed Goose	151, 162
Barn Owl	134
Barn Swallow	20–21
Baya Weaver	100–101
Bay-backed Shrike	105
Black Bulbul	28
Black Drongo	30–31
Black Francolin	36
Black Hooded Oriole	251
Black Kite	148
Black Redstart	18
Black-crowned Night Heron	70
Black-headed Ibis	238–239
Black-headed Jay	192
Black-Lored Tit	247
Black-naped Monarch	82
Black-necked Stork	77
Black-winged Kite	193
Black-winged Stilt	64
Blood Pheasant	212
Blue Whistling Thrush	35
Blue-tailed Bee-eater	166
Blue-throat	98
Brahminy Kite	229
Brahminy Starling	113
Bronze-winged Jacana	34
Brown Rock Chat	104
Brown-fronted Woodpecker	53
Brown-headed Barbet	169
Brown-headed Gull	195

C

Cattle Egret	234
Chestnut-bellied Nuthatch	81
Chestnut-bellied Sandgrouse	128
Chestnut-tailed Starling	180
Chukor	194
Cinnamon Bittern	136
Common Babbler	114
Common Crane	203
Common Goldenback	252
Common Greenshank	129
Common Hawk Cuckoo	114, 183, 185, 190–191
Common Hoopoe	226
Common Iora	249
Common Kestrel	225
Common Kingfisher	84
Common Moorhen	37
Common Myna	57, 116–117
Common Pigeon	186–187
Common Pochard	156, 157
Common Quail	108–109
Common Redshank	125
Common Rosefinch	221
Common Sandpiper	111
Common Snipe	118
Common Starling	24
Common Tailorbird	94
Common Teal	155
Coppersmith Barbet	165
Cotton Pygmy Goose	155
Crested Kingfisher	58
Crested Serpent Eagle	149
Crimson Sunbird	220

D

Dabchick (Little Grebe)	119
Dalmatian Pelican	243
Darter	48–49
Demoiselle Crane	151, 200–201
Dusky Crag Martin	15
Dusky Eagle Owl	144–145

E

| Egyptian Vulture | 236–237 |
| Eurasian Collared Dove | 127 |

Eurasian Coot 40
Eurasian Curlew 143
Eurasian Marsh Harrier 142
Eurasian Spoonbill 240

F

Frogmouth, Sri Lanka 115
Fulvous Whistling Duck 156

G

Gadwall 156
Garganey Duck 155
Glossy Ibis 147
Golden Oriole 251
Golden-fronted Leafbird 168
Great Barbet 171
Great Cormorant 46–47
Great Egret 242
Great Hornbill 74–75
Great Indian Bustard 7, 153
Great White Pelican 243
Greater Adjutant 78
Greater Coucal 228
Greater Flamingo 241
Greater Goldenback 252
Greater Racquet-Tailed Drongo 32–33
Greater Yellownape 170
Green Bee-eater 166
Green Sandpiper 111
Green-backed Tit 248
Grey Francolin 133
Grey Heron 202
Grey Hornbill 197
Grey Junglefowl 199
Greylag Goose 163
Grey-winged Blackbird 29

H

Himalayan Goldenback 252
Himalayan Monal 214–215
House Crow 38–39
House Sparrow 96–97

I

Indian Cormorant 44
Indian Nuthatch 81
Indian Peafowl 216–217
Indian Pitta 208
Indian Pond Heron 139

Indian Robin 19
Indian Roller 86–87
Indian Silverbill 92
Indian Skimmer 65
Indian Spot-billed Duck 158
Indian Spotted Eagle 150
Indian Thick-knee 135
Indian Yellow Tit 247
Intermediate Egret 235

J

Jacobin Cuckoo 62
Jungle Babbler 182–183
Jungle Crow 41
Jungle Myna 27

K

Kalij Pheasant 72
Knob-billed Duck 159

L

Large Pied Wagtail (White-browed Wagtail)
    54–55
Large-tailed Nightjar 132
Laughing Dove 120–121
Lesser Adjutant 78
Lesser Flamingo 241
Lesser Florican 7, 67
Lesser Goldenback 252
Lesser Racket-tailed Drongo 32
Lesser Whistling Duck 156
Lesser Yellownape 170
Little Cormorant 44
Little Egret 198, 235
Little Grebe (Dabchick) 119
Little Ringed Plover 102
Little Stint 95
Little Swift 15
Long-tailed Broadbill 209
Long-tailed Shrike 184–185

M

Malabar Grey Hornbill 197
Malabar Trogon 211
Mallard 158

N

Northern Pintail 157
Northern Shoveler 157

257

O

Orange-headed Thrush 224
Oriental Honey Buzzard 146
Oriental Magpie-robin 56
Oriental Pied Hornbill 69
Oriental Skylark 103
Oriental Turtle Dove 130
Oriental White-eye 246
Osprey 68

P

Paddyfield Pipit 99
Painted Stork 76
Pallas' Fish Eagle 151
Partridge, Chukar 194
Peregrine Falcon 138
Pheasant-tailed Jacana 60–61
Pied Avocet 66
Pied Bushchat 51
Pied Kingfisher 58
Plum-headed Parakeet 176
Purple Heron 202
Purple Sunbird 16–17
Purple Swamp Hen 88
Purple-rumped Sunbird 245

R

Red Avadavat 219
Red Junglefowl 230–231
Red-billed Blue Magpie 89
Red-billed Leiothrix 207
Red-crested Pochard 158
Red-naped Ibis 45
Red-rumped Swallow 20
Red-vented Bulbul 22–23
Red-wattled Lapwing 131
Red-whiskered Bulbul 106
River Tern 196
Rose-ringed Parakeet 174–175
Rosy Starling 26
Ruddy Shelduck 160–161
Rufous Sibia 223
Rufous Treepie 140–141

S

Sarus Crane 204–205
Satyr Tragopan 213

Scaly-breasted Munia 91
Scarlet Minivet 222
Shikra 30, 188–189
Sirkeer Malkoha 137
Small Pratincole 179
Southern Coucal 228
Southern Grey Shrike 181
Spotted Dove 126
Spotted Forktail 59
Spotted Owlet 112
Streaked Laughing Thrush 110
Striated Laughing Thrush 124

V

Verditer Flycatcher 83

W

Wedge-tailed Green Pigeon 172
Western Reef Egret 198
White Spotted Fantail Flycatcher 52
White-breasted Waterhen 63
White-browed Fantail Flycatcher ... 52
White-browed Wagtail (Large Pied Wagtail)
     54–55
White-cheeked Barbet 169
White-crested Laughing Thrush 123
White-eared Bulbul 107
White-rumped Vulture 152
White-throated Fantail Flycatcher ... 52
White-throated Kingfisher 85
White-throated Laughing Thrush ... 122
Wigeon 157
Wire-tailed Swallow 20
Wood Sandpiper 111
Woolly-necked Stork 73

Y

Yellow Wagtail........................... 250
Yellow-billed Babbler.................. 182
Yellow-crowned Woodpecker 53
Yellow-footed Green Pigeon 173

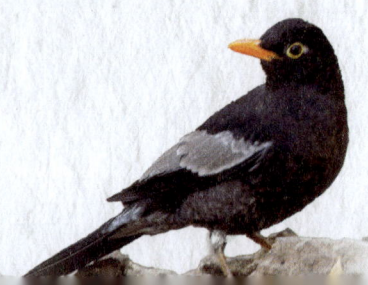